Mad Skills
Exercise Mixtape
Volume 1

100+ Illustrated At-home Workouts

Ben Musholt

First edition published in 2020 by BPM Rx, Inc.

ISBN: 9798670628532

www.BPMRx.com
www.BenMusholt.com

This book is dedicated to my Mother.
I'm grateful for your inspiration to live a life of
exercise, health, and adventure.

DISCLAIMER

The material contained in this book is for informational purposes only. BPM Rx Inc. and Ben Musholt advise that the exercises and workouts described in this book can be strenuous, and may not be suitable for all individuals. The author makes no claim to the safety of the movements or techniques in this book, and advises consultation with a qualified professional to determine if they are appropriate for you. It is strongly recommended that the reader consult with a physician before engaging in any of the physical activities described in this book, or any other exercise routine. The publisher and author disclaim any and all liability for any injury or conditioned sustained via performance of the exercises in this book, and may NOT be held liable for any damages from the practice of said exercises.

Your health and safety are most important.

Be smart: Consult with professionals, train with caution, and use appropriate exercise progressions.

Intro

Welcome to the Mad Skills Exercise Mixtape – Volume One. This companion to the *Mad Skills Exercise Encyclopedia* covers over 100 illustrated workouts that you can perform at home. The first half of the book (Side A) contains routines that can be performed with common items like kettlebells, dumbbells and medicine balls. The second half of the book (Side B), expands to include pull-up bars, gymnastic rings, parallettes, and stability balls. The purpose of this "mixtape" is to provide exposure to numerous exercise combinations that fit together into effective, at-home workouts.

Workout Structure

The workouts that you'll encounter all stick to a common training structure. The format is a three-tiered system of the warm-up, circuit training, and cool-down. The warm-up generally entails two bodyweight or light-weight exercises to get your heart rate up and prepare you for more intense exercise. Use the warm-up as a time to prime your nervous system and get your joints ready for action.[1]

The circuit training portion of each workout is the heart and soul of mixtape. In this middle section, you'll find three to four exercises that address leg strength, upper body pulling strength, and upper body pushing strength. By hitting these three categories, and varying the type of leg strengthening between sessions, circuit training like this provides a powerful whole-body workout.

The last section of each workout adds another two bodyweight movements to the session. These final exercises are often different calisthenics, like push-up variations or core strengthening movements. Think of these as the finishing touches to each workout. They will help you cool down after the more intense exercises of the circuit. They may also help address any body regions that might not have been targeted by the previous three to four exercises.

---

1 By the way, don't feel limited to only perform the two movements listed in the warm-up section. Add enough movement until you feel your body is sufficiently prepared for heavier exercise.

Intro

2-3-2 Method

2 Warm-up Exercises

3 (or 4) Circuit Exercises

2 Cool-down Exercises

Use What You've Got

Don't be discouraged if you don't have every piece of equipment displayed in the book. It can take years to build out your home gym—there's no reason to go broke purchasing all of the gear at once! The best recommendation is to be flexible and creative in your use of what exercise tools you *do* have.

For many movements, a dumbbell can be a great substitute for a kettlebell. If you don't have a weight bench or a plyo box, a stairwell can work well for jumps and split squats. A piece of sturdy furniture can even do the trick for certain movements like reverse hypers and hip thrusts. If you don't have access to a pull-up bar, head over to the local park and use the jungle gym for that portion of the workout. Likewise, if you don't have a sandbag, load up a duffle bag or a backpack. Bottom line: Be open-minded, and use what you've got.

Why You Won't See Specific Reps, Sets, or Weight Recommendations

Once you dive into the workouts you will notice that they don't have associated reps and sets or prescribe a certain weight to lift. Why have these been omitted? It's because each reader is starting from a different point and has access to a different set of equipment. Perhaps you don't have a 50 lb kettlebell or your dumbbells don't go up to 25 lbs. Maybe you are just starting out and aren't ready for the intensity that someone else can tolerate.

Prescribing a workload at a specific resistance level is bound to be too much for some, and not enough for others. The diagrams are meant to illustrate the variety of ways that movements can be pieced together for an effective at-home workout. If you want a personalized approach to fitness, you'll need to meet one-on-one with a coach.

However, that doesn't mean that you are totally on your own here. By sticking to a few simple parameters, you can adjust each workout into a productive session. In terms of general guidelines, here is a basic framework to follow:

Warm-up

The initial phase of your workout should last between *5 to 10 minutes*. You want it to be long enough to prepare you for action, but not so long that it wears you out for the bulk of the session. In general, a good target is to perform **50 to 100 reps** of each motion. An example could be 100 jumping jacks, and 50 prisoner lunges. It could also be 50 mountain climbers, and 100 twisting jumps. If the movement is locomotive, like a bear crawl or crab walk, set a target distance of 15 to 30 feet and run it for a few lengths.

INTRO

There is always the exception though, so be mindful and adjust as necessary. Burpees are a good example. You might find them in the warm-up, but trying to do 50 to 100 would be overkill. It might make more sense to do 10 to 20 burpees. Similarly, beginners might be toasted after 25 air squats, so doing more would only limit their abilities in the circuit training portion. Use your head, and understand that this part of the workout is only meant to get you ready for the next portion of the session.

Additionally, don't think you have to perform each exercise distinct from the other one. The two warm-up movements can be done sequentially, or you can alternate back and forth until you are sufficiently prepped.

Circuit Training

Recall that each circuit is going to consist of three to four movements. To turn these exercises into an effective circuit, you want to **cycle through the movements for three to five "sets"**. If you are a beginner, or are pressed for time, cycle through the movements three times. If you want a heavier-duty workout, push yourself to complete five or more cycles. Four rounds through seems to be a sweet spot. When a four-round circuit is combined with the warm-up and cool-down, you should be able to complete the workout in about 30 minutes.

Now, how many repetitions of each exercise should you perform? As a rule of thumb, **5 to 12 repetitions of an exercise** are a good target. Bodybuilders might use higher rep ranges, and power lifters might use lower ones, but they have specific training goals in mind. For the purposes of an at-home fitness regimen, 5 to 12 reps are a safe target. Of course, the caveat is that you have to be using enough resistance for the movement to be effective.[2] The idea is that you should be fatigued at the end of the target rep range, but still have enough gas to complete the motion with good form. Danger happens when you are too spent to safely lift the weight anymore.

2 Some resisted exercises like kettlebell swings naturally lend themselves higher rep ranges. A 15, 20, or even 30-rep set of kettlebell swings is fine in some scenarios.

Intro

What about bodyweight or static exercises? Once you are strong enough to crank more than a dozen pull-ups or other bodyweight movements, you should start thinking about adding external weight. Wearing a weight vest or holding a dumbbell can provide the additional stimulus for continued strength development. In terms of static exercises like L-sits, planches, and levers, aim to hold the position for 5 to 10 seconds. Exercises that specifically target the core, like planks, can be held for 10 to 30 seconds.

How long should you wait between finishing one exercise and starting the next one? Let yourself catch your breath enough that you can be present and focus on the quality of the next movement. Sometimes 30 seconds is enough. Sometimes you will need 90 to 120 seconds (or more) before you are ready to move on to the next movement. Rotating through a circuit instead of cranking multiple sets of a single exercise allows you move through the volume of exercise at a slightly faster pace.

Cool-down

After grinding through the circuit, your cool-down needs to be less intense. Keep things simple and try to **perform three sets of each cool-down exercise**. If the movement is repetitive, shoot for 10 to 20 reps. If the exercise is a static hold, follow the guidelines above: 5 to 10 seconds for bodyweight strength skills and 10 to 30 seconds for core-specific holds.

> Appendix A at the back of the book gives names for each of the movements in the workout. It also provides a designation of "reps", "hold", or "distance" if there is any confusion for how a movement should be performed.

Intro

Movement Advice

Don't be sloppy.

You've only got one body, so don't go thrashing it about! As you perform an exercise, imagine yourself as a dancer with exquisite poise from the top of your head all the way to your tiptoes. If you were to record yourself on video, how would your body look? Would it appear centered, symmetric, and balanced? If not, focus on the quality of your movement and posture before adding resistance or difficulty.

Listen to your body.

As you work your way through the workouts in this book, you are going to encounter a wide variety of new movements. As you try them out, pay attention to how your body feels. If a skill seems seriously awkward, it could be that your alignment is way off, or you aren't strong enough for it yet.

If you have pain with a movement, then something isn't right. Try to adjust your stance, positioning, or movement pattern. If little tweaks don't help, get it checked out. Maybe a physio needs to address some underlying injury. A visit with a fitness coach could help adjust your form or provide a substitute movement.

Trust your gut. If a movement doesn't jibe with your body, swap it for an alternative.

Intro

Be smart about loading.

Injuries related to fitness are often the result of doing too much too soon. Jump into a workout routine after months off, and BOOM an injury flares up. Increase the resistance or a movement's degree of difficulty too fast, and you are setting yourself up for disaster. Being cautious about how you introduce and increase load is an important trait for anyone who is working out at home.

For example, if you can't perform a movement through its target range of motion without resistance, then don't go adding extra load. Master the bodyweight version before adding more challenge. Master air squats before dumbbell front squats. Master split jumps before resisted split jumps. You get the picture.

In a similar way, don't advance to single limbed skills until you have sufficient strength with the double limbed version. Only attempt single arm hangs after you can perform a double arm hang for a healthy amount of time. Only attempt pistol squats versions once you can move through the array of split squats with confidence.

Another common-sense recommendation is that if you can't support yourself in the beginning position of the movement, don't attempt the rest of the motion. Inverted skills are the best reference point here. If you can't safely support your torso through your shoulders at the top of a pike or jackknife push-up position, don't think about trying the full movement. Your head and neck are too valuable.

---

3 *Open chain* exercises like dumbbell shoulder presses or bicep curls are an exception to the "double before single limb" rule.

Intro

Understand how to use exercise progressions.

As someone who plans to train at home, it will be helpful to know how to adjust the exercises in this book to fit your ability level. Some movements may be way too easy. Some may be way too hard. Rather than skip those sections of each workout, figure out how you could make the movement easier or harder to match your ability level.

Common progressions include:

- **Unloaded » Loaded**
- **Less resistance » More resistance**
- **Assisted » Unassisted**
- **Slow » Fast**
- **Kipping » Strict**
- **Shortened range of motion » Full range of motion**
- **Symmetric double limb » Asymmetric double limb » Single limb**
- **Shorter levers » Longer levers**
- **Simple » Complex**
- **Single plane » Multi-plane movements**

Appendix B at the end of the book has a number of common progressions to get you started.

Intro

Effort = Outcomes.

When your goal is to build strength and muscle, then your body needs the stimulus to add muscle mass and connective tissue capacity. Training at an intensity that is below this threshold is fine, but it won't lead to the gains you seek. That means that when you settle in for the circuit training portion of each session, you need to put in the work. Go hard, but be safe about it

This idea is summarized by the principle of *progressive overload*. By gradually increasing the total workload between training sessions, your body will adapt through improved strength.

Note how this cycles back to why you won't find specific reps/sets or weight prescriptions in this book. It's up to YOU to continually push the needle on your training. It's up to you to gradually add more weight to each exercise. In the absence of more resistance—maybe your home gym isn't fully complete yet—increase your overall workload via more reps or sets of the movements.

If you don't put in the effort, don't expect the outcomes.

Are you someone who needs more accountability
on your fitness journey?
Head over to **benmusholt.com/coaching** to learn more about
virtual coaching options

Get After It

Have fun leafing through the workouts in these pages. There is no need to do them in any certain order. If you find a workout that you enjoy, earmark the page so that you can repeat it again.

While exploring the exercise combinations, take comfort in the fact that you are expanding your movement repertoire and becoming a more well-rounded athlete. A troublesome aspect of life is how we tend to lose movement skills with age. It's like our movement abilities sprout forth from infancy, and grow into a full-bodied tree in early adulthood. Sadly, over time the branches of the movement tree start shear off, and we become left with only a few skills. We stop jumping, hanging, twisting, and enjoying the many ways we can use our bodies.

Use the workouts in this book to improve your fitness, muscle mass, and body composition. Use them to look better, feel stronger, and move with greater confidence. Use them to become a more capable version of yourself. That's the *Mad Skills* way.

Side A

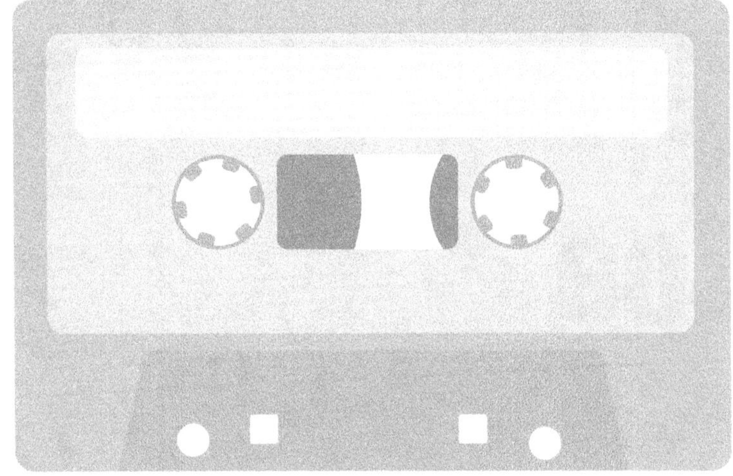

SIDE A

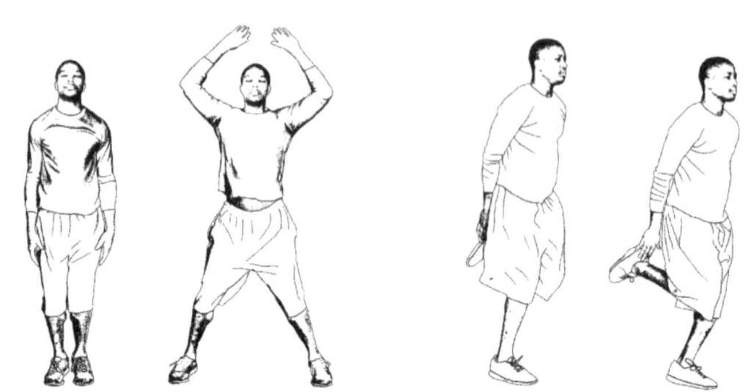

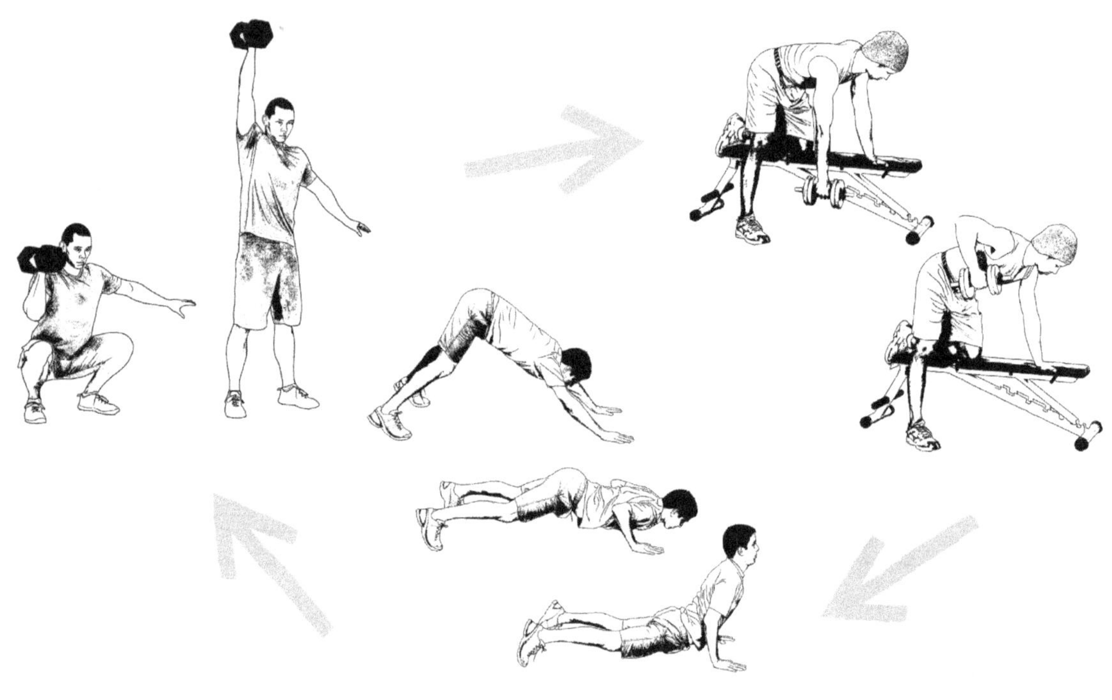

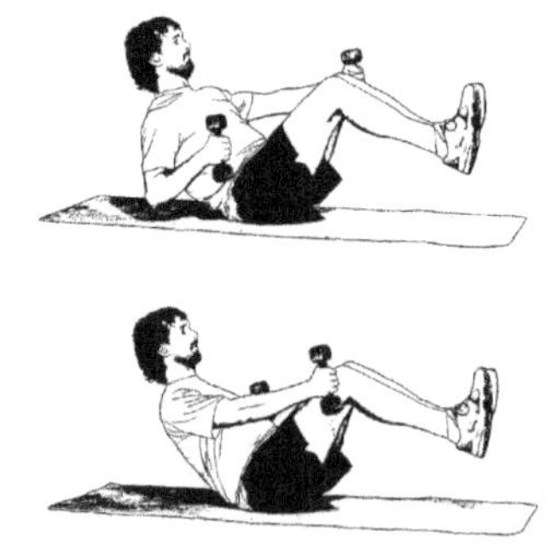

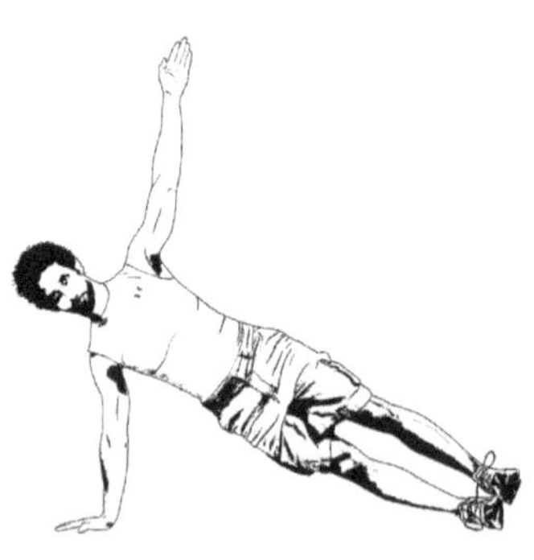

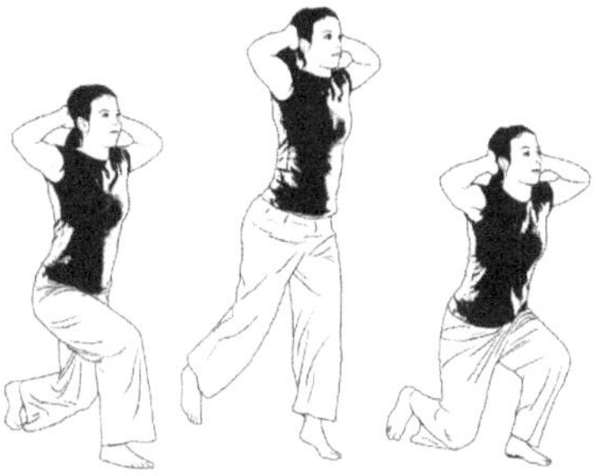

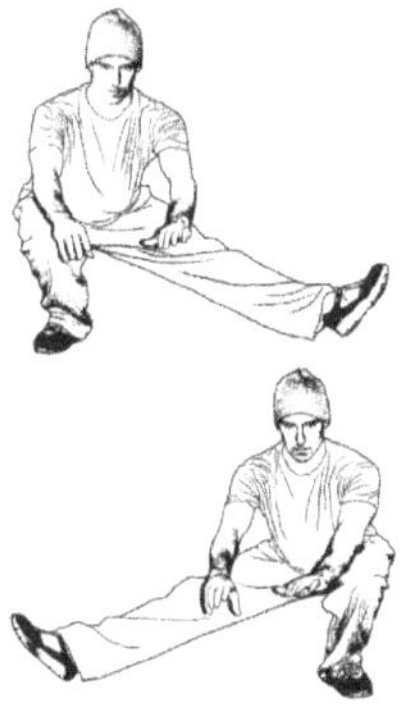

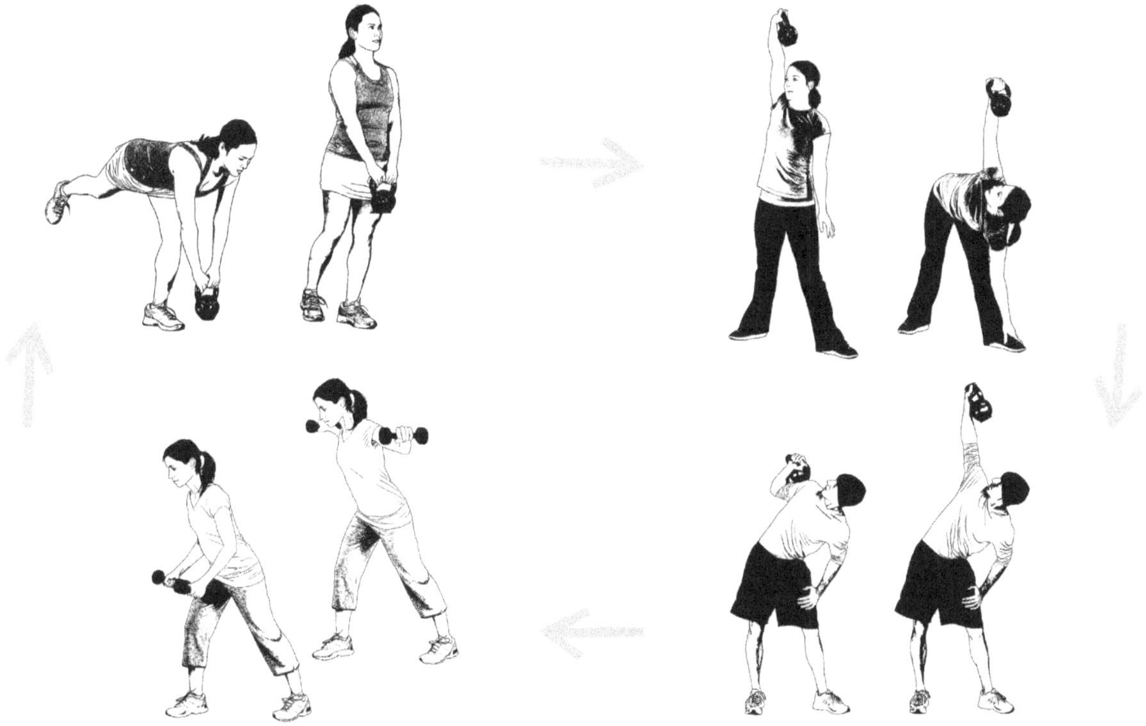

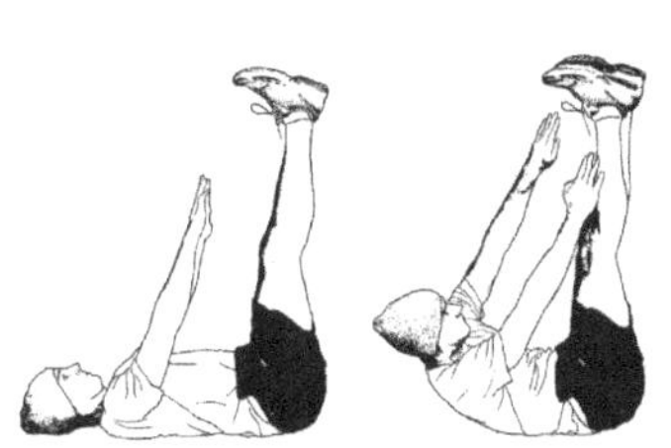

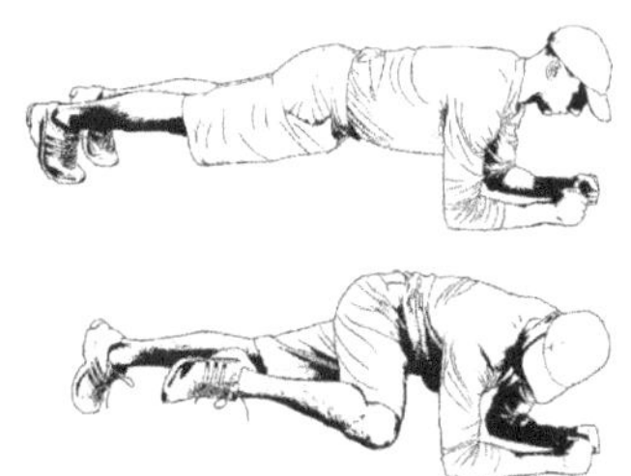

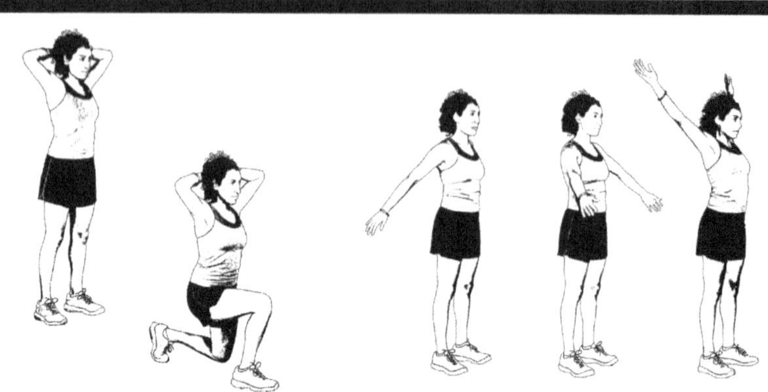

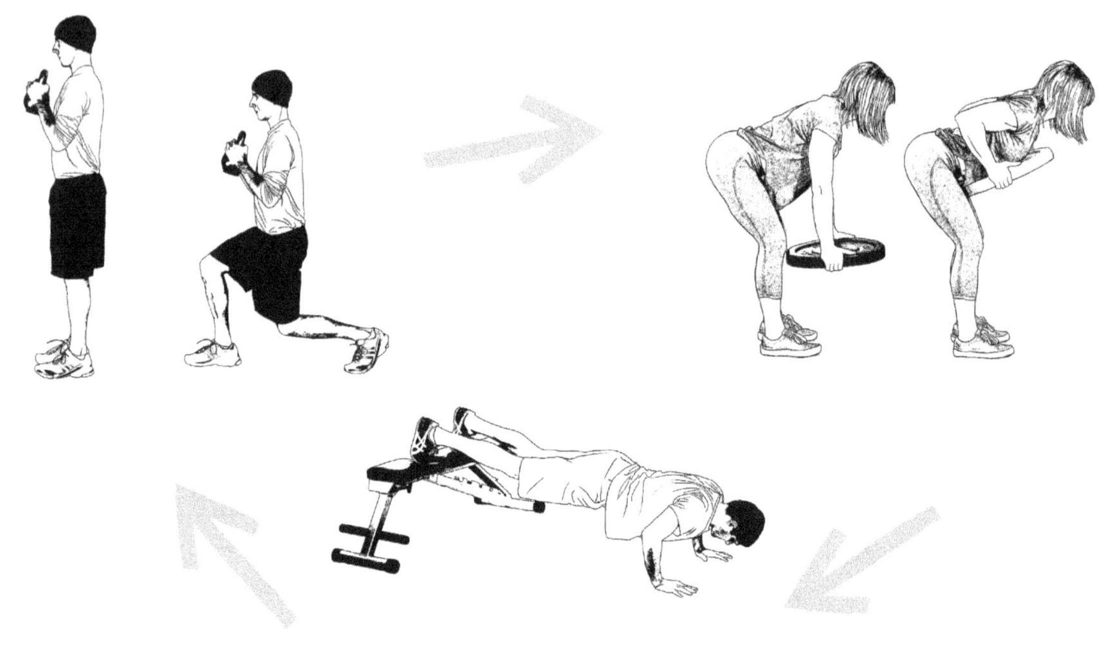

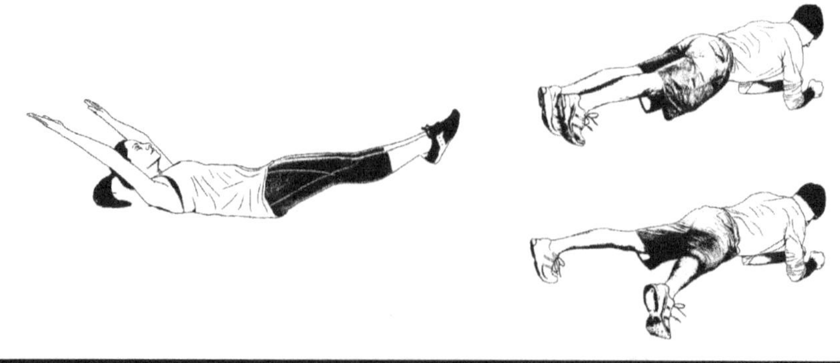

SIDE A

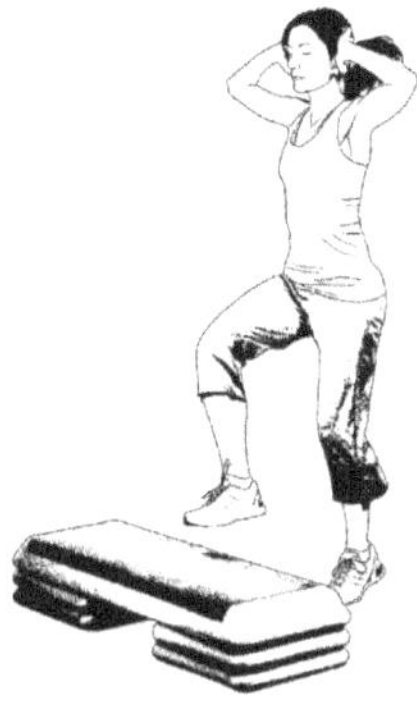

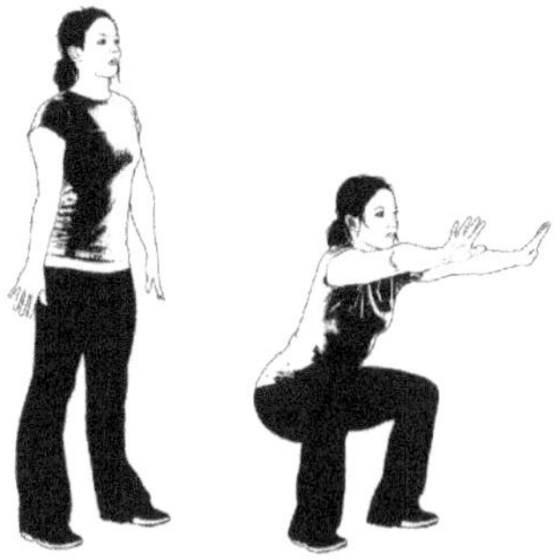

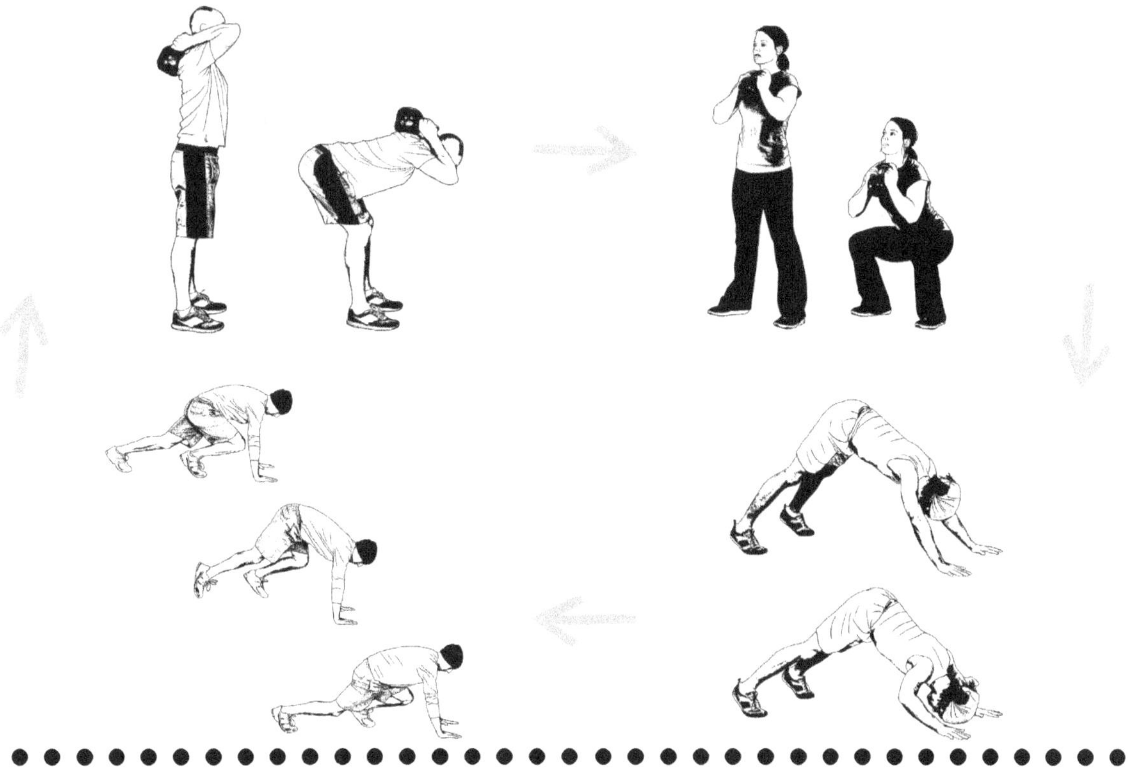

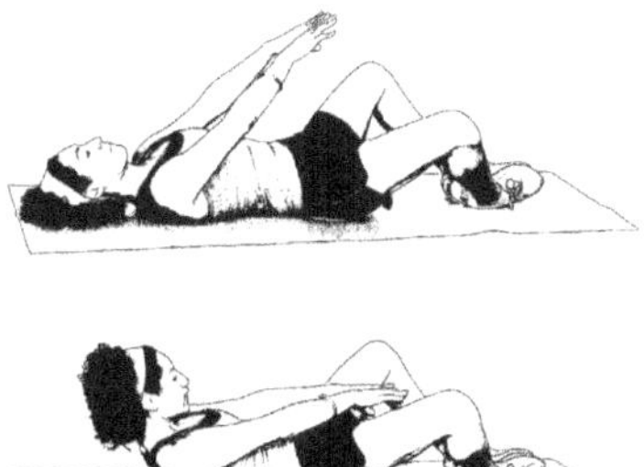

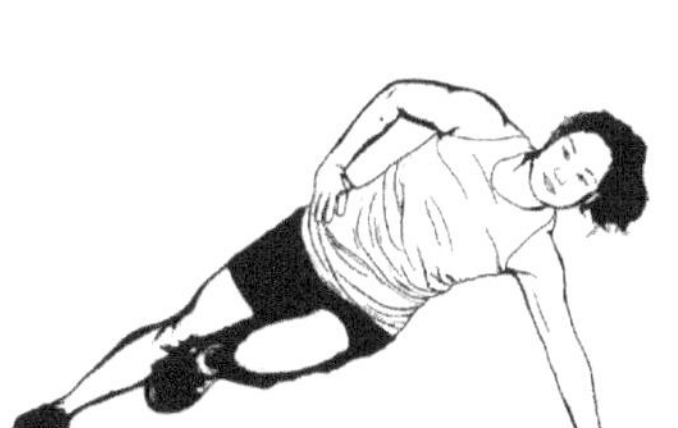

SIDE A

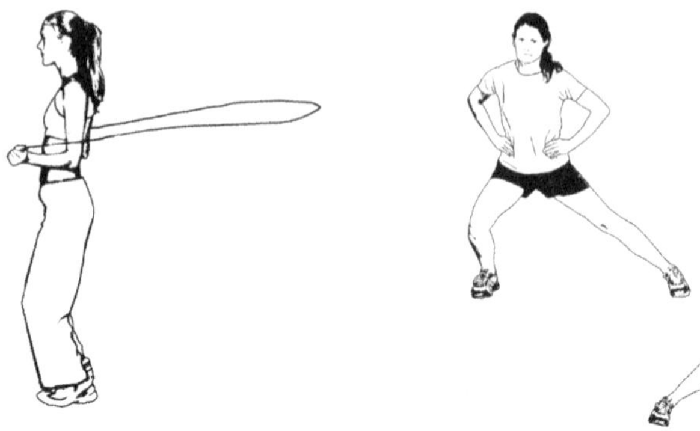

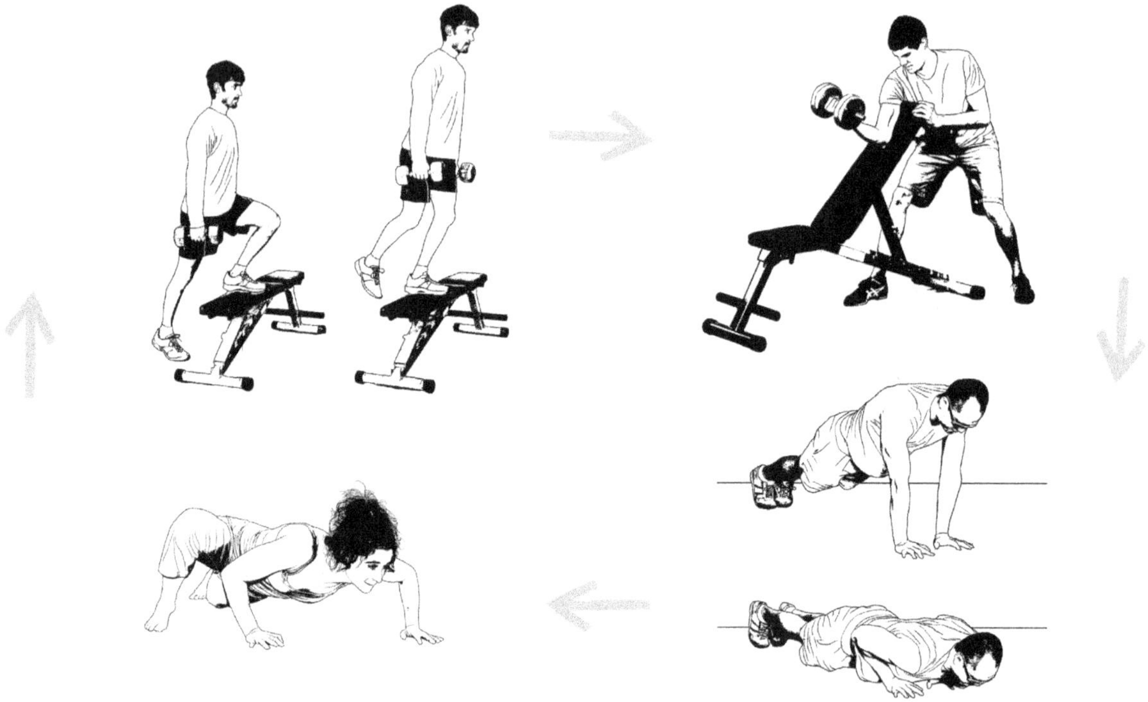

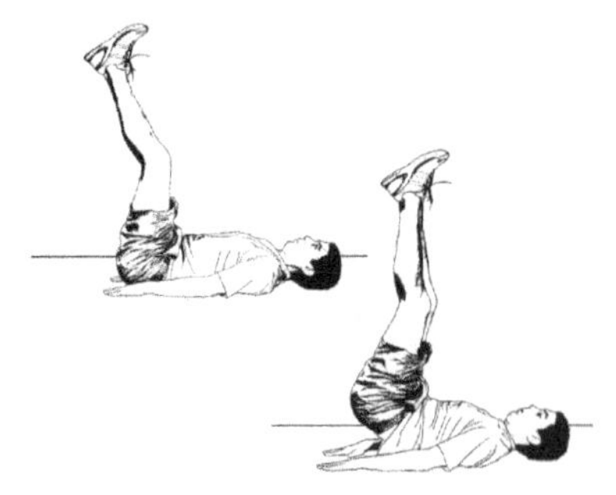

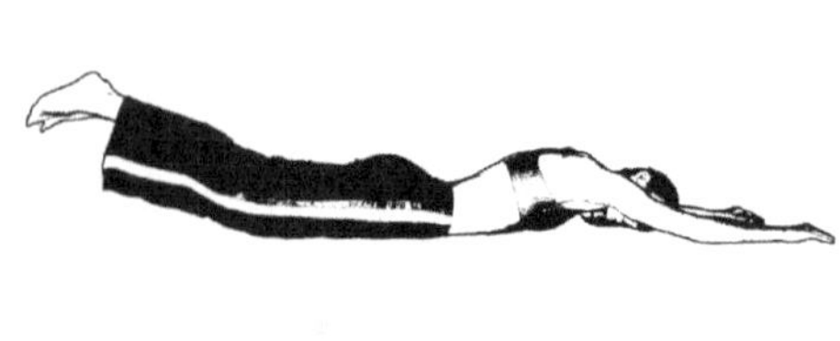

SIDE A

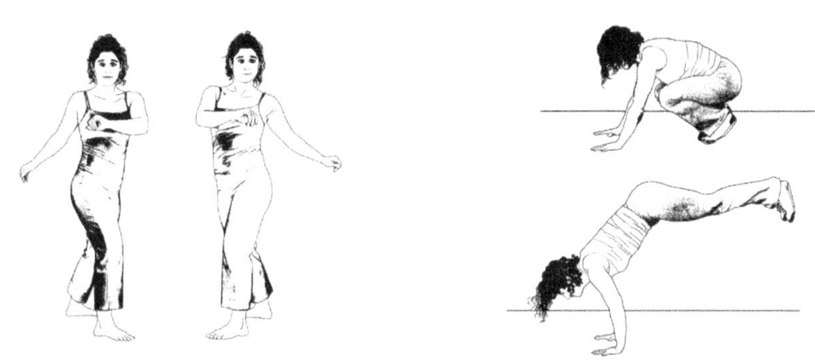

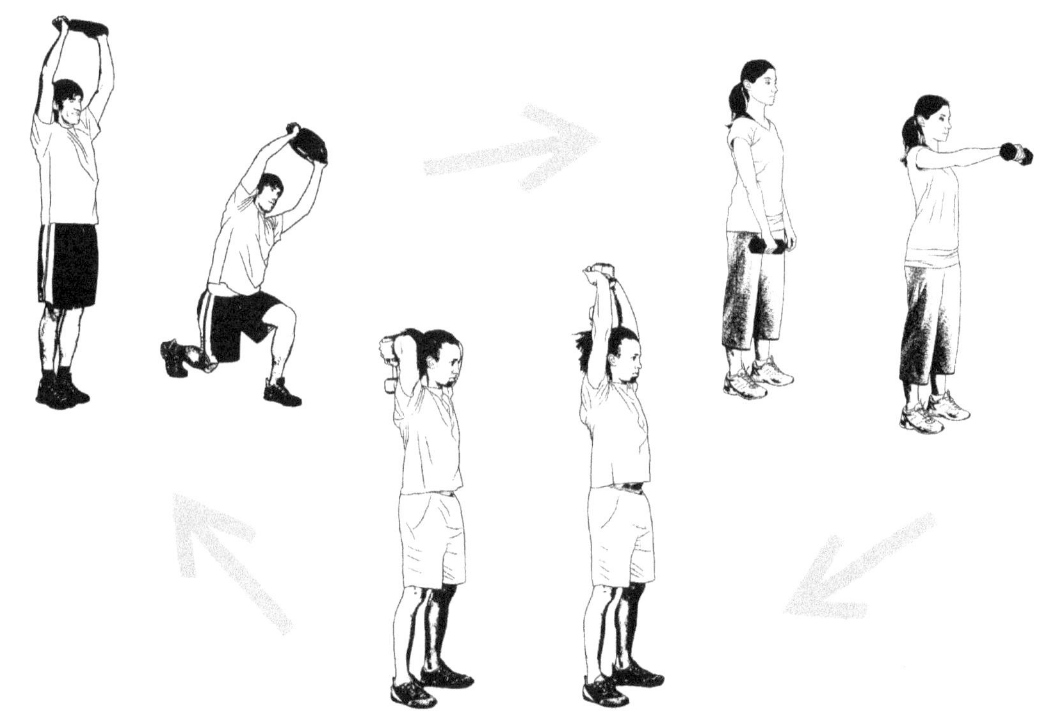

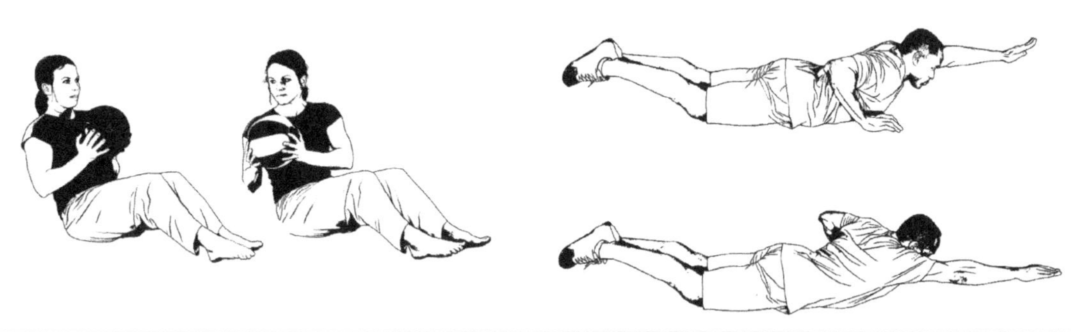

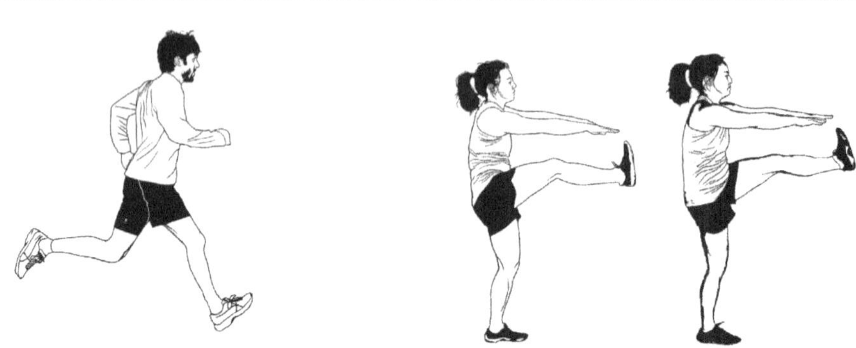

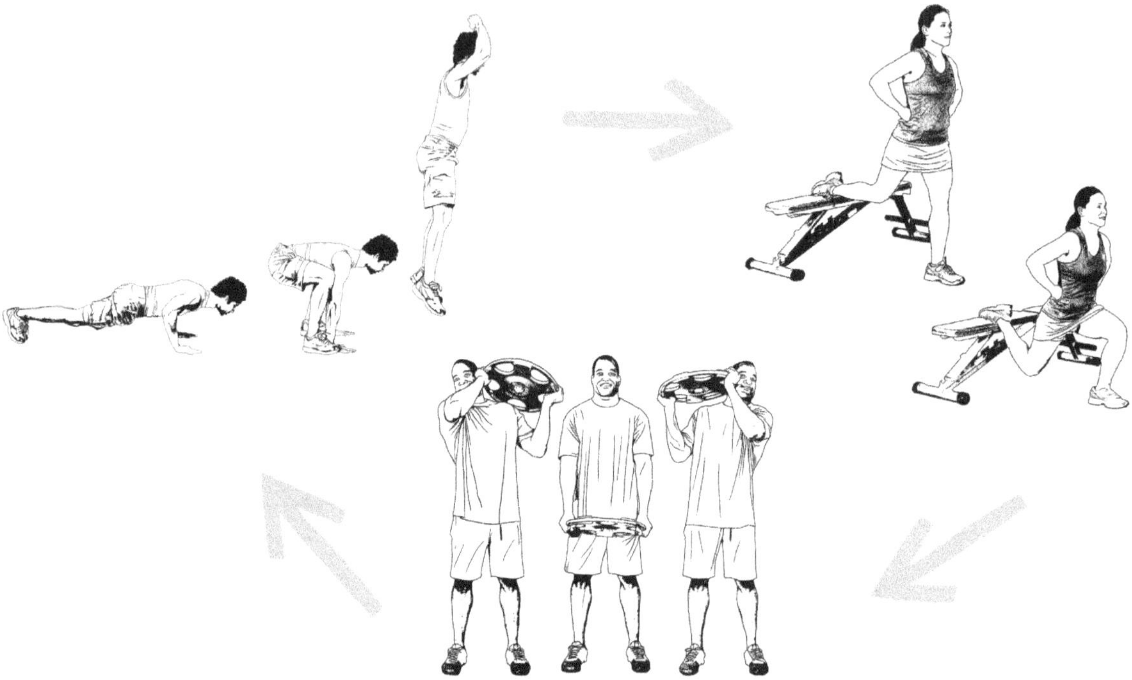

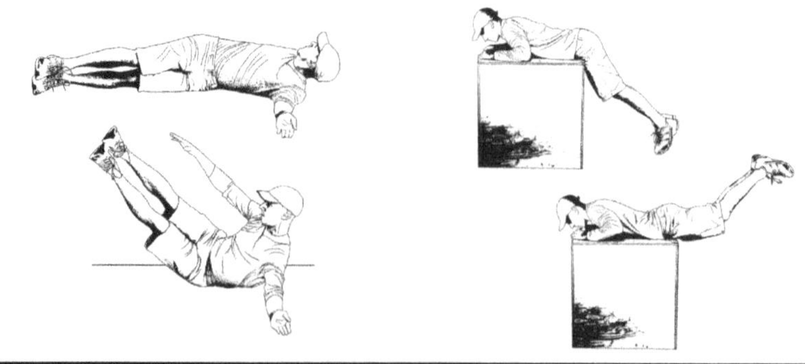

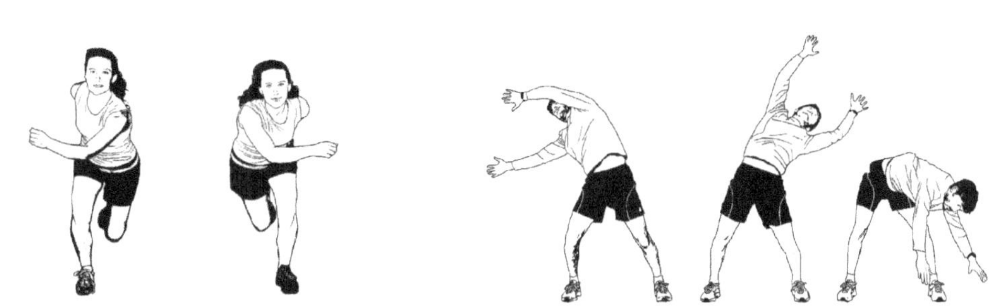

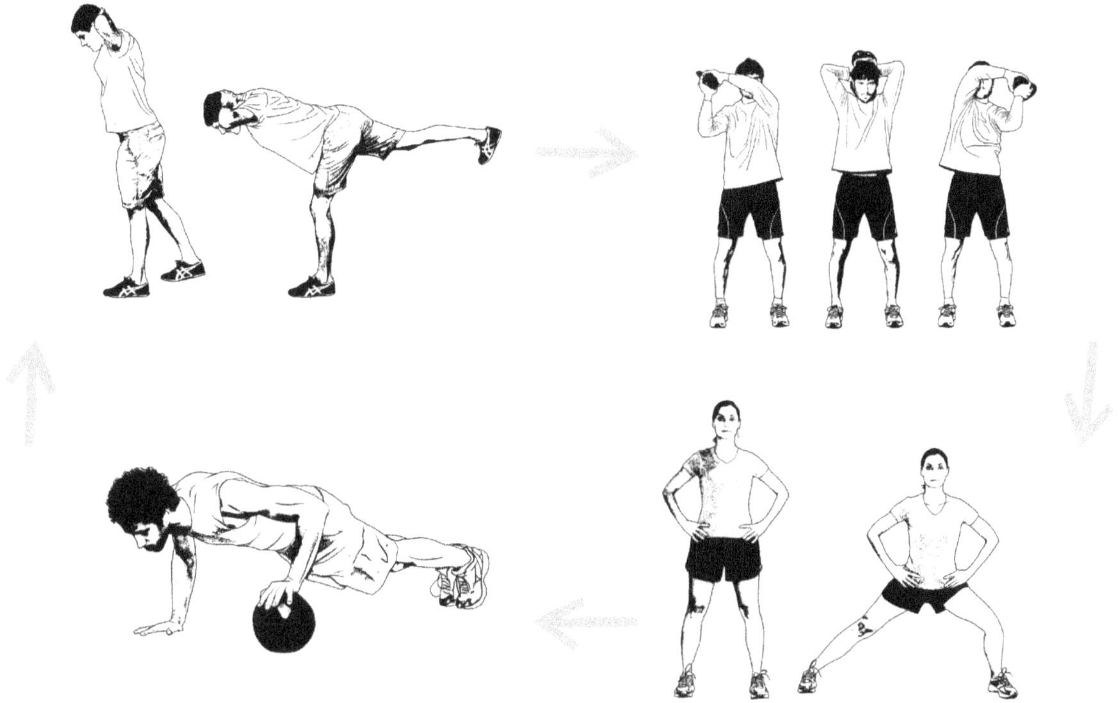

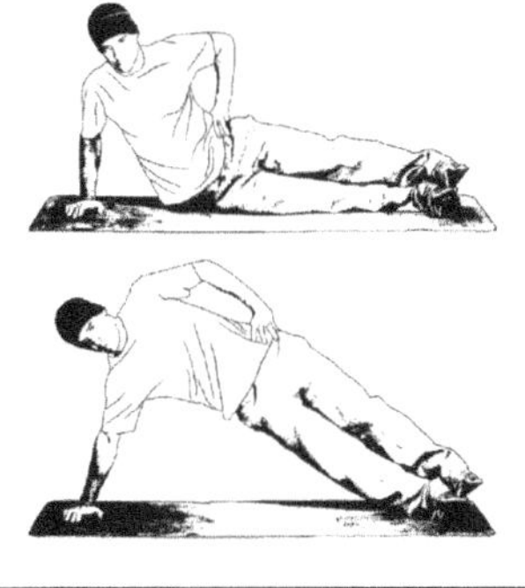

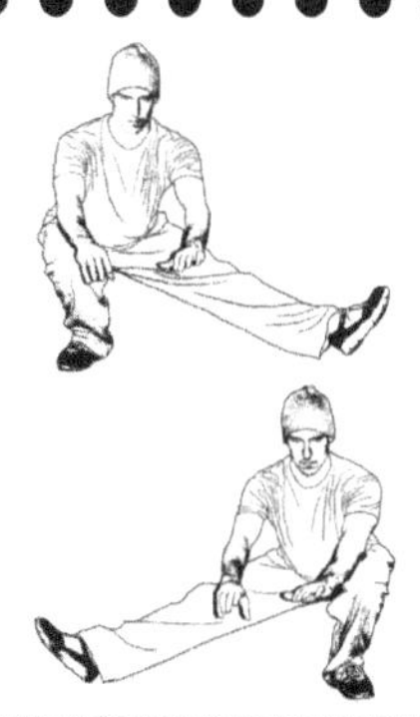

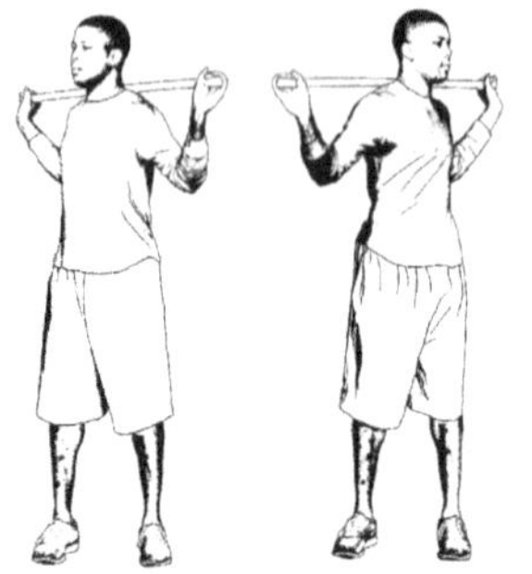

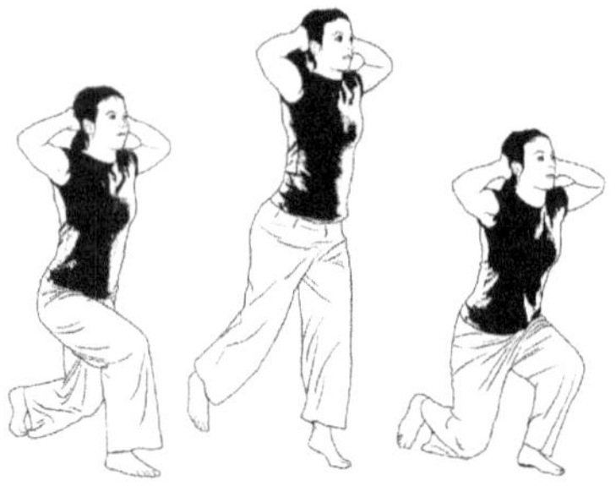

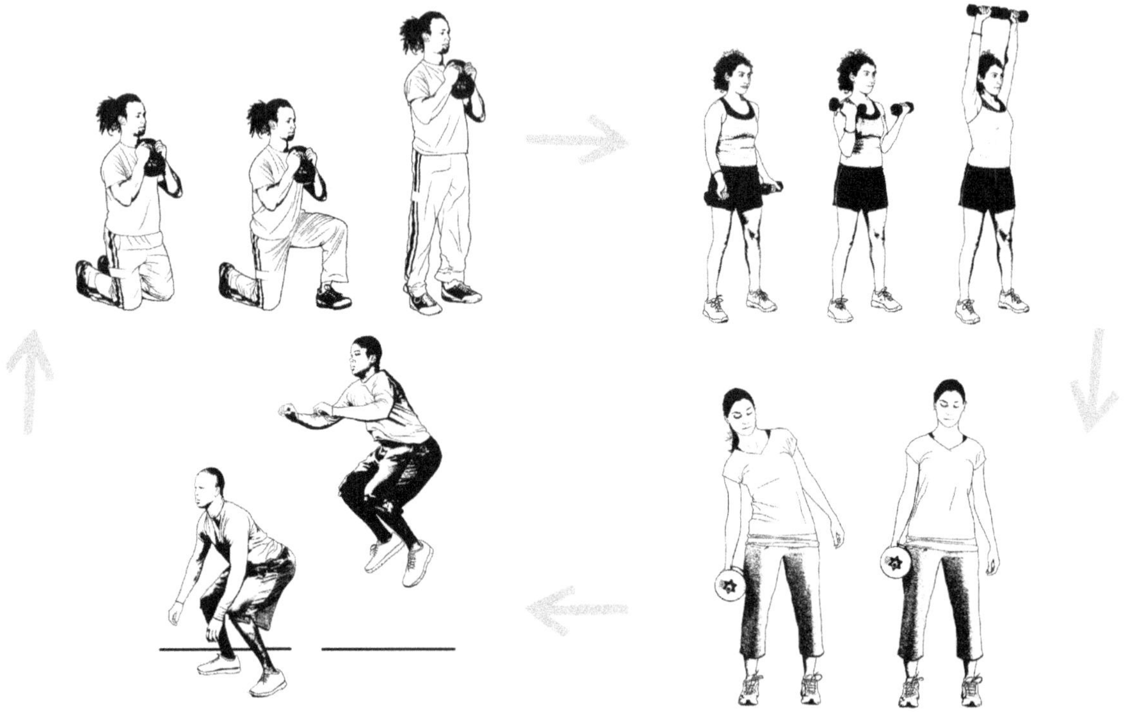

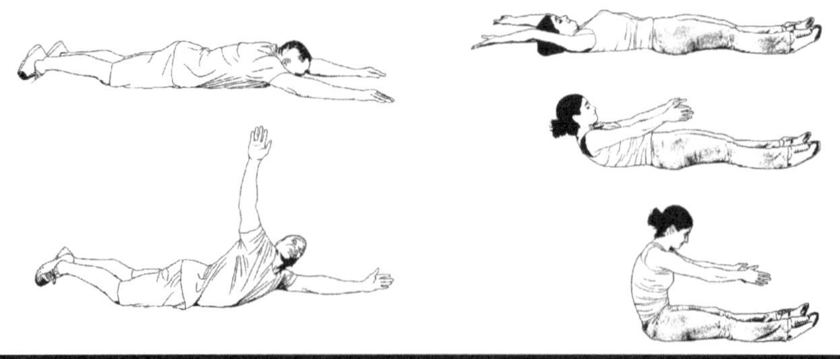

SIDE A

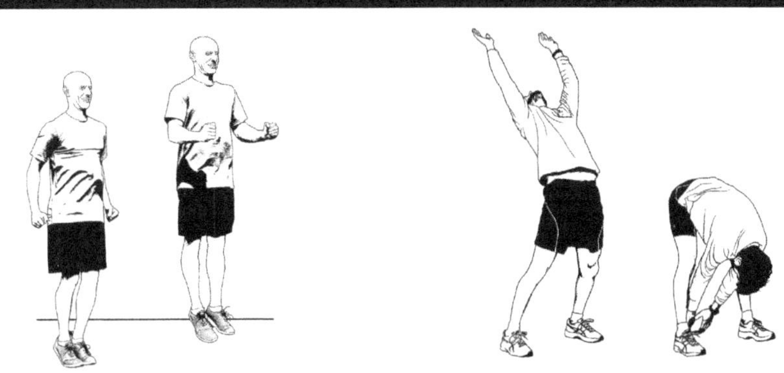

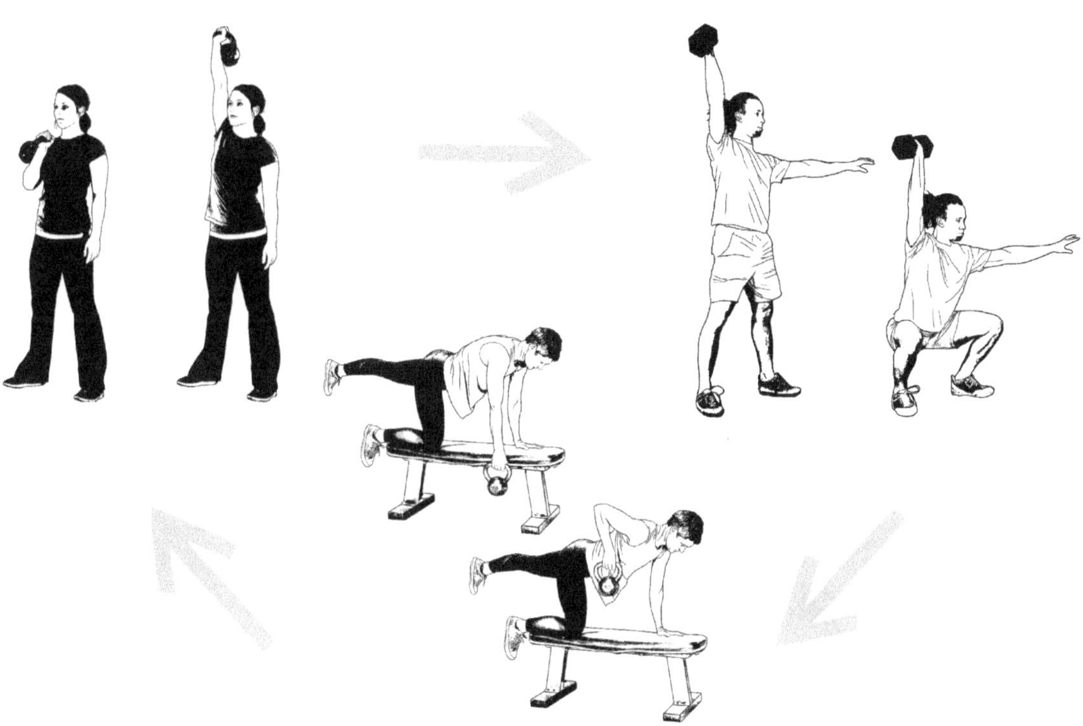

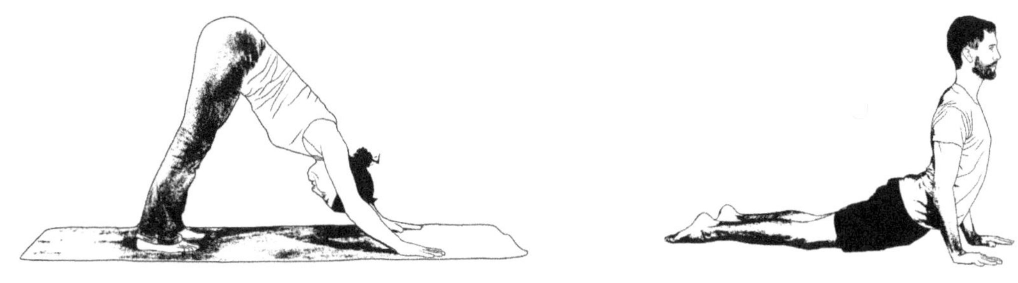

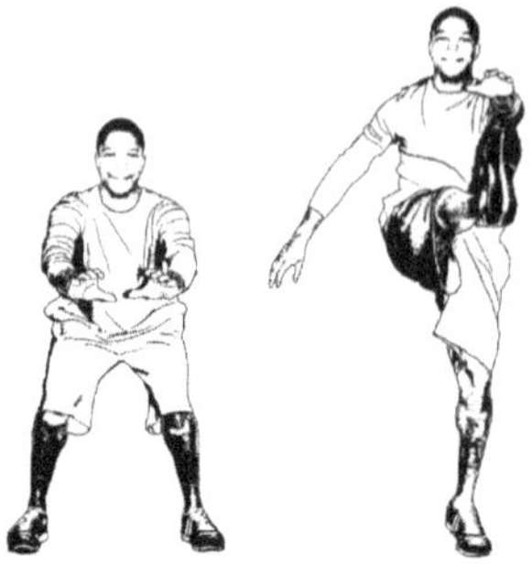

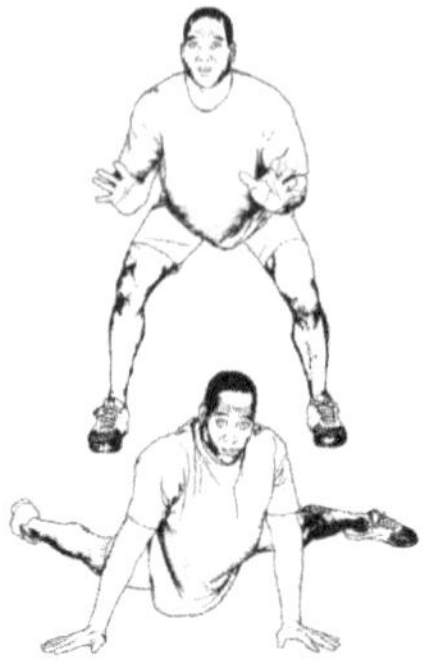

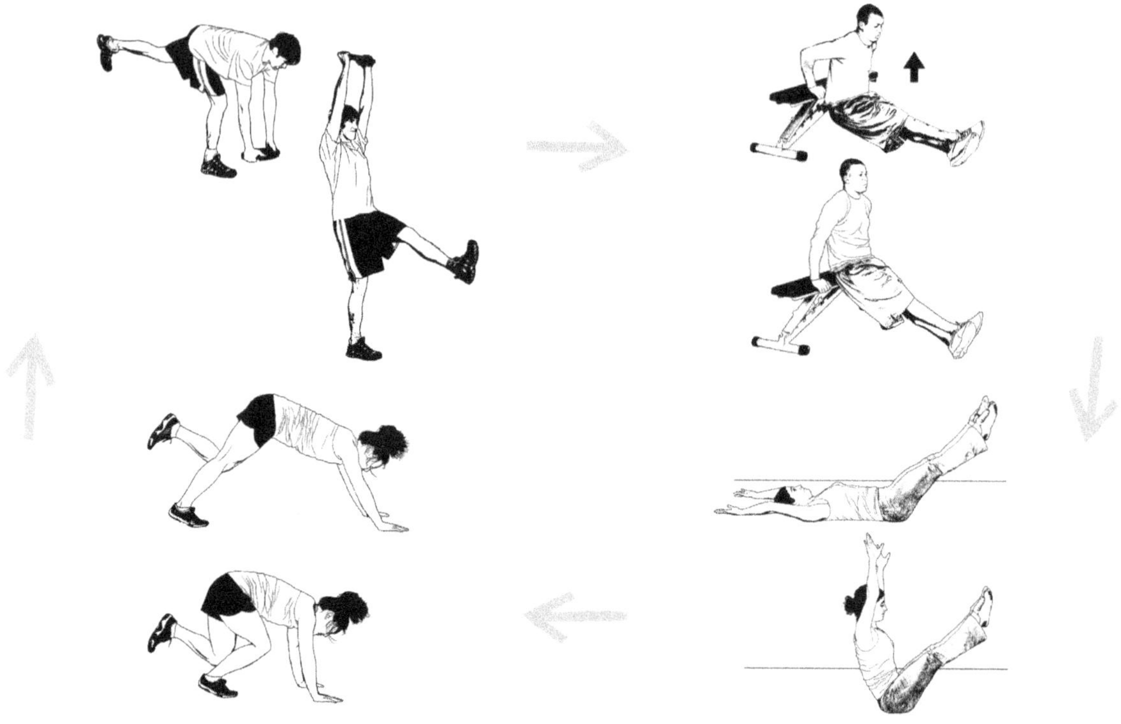

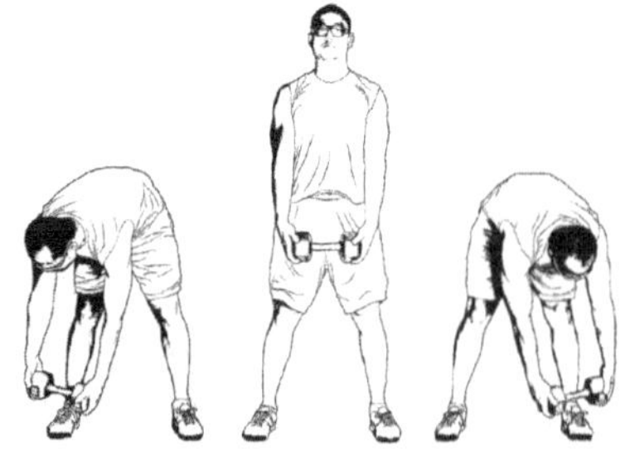

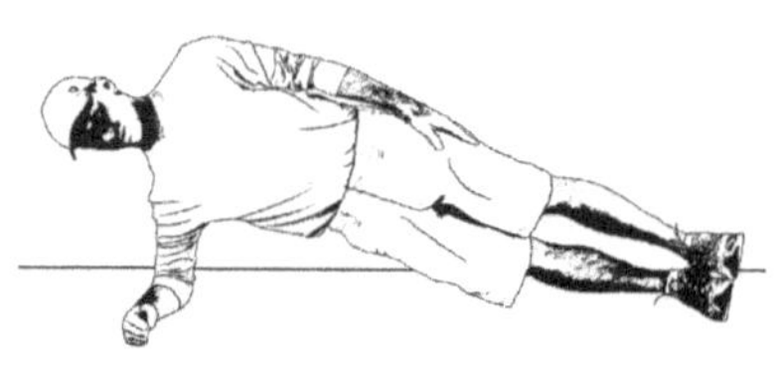

SIDE A

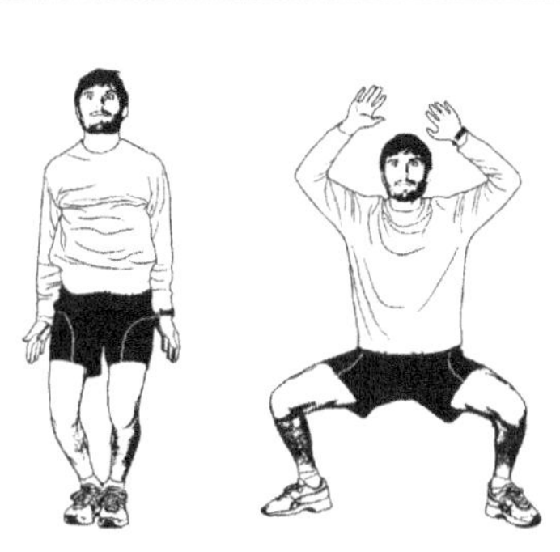

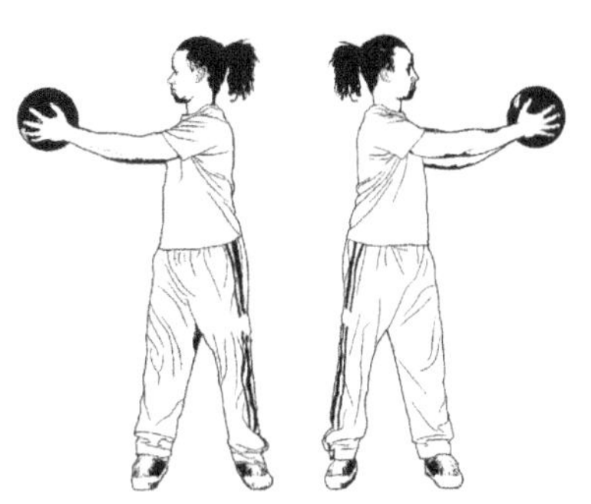

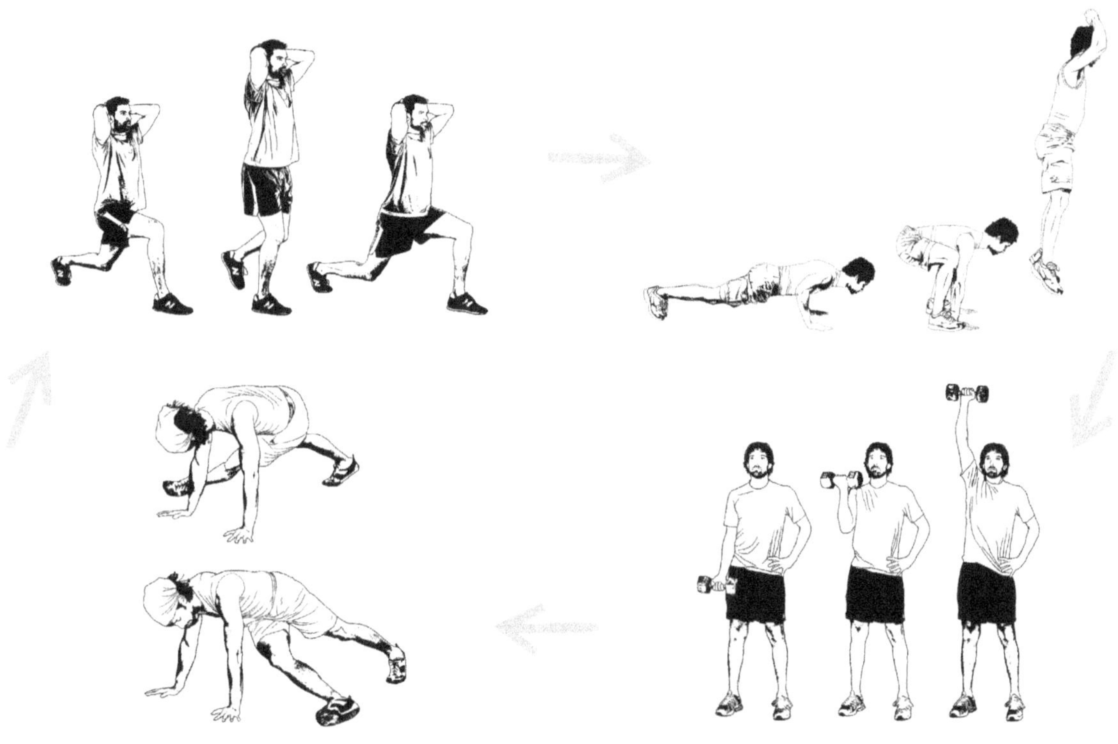

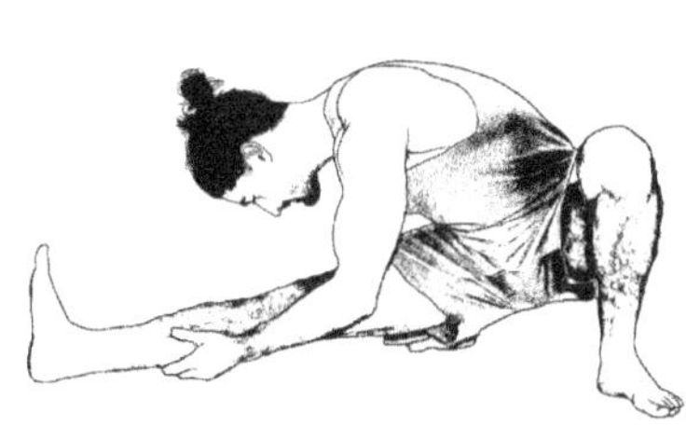

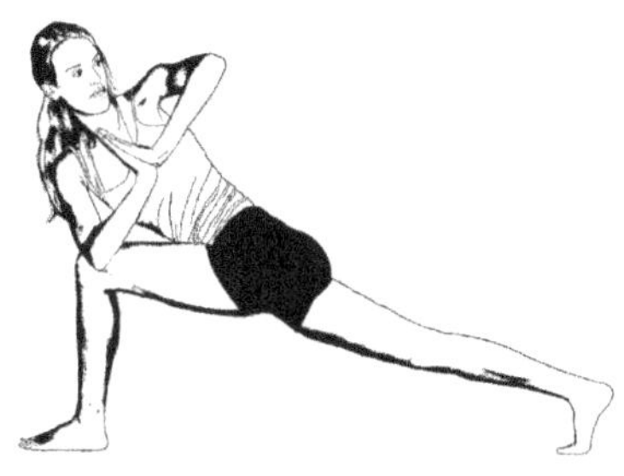

SIDE A

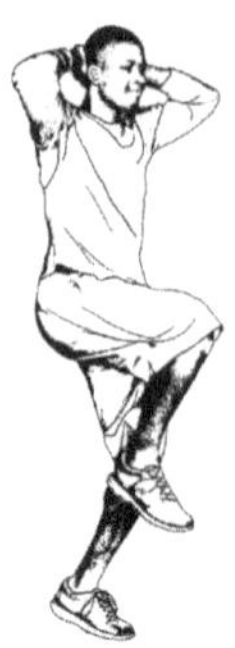

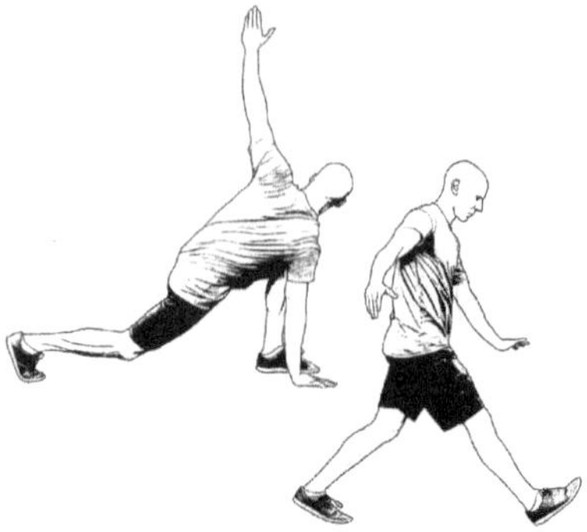

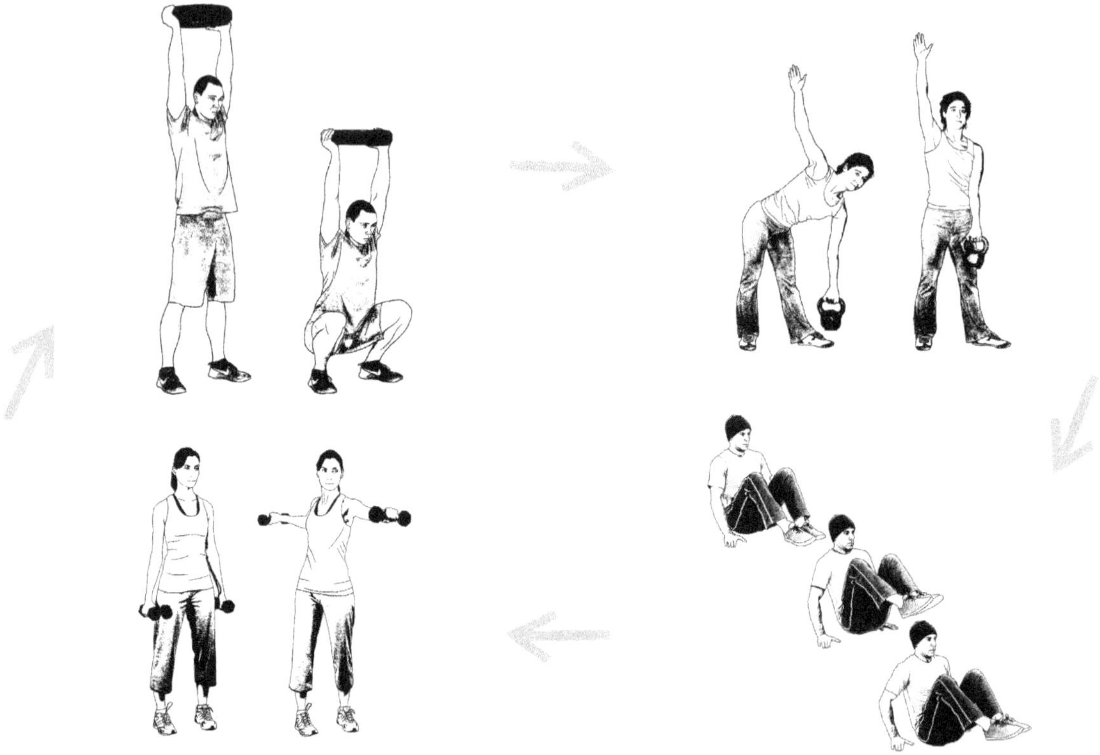

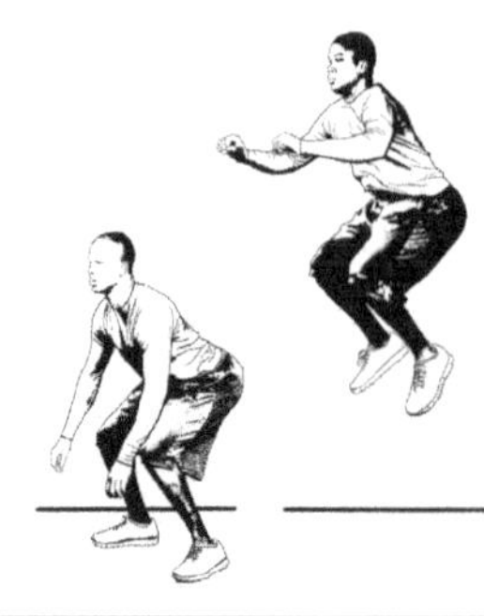

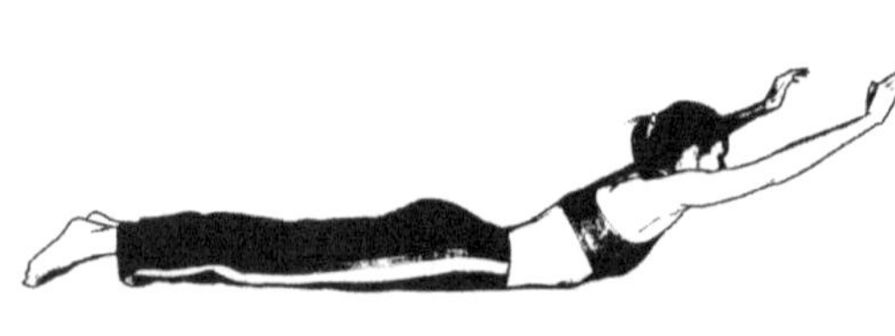

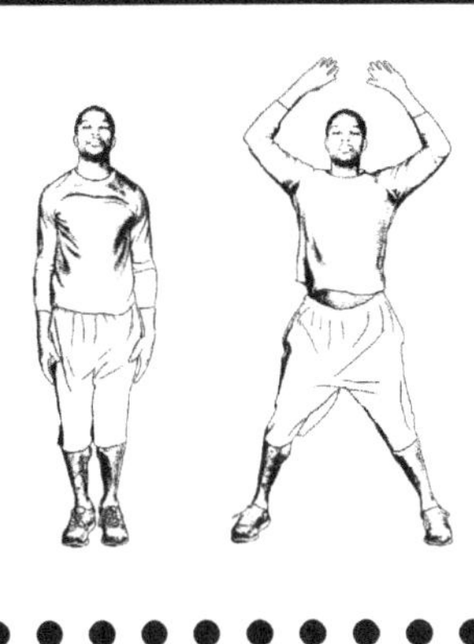

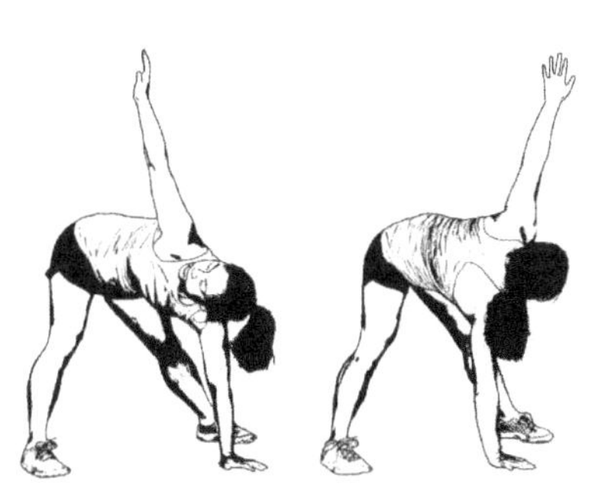

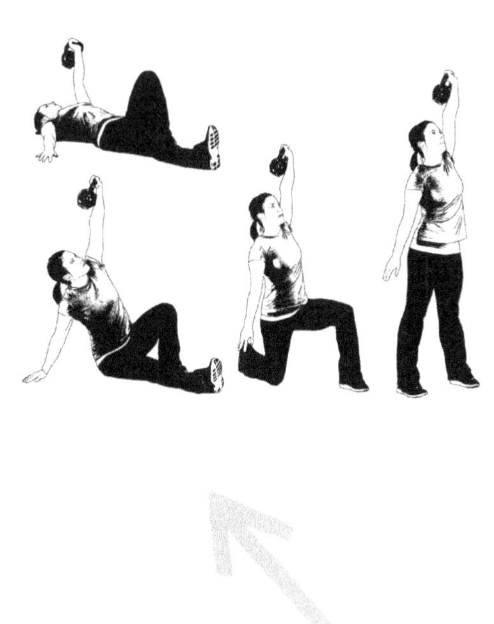

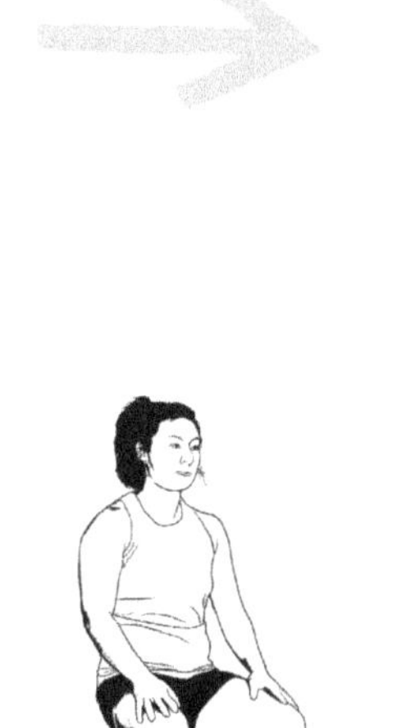

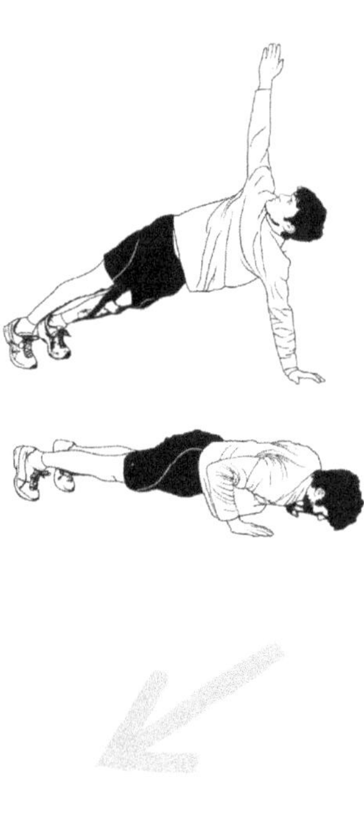

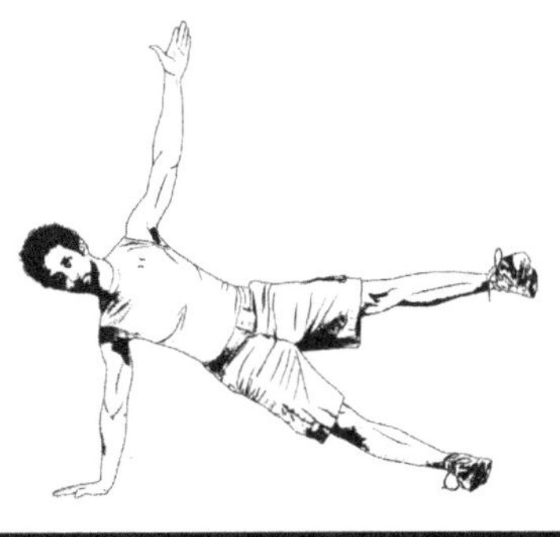

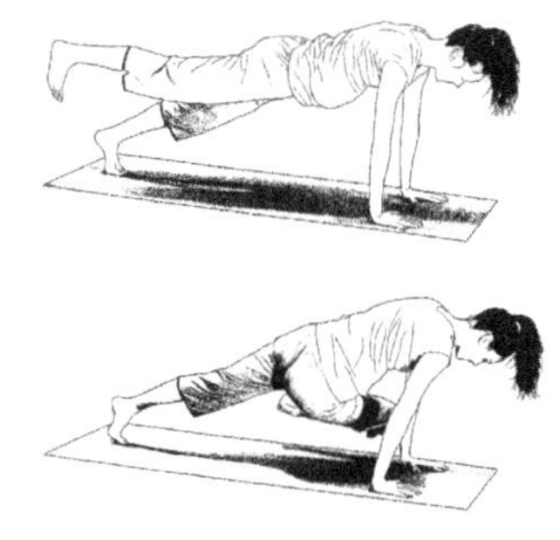

SIDE A

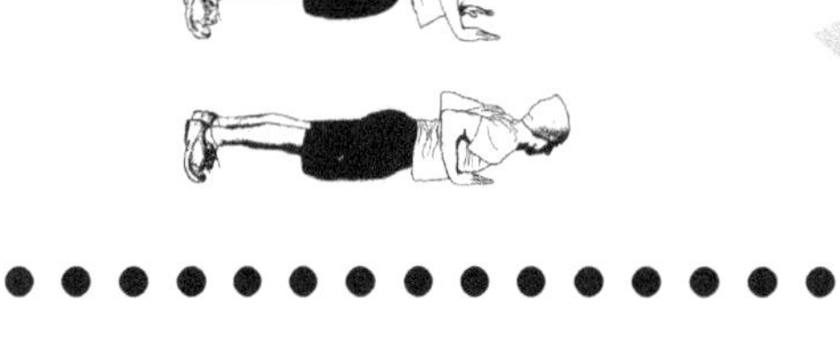

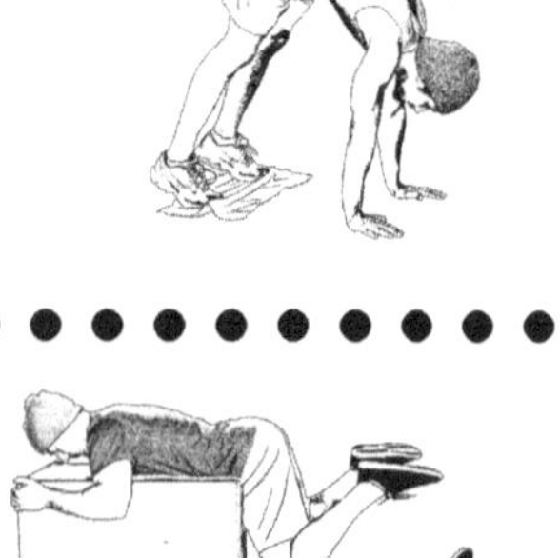

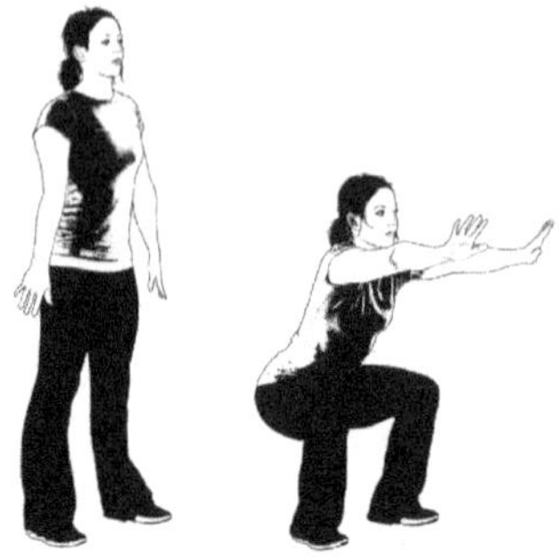

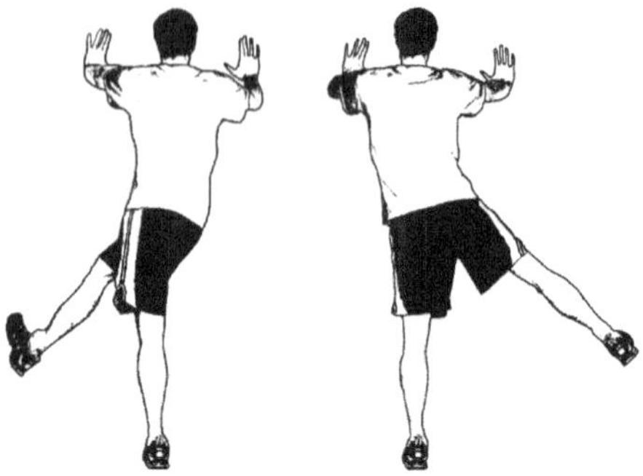

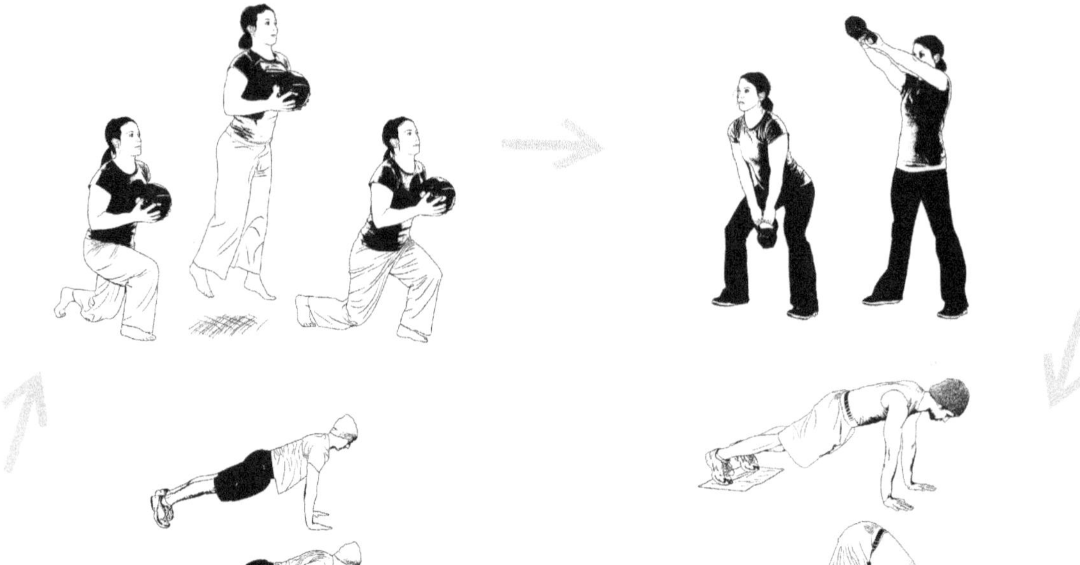

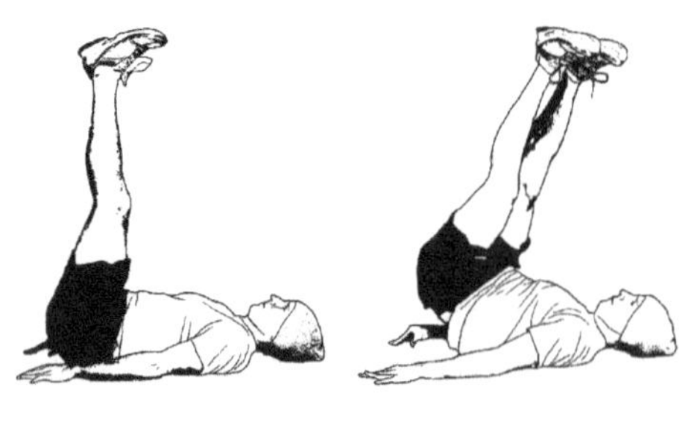

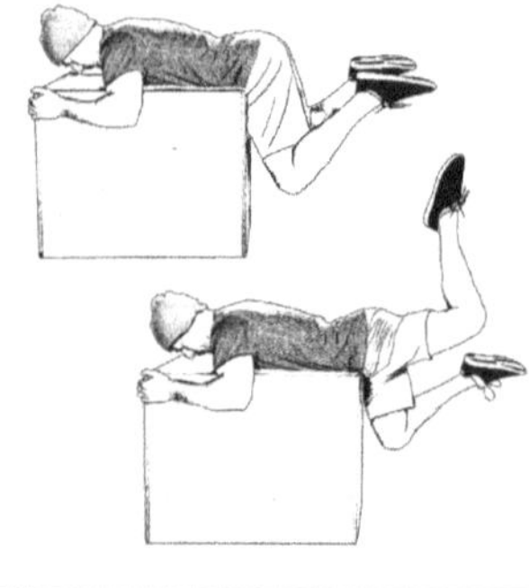

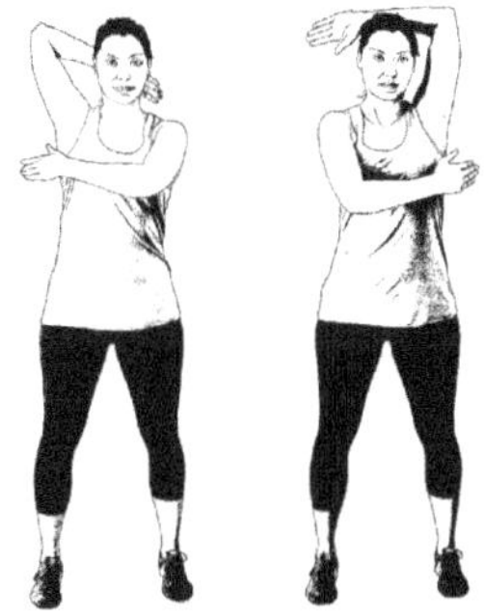

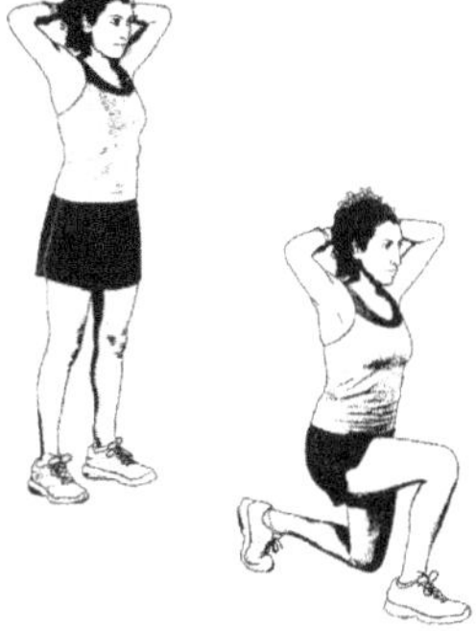

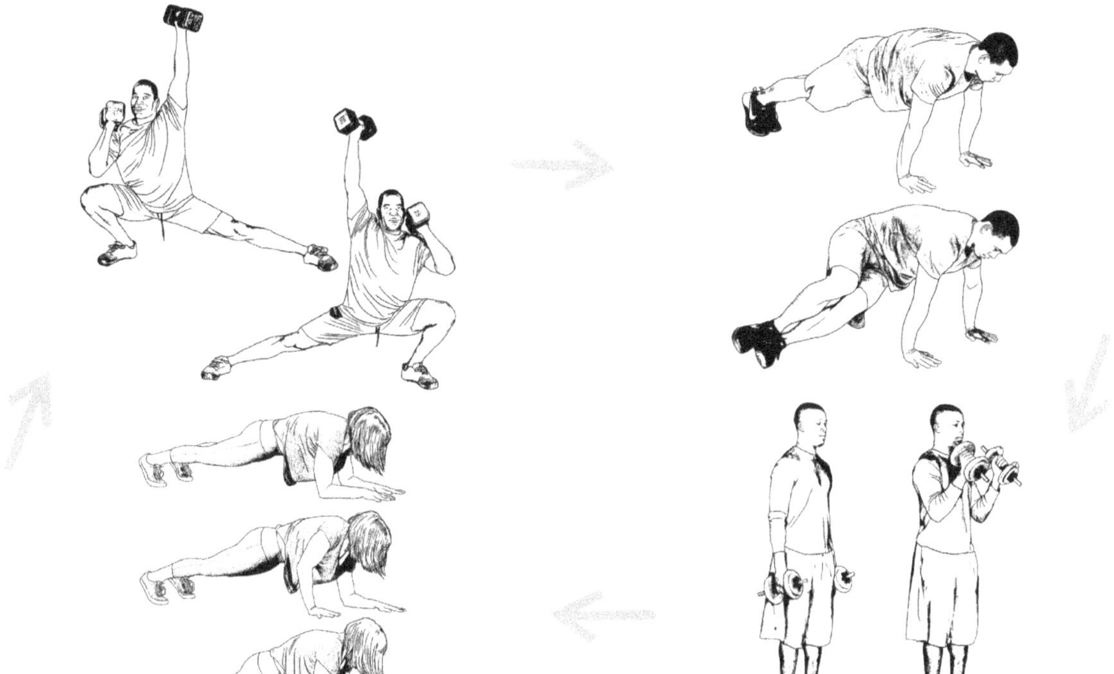

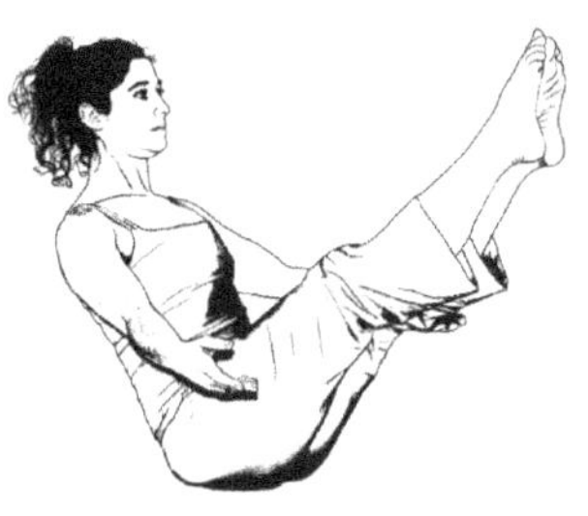
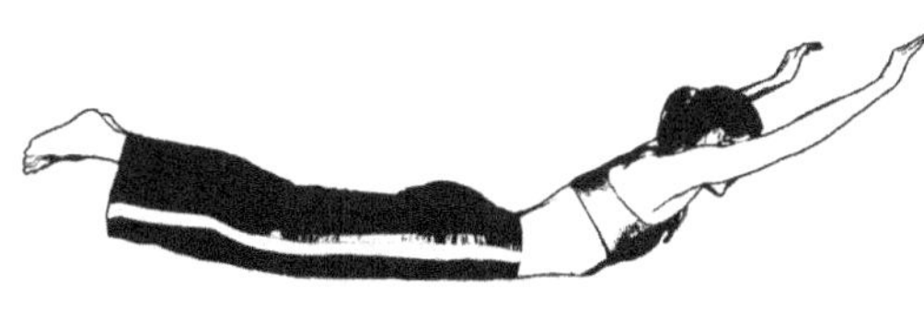

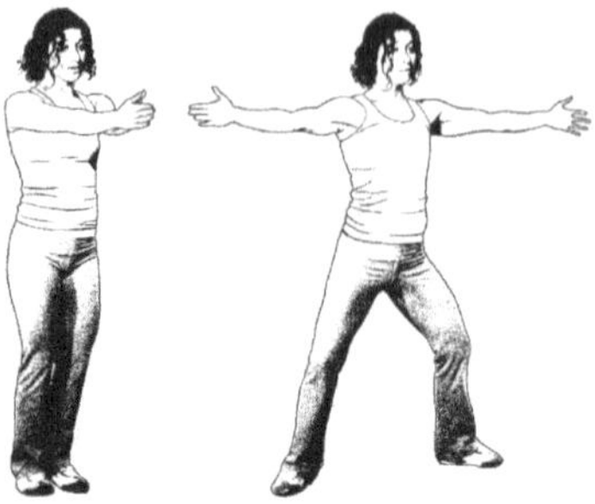

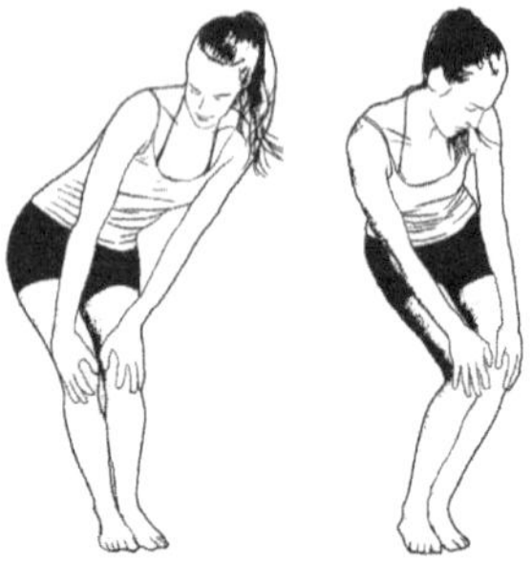

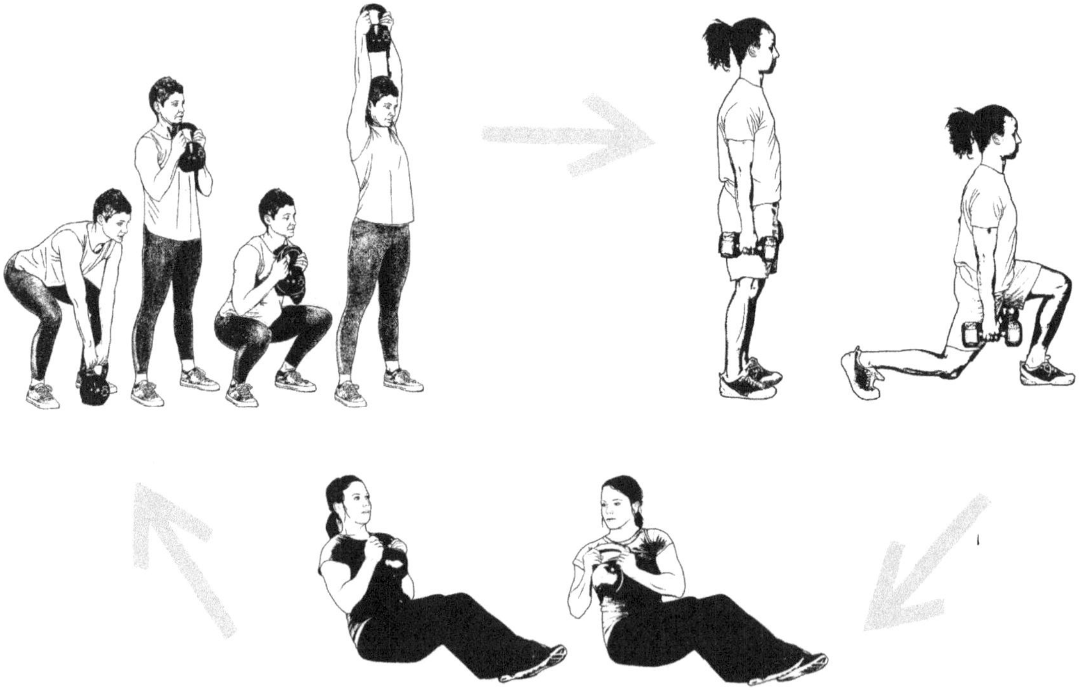

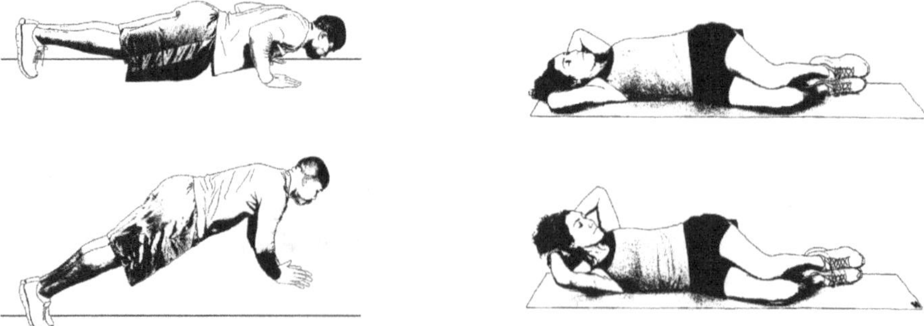

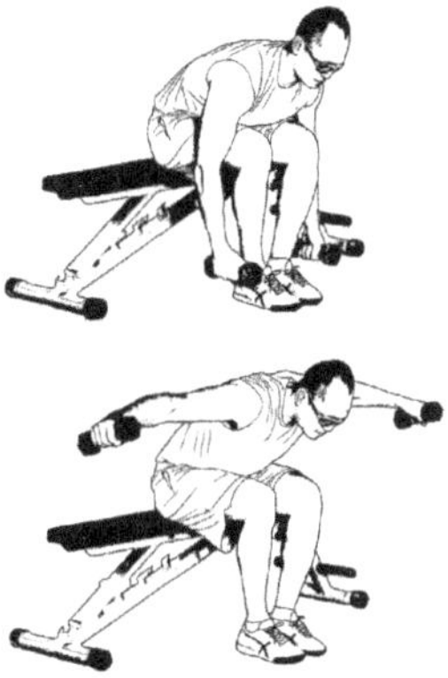

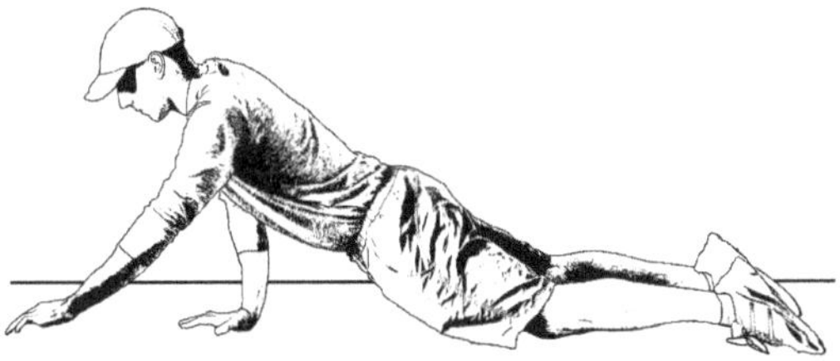

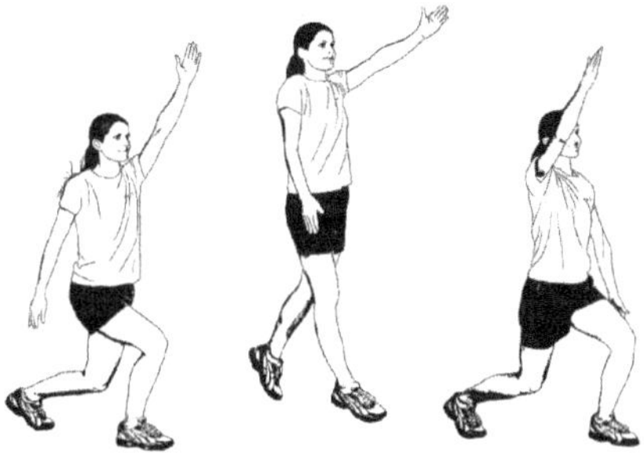

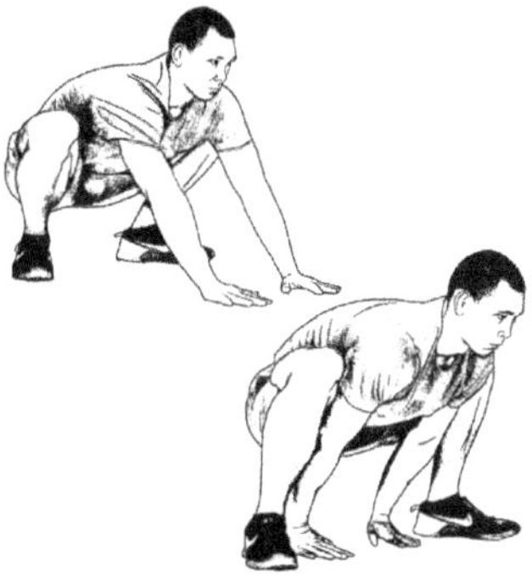

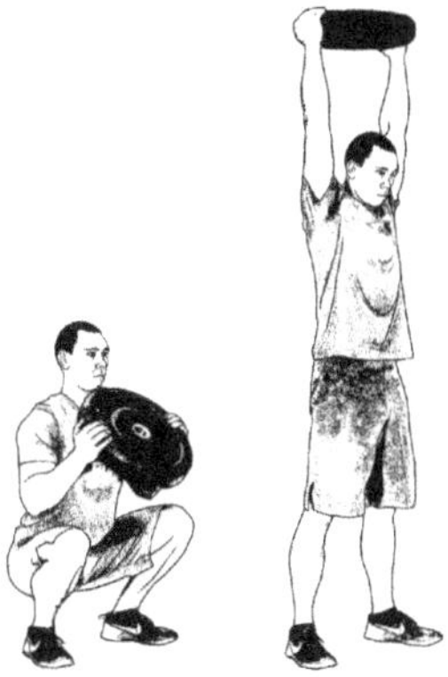

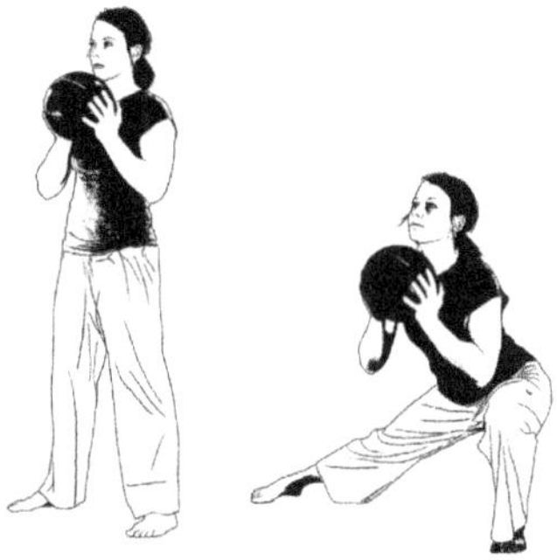

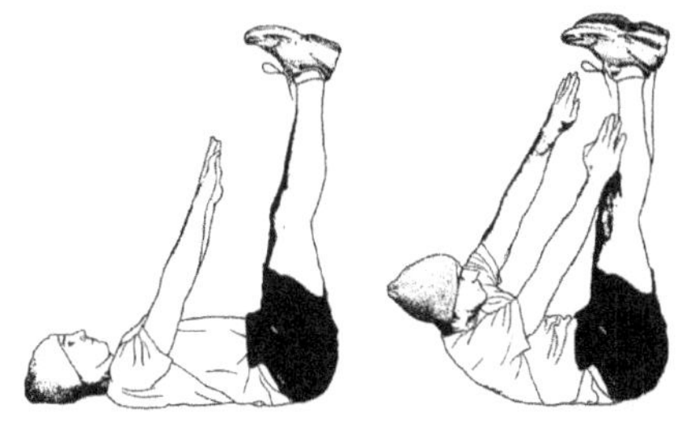

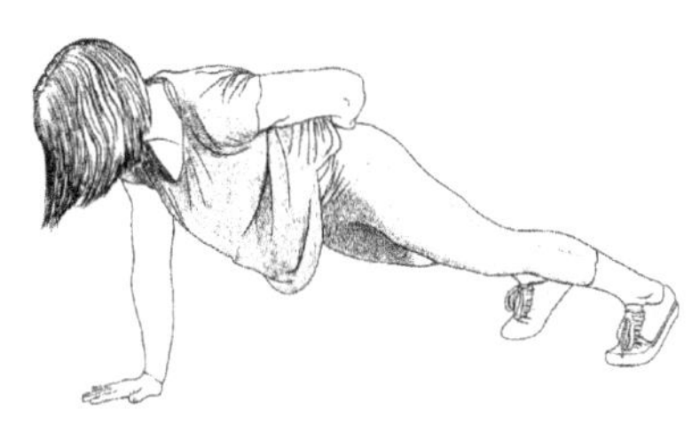

SIDE A

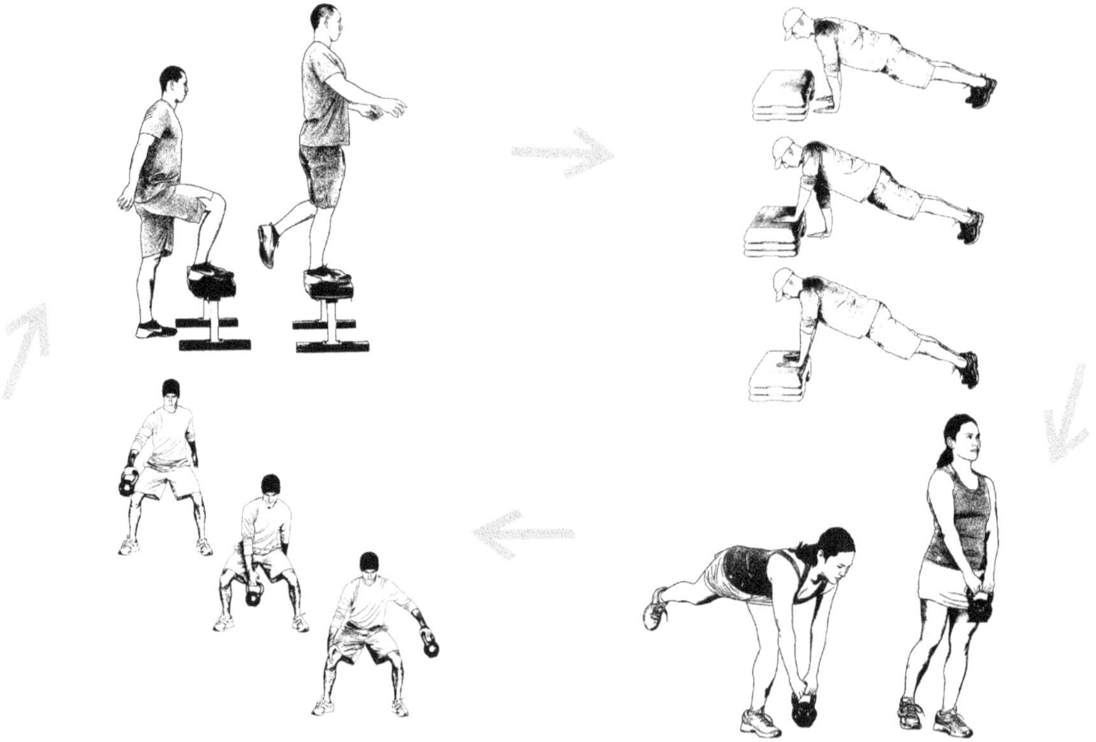

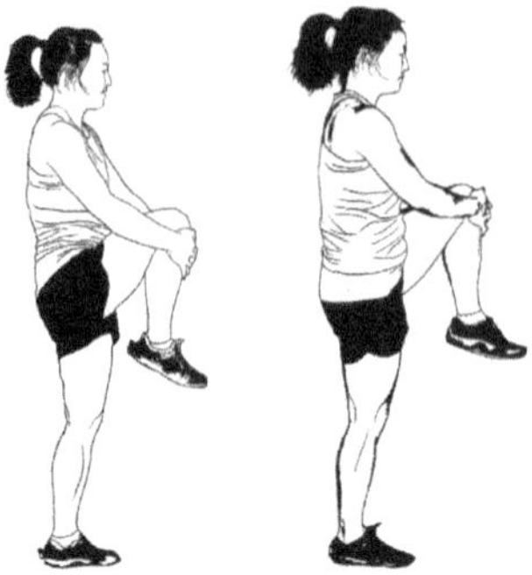

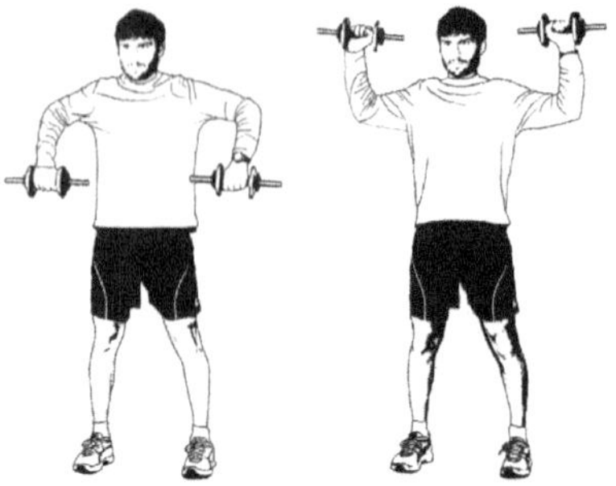

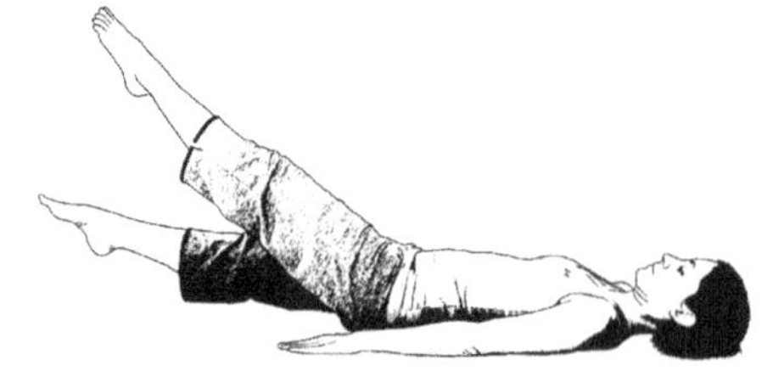

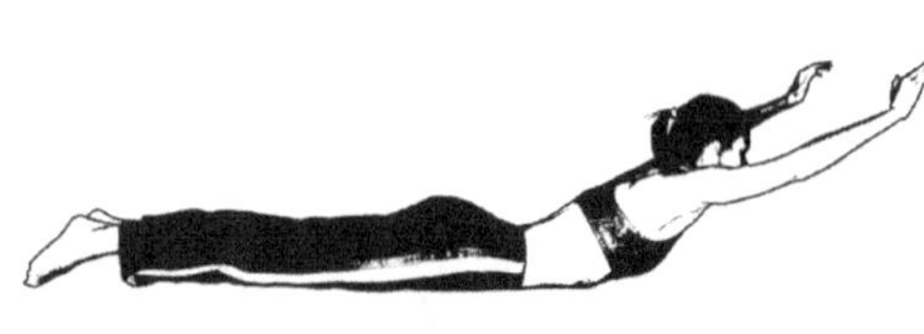

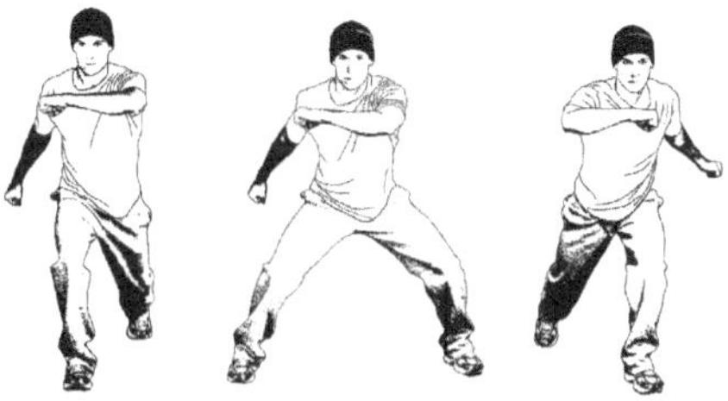

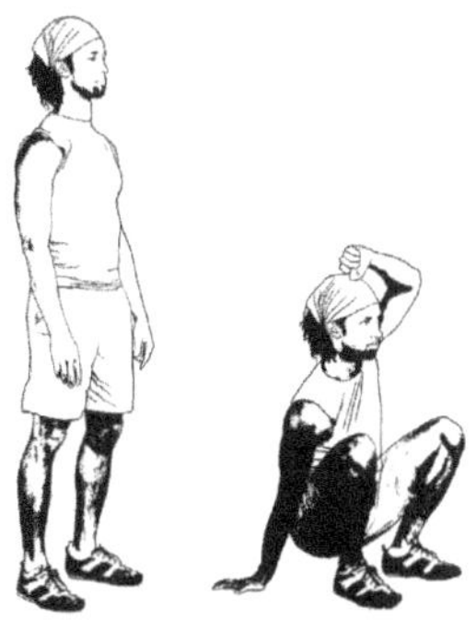

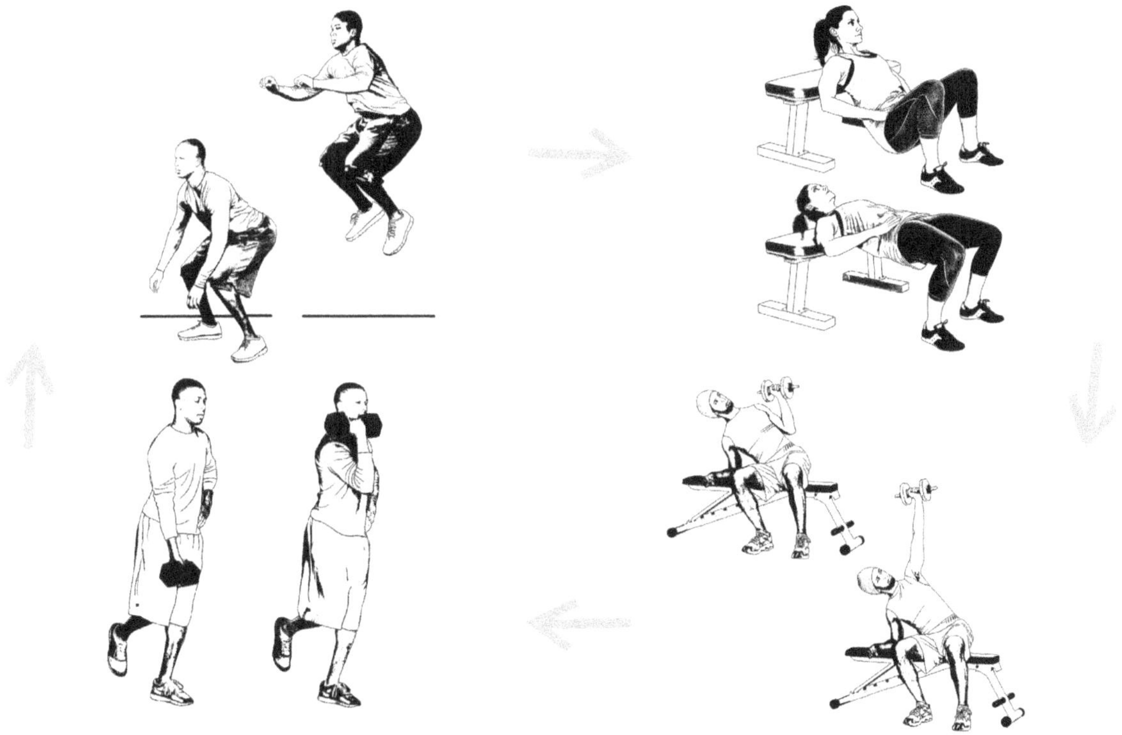

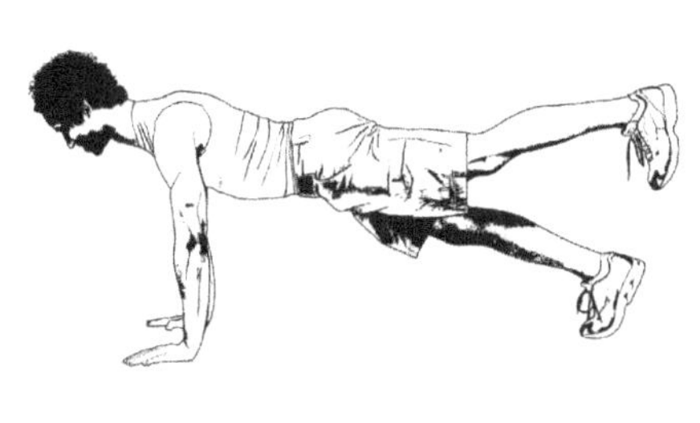
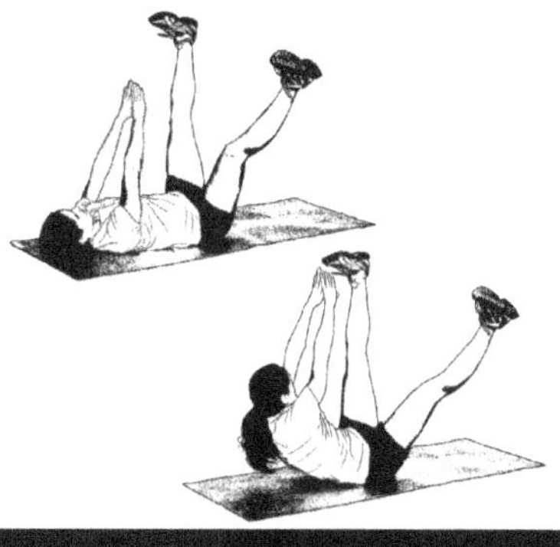

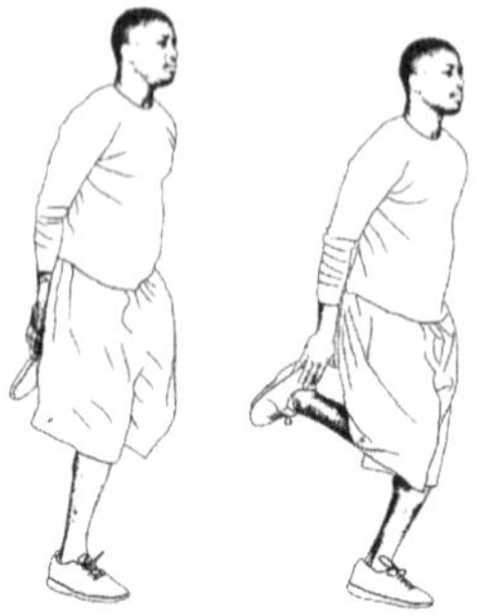

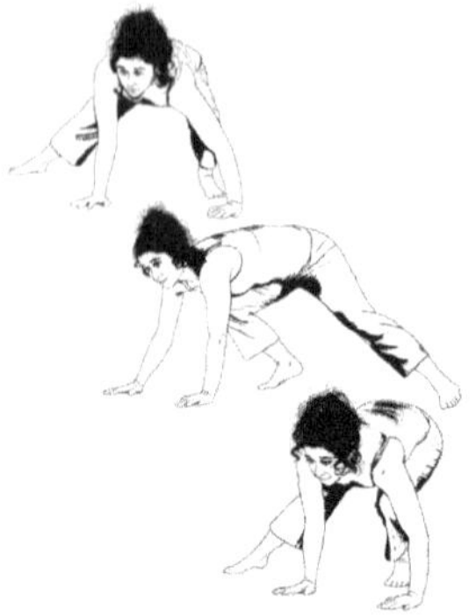

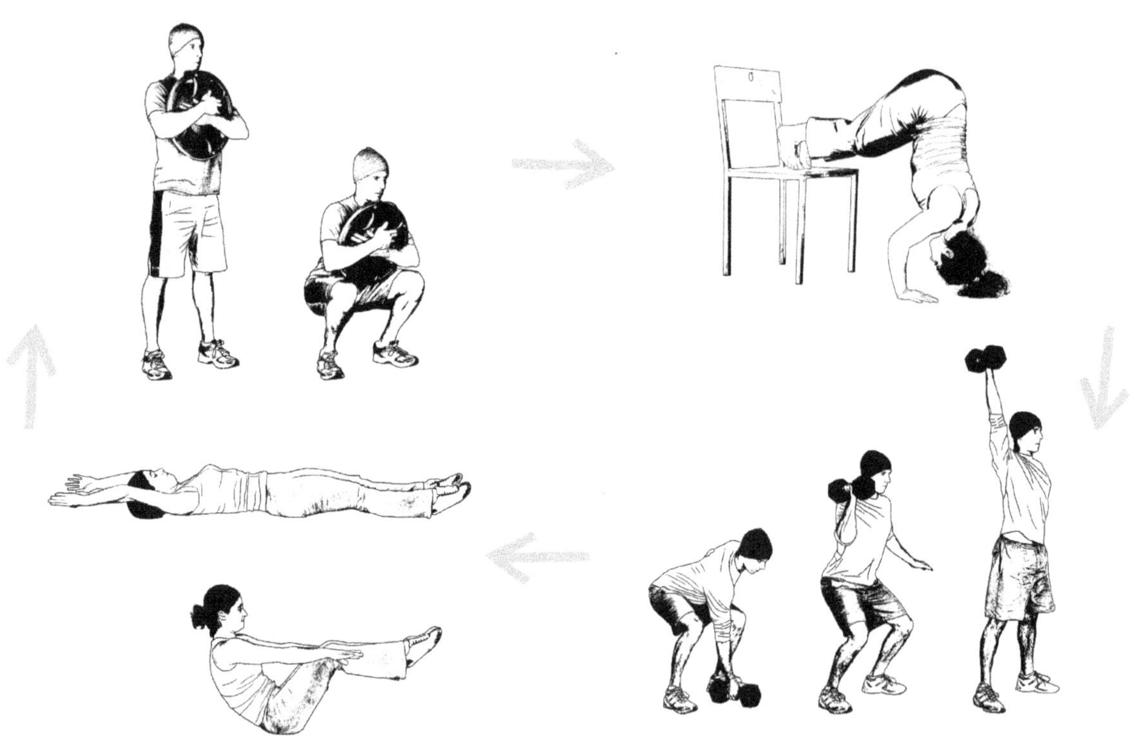

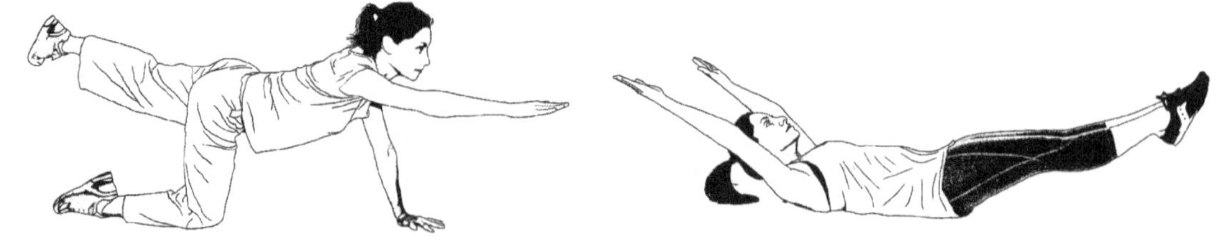

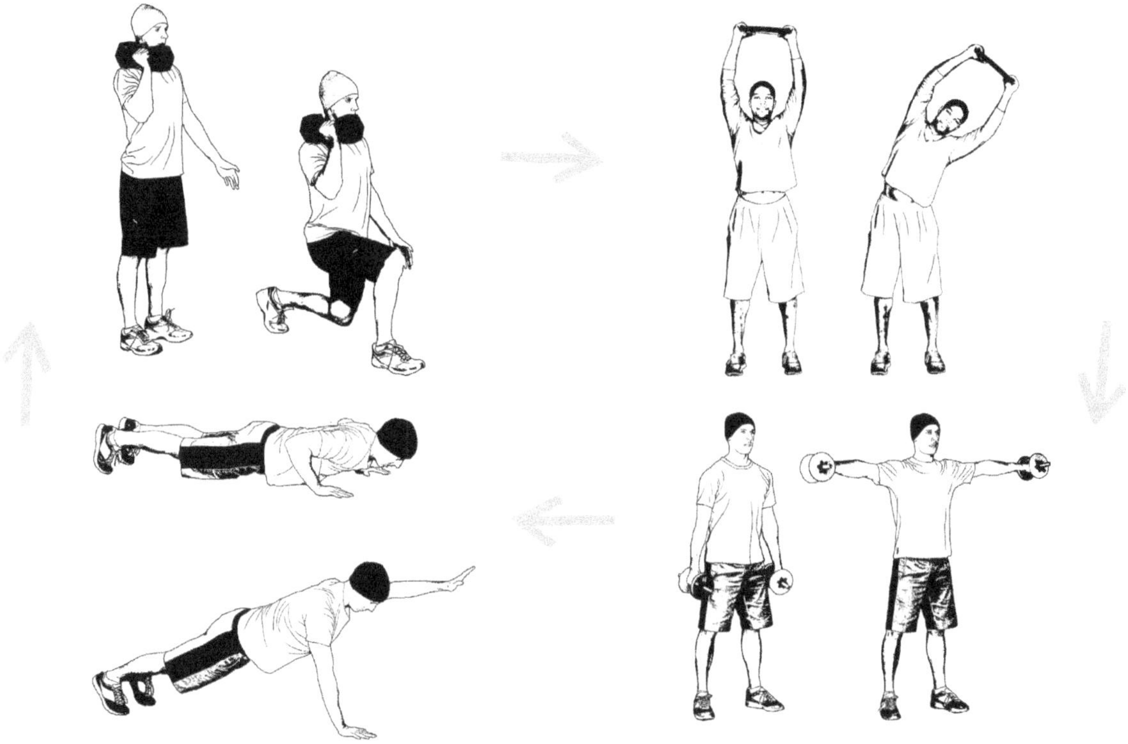

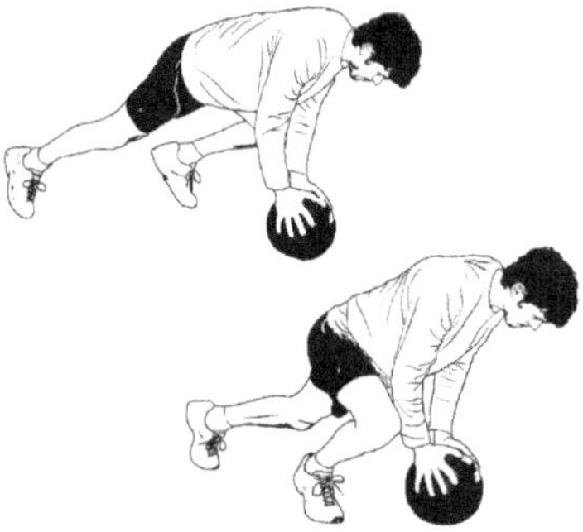

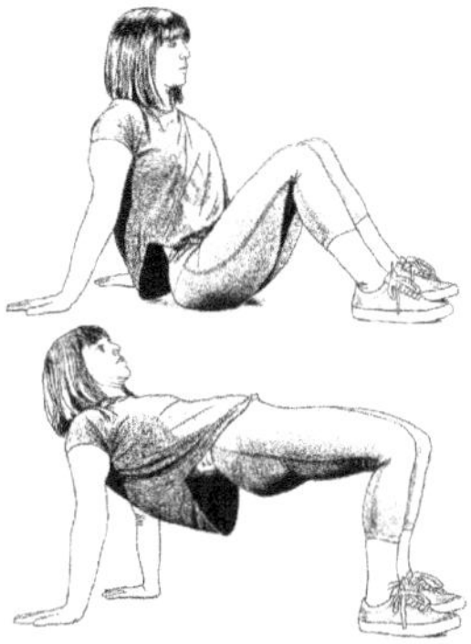

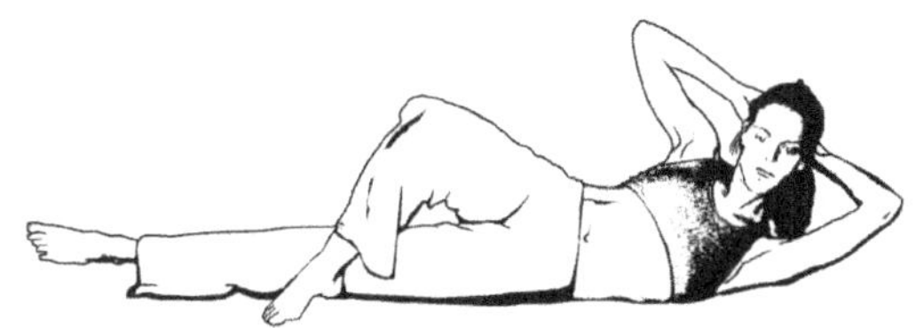
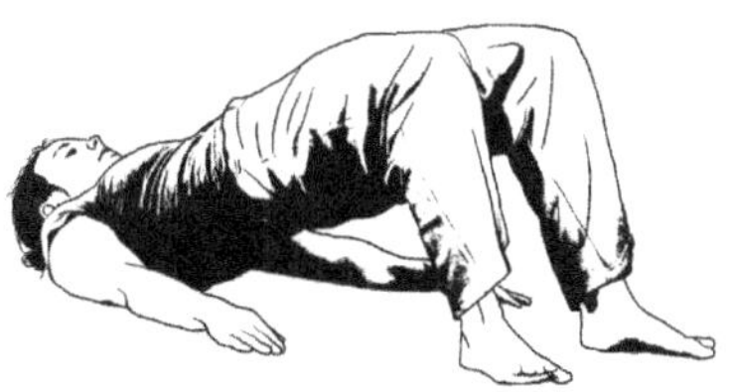

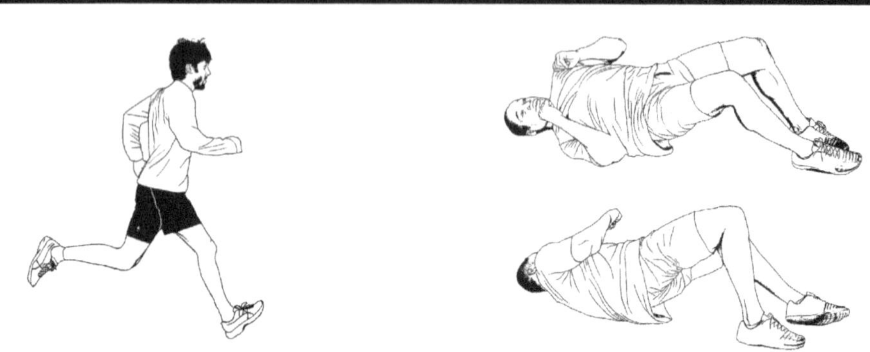

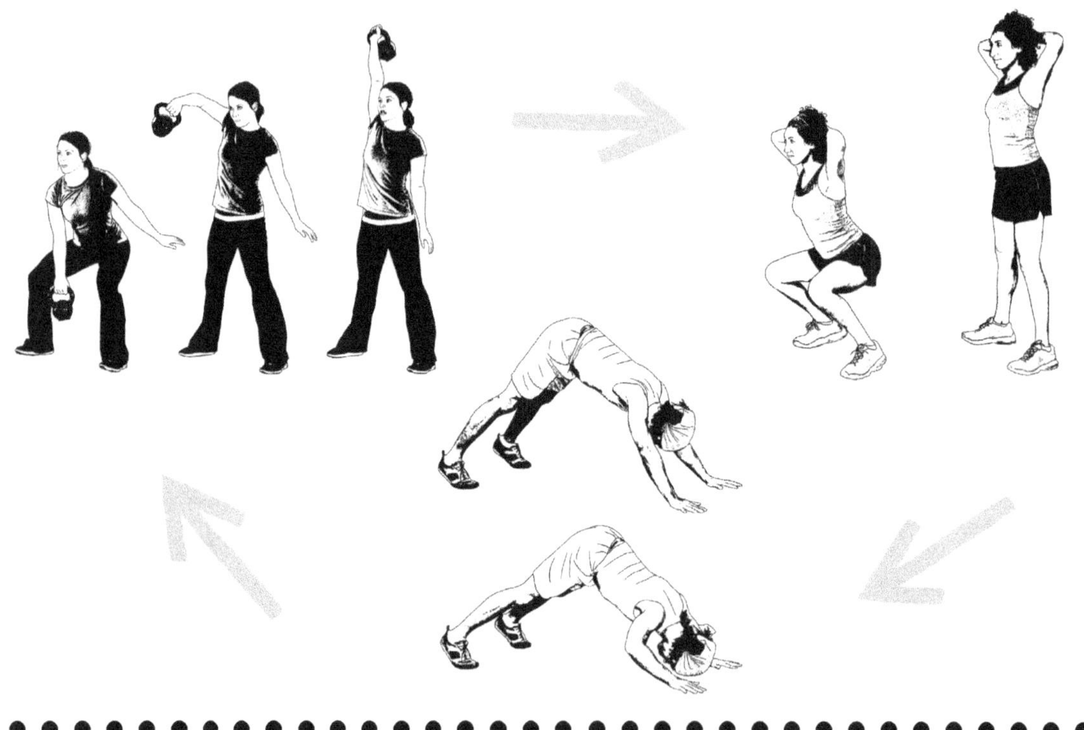

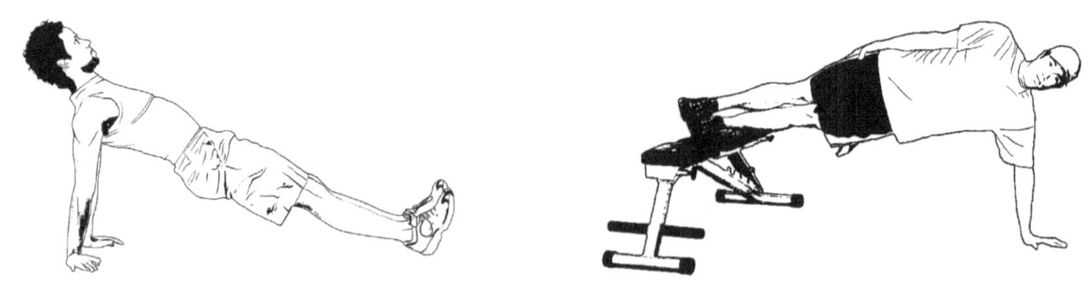

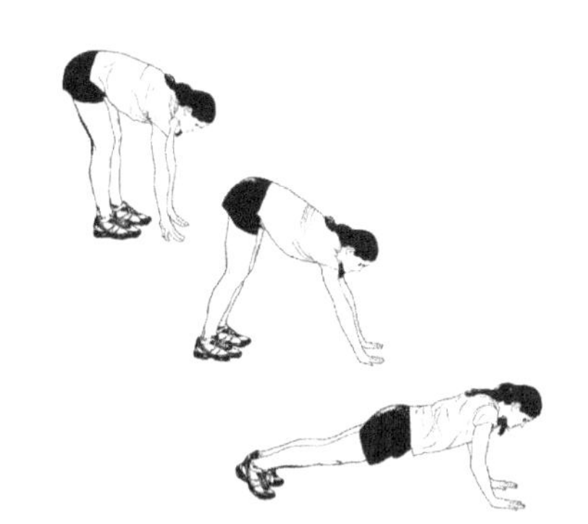

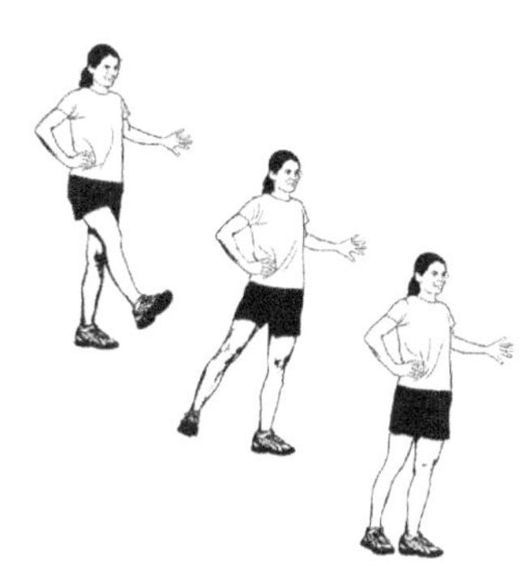

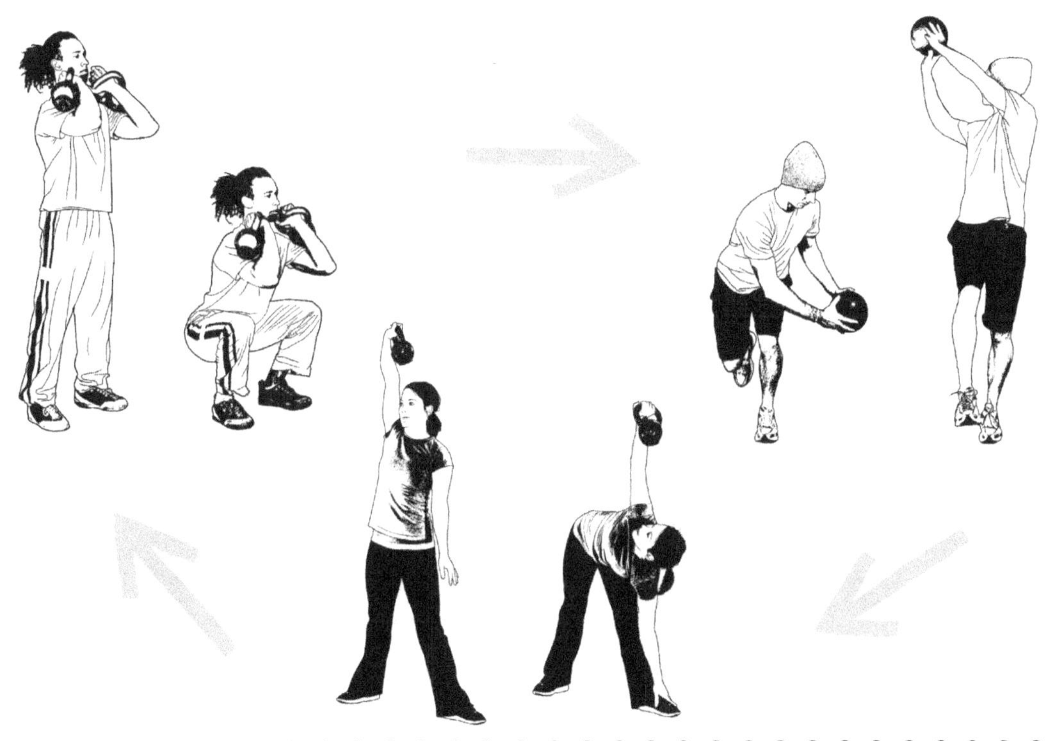

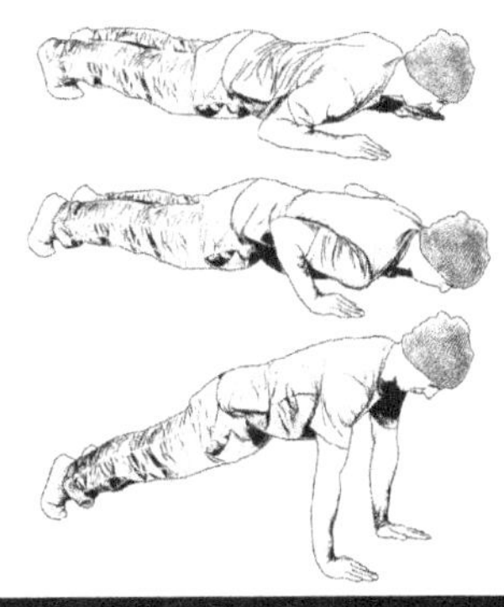

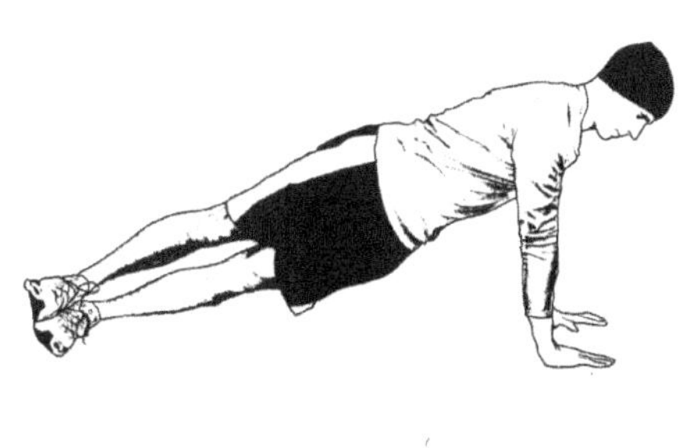

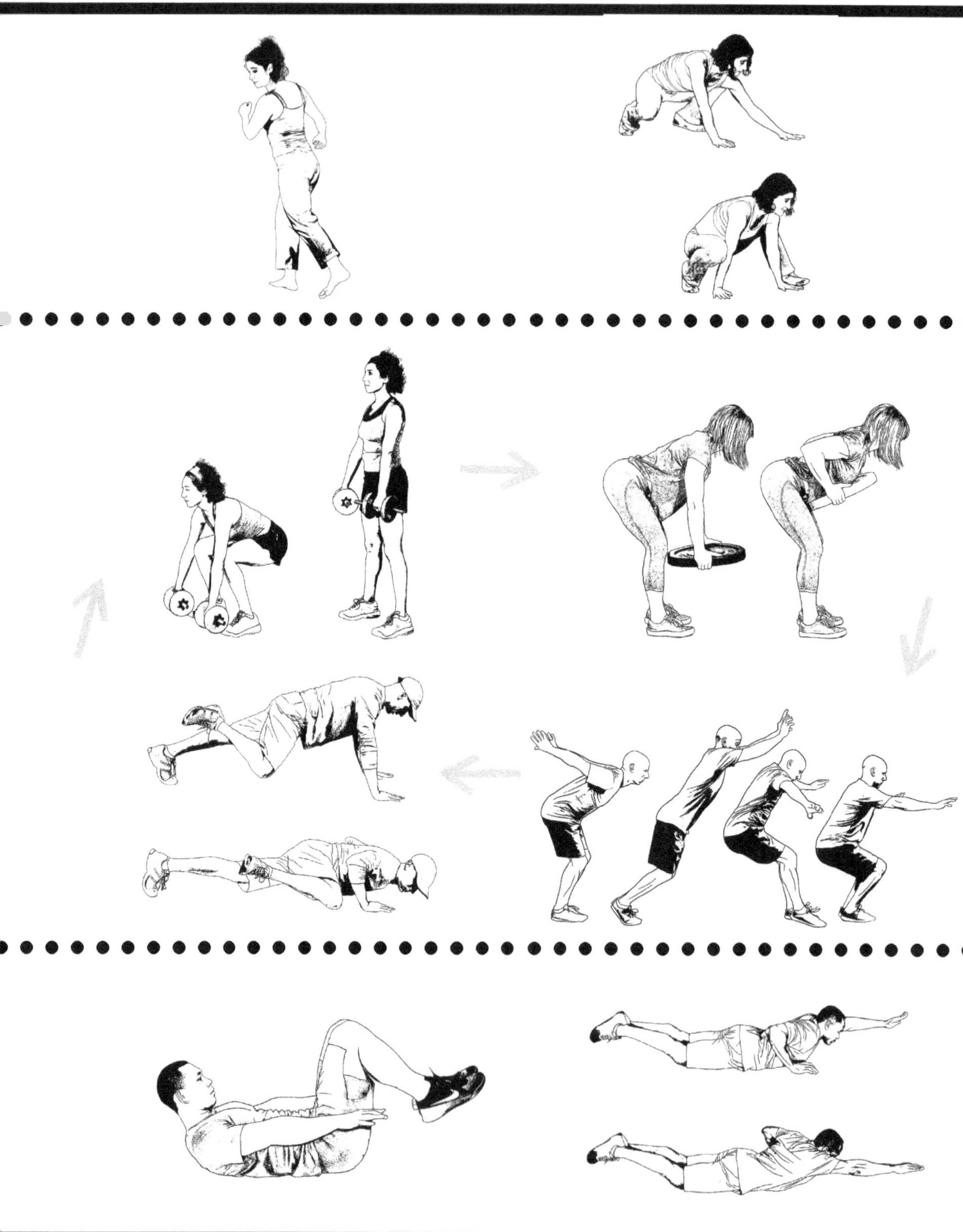

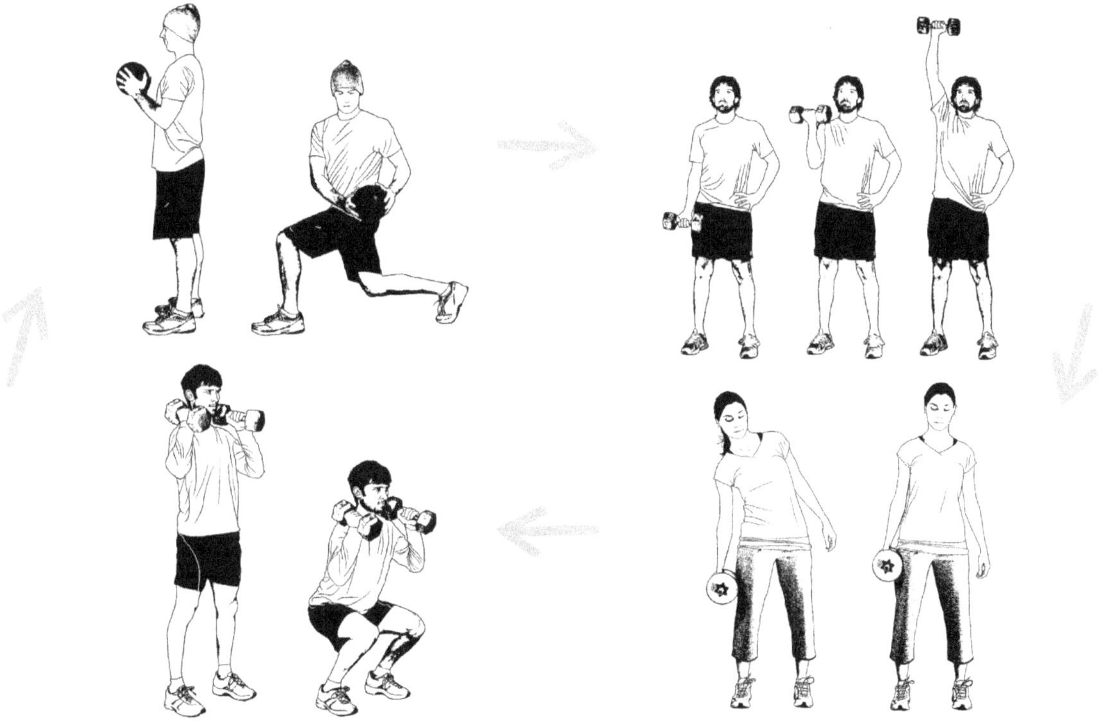

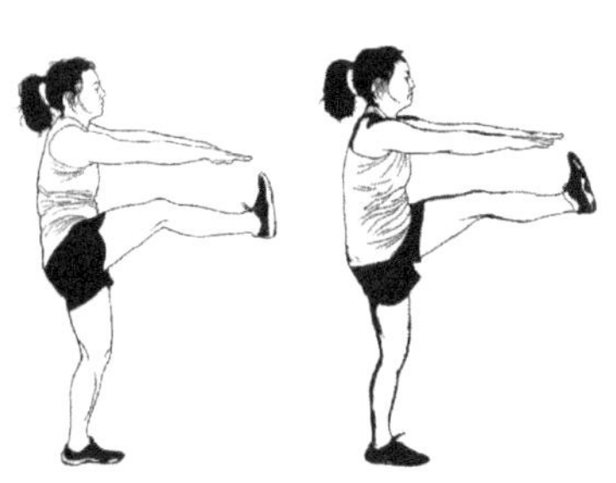
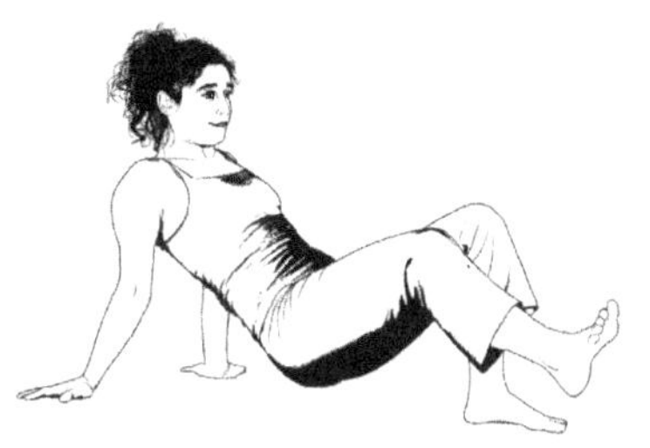
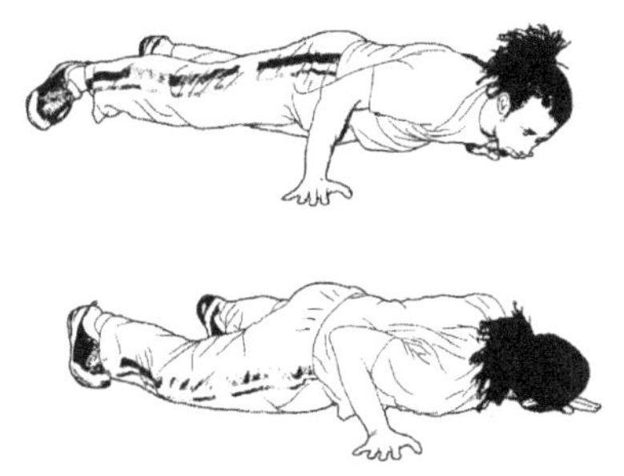
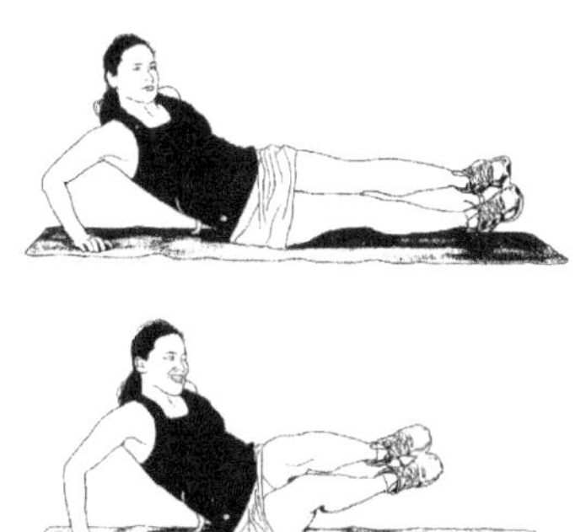

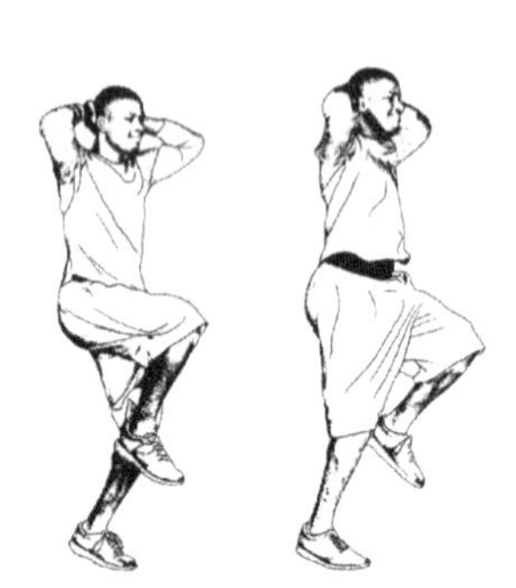

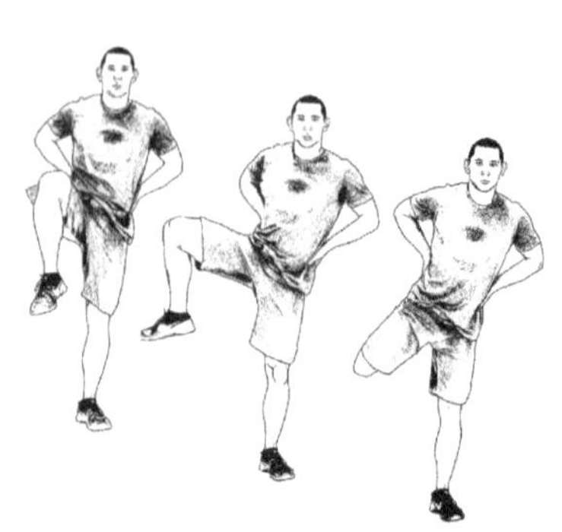

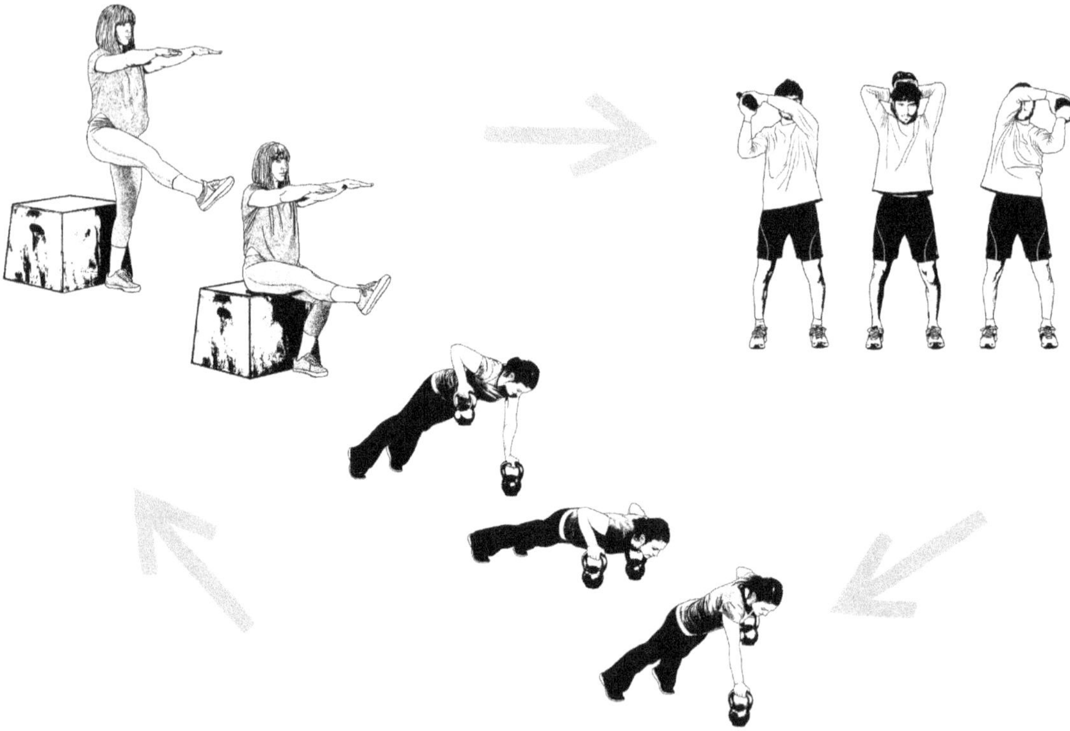

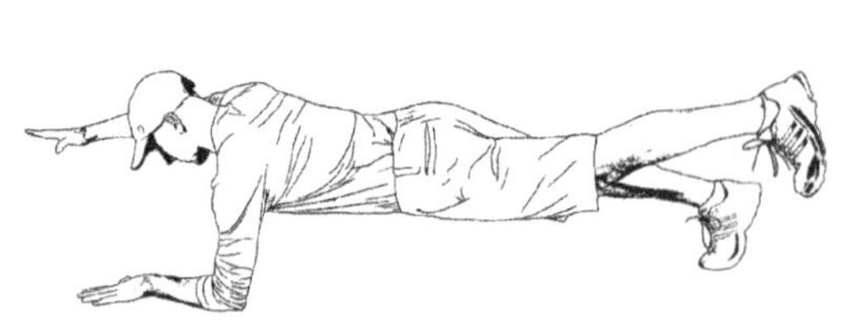

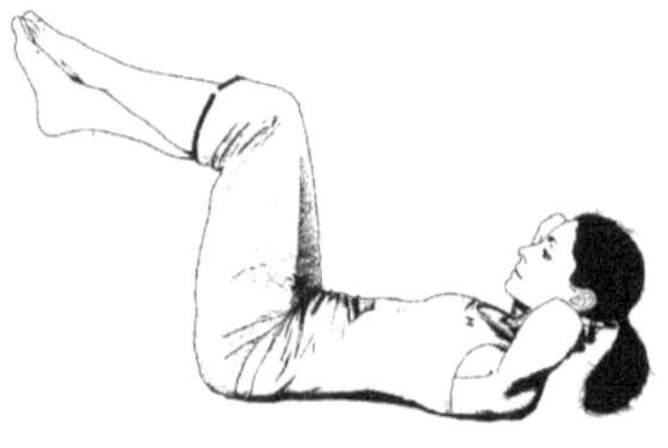

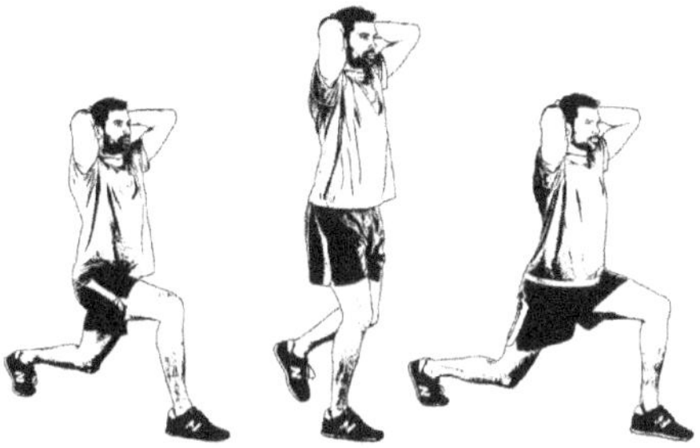

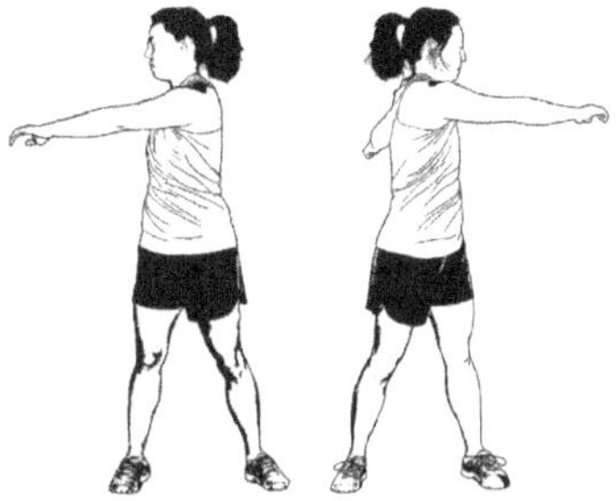

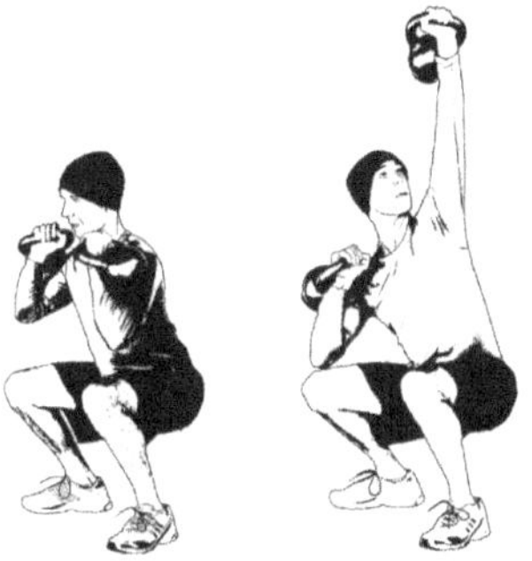

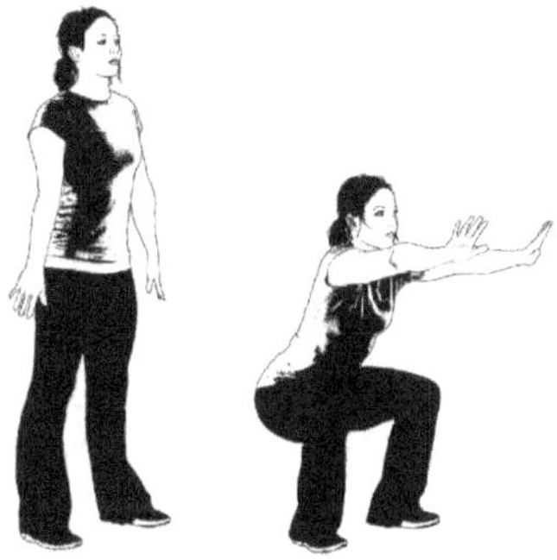

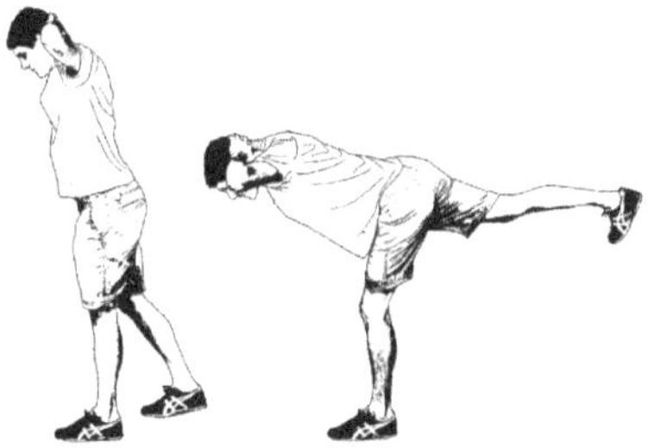

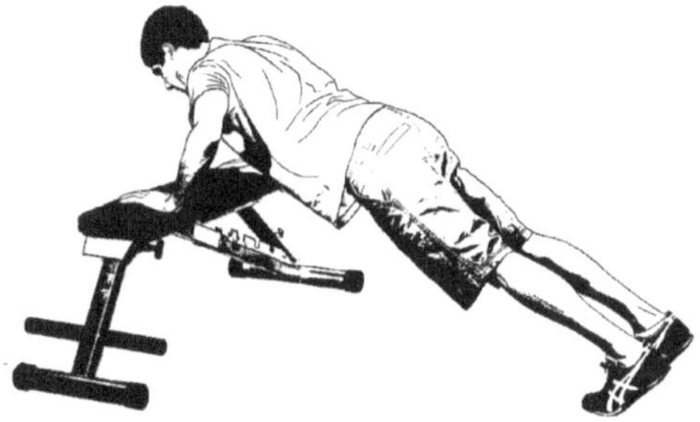

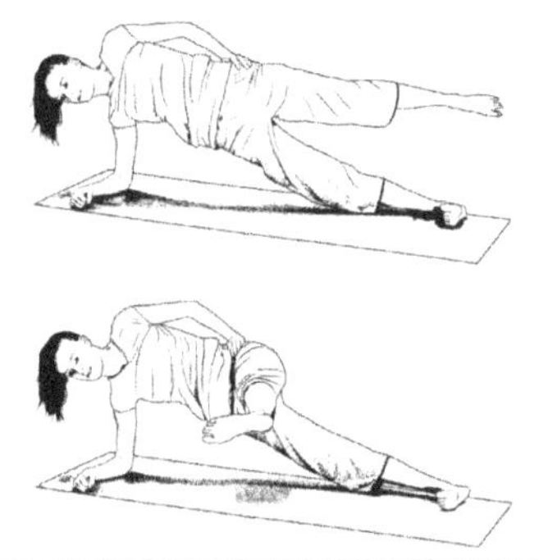
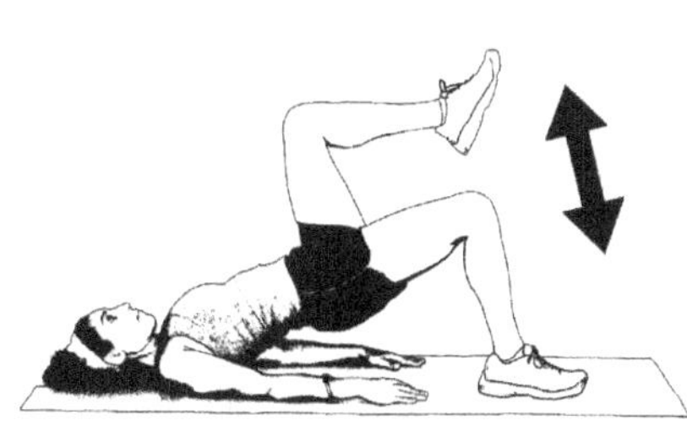

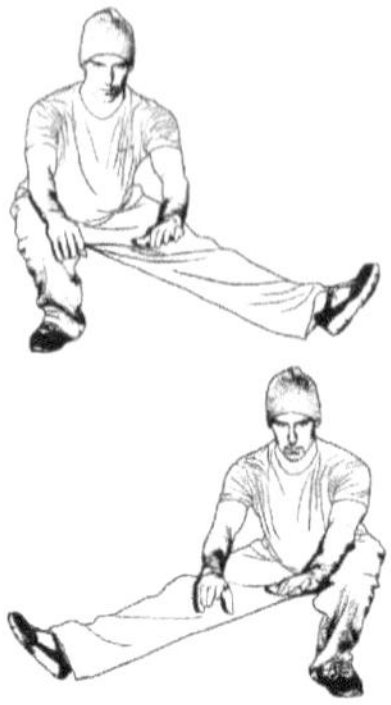

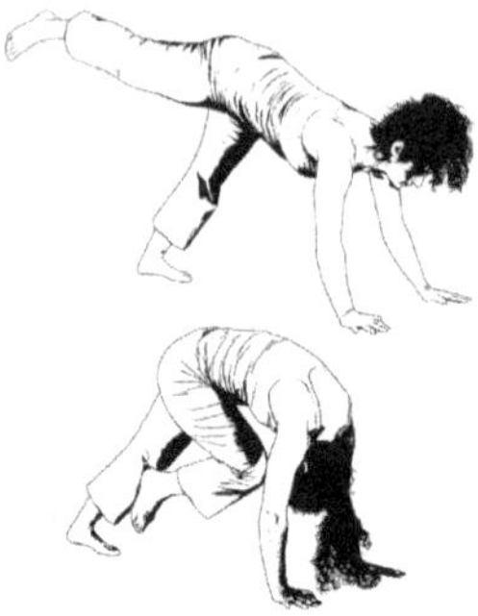

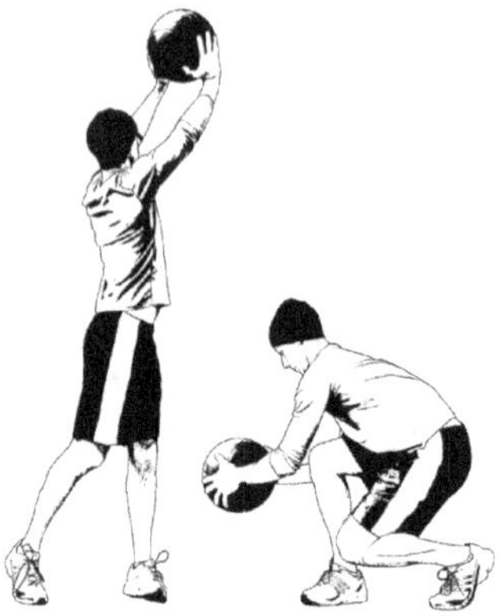

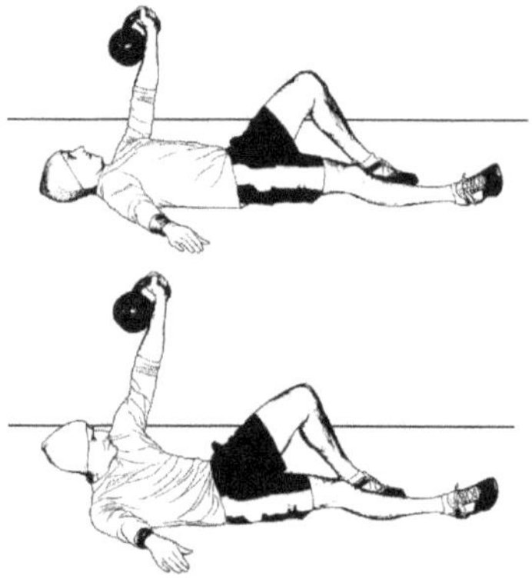

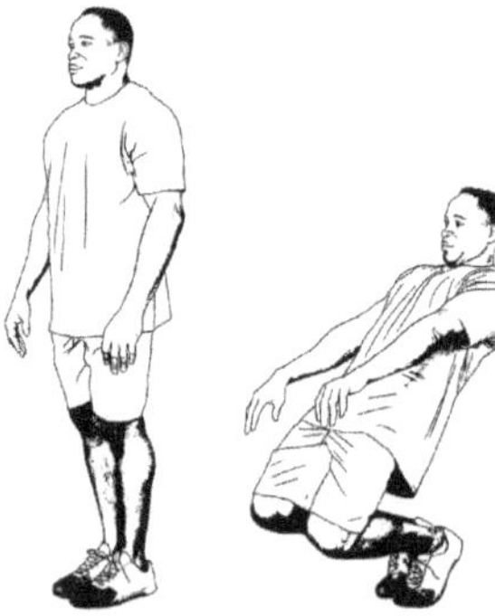

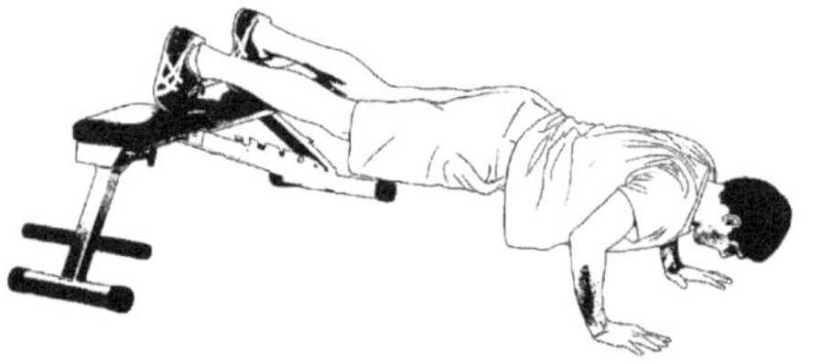

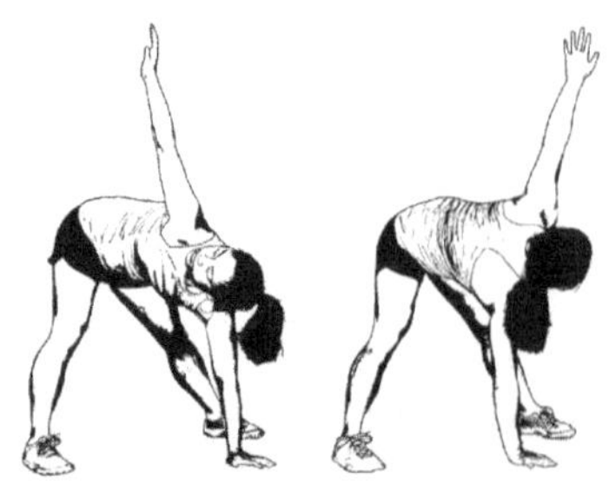

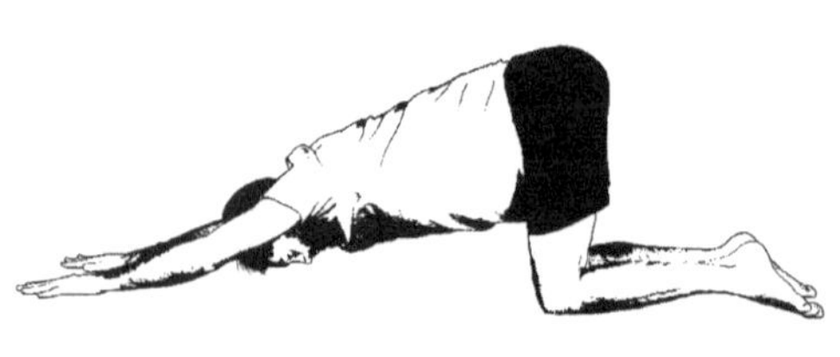

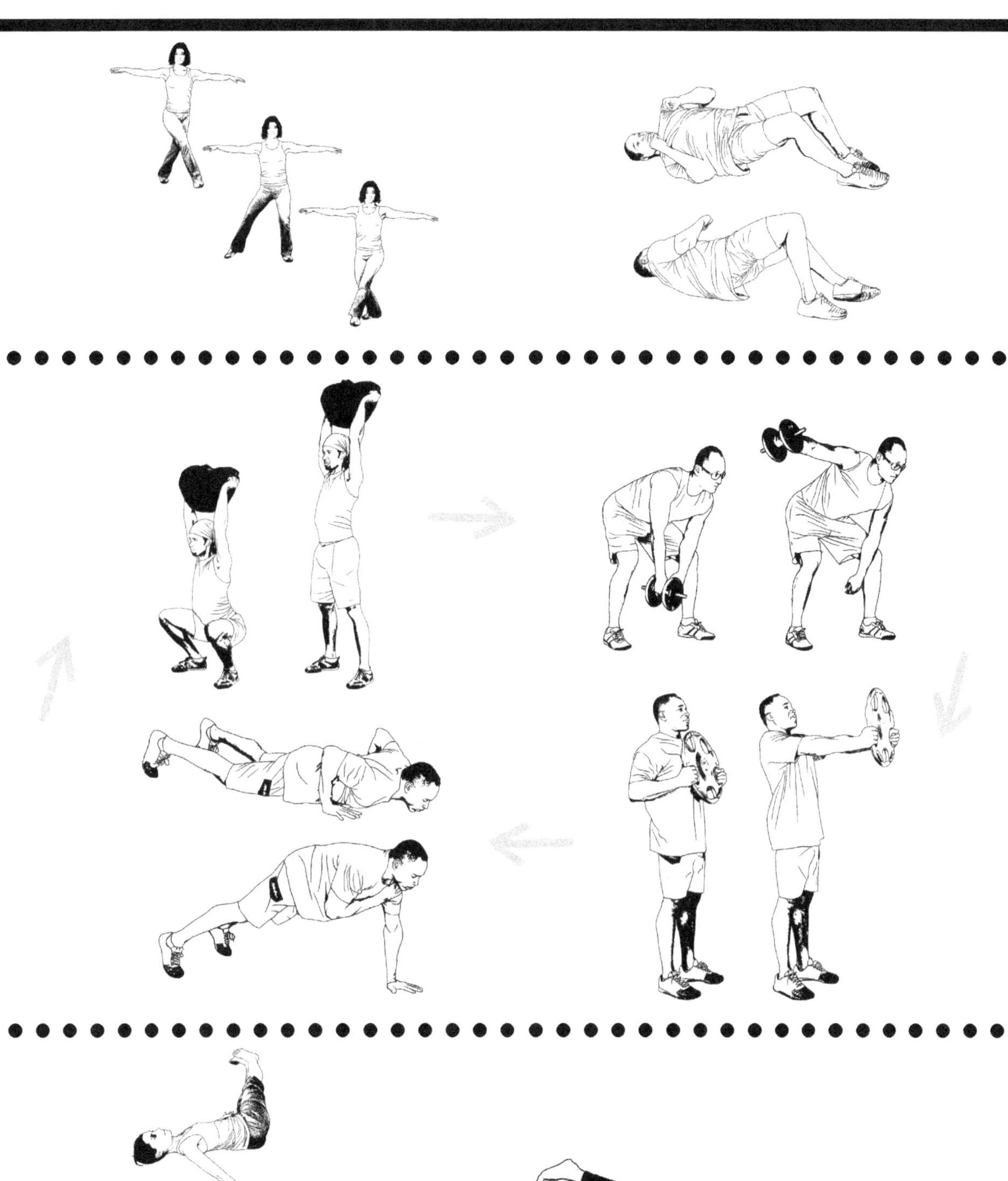

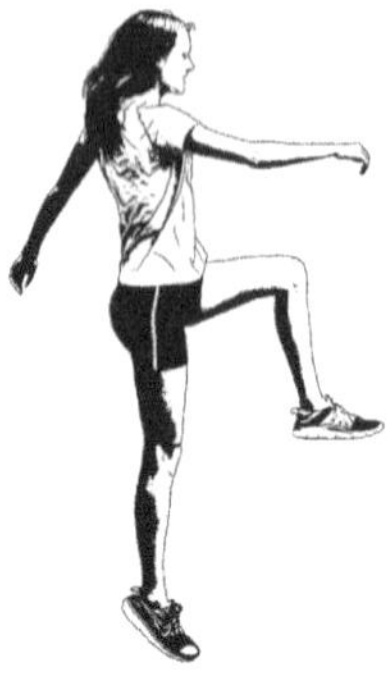

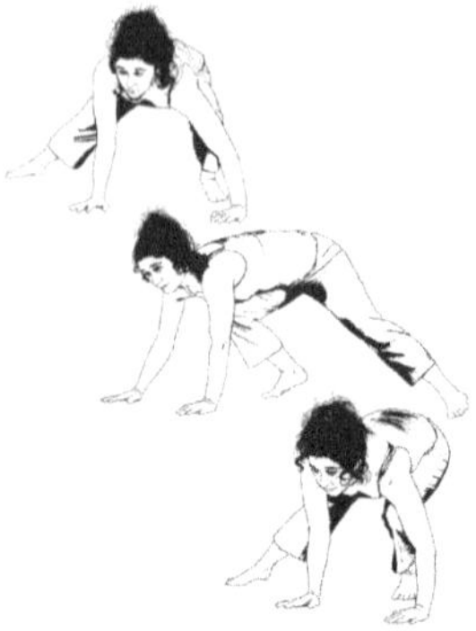

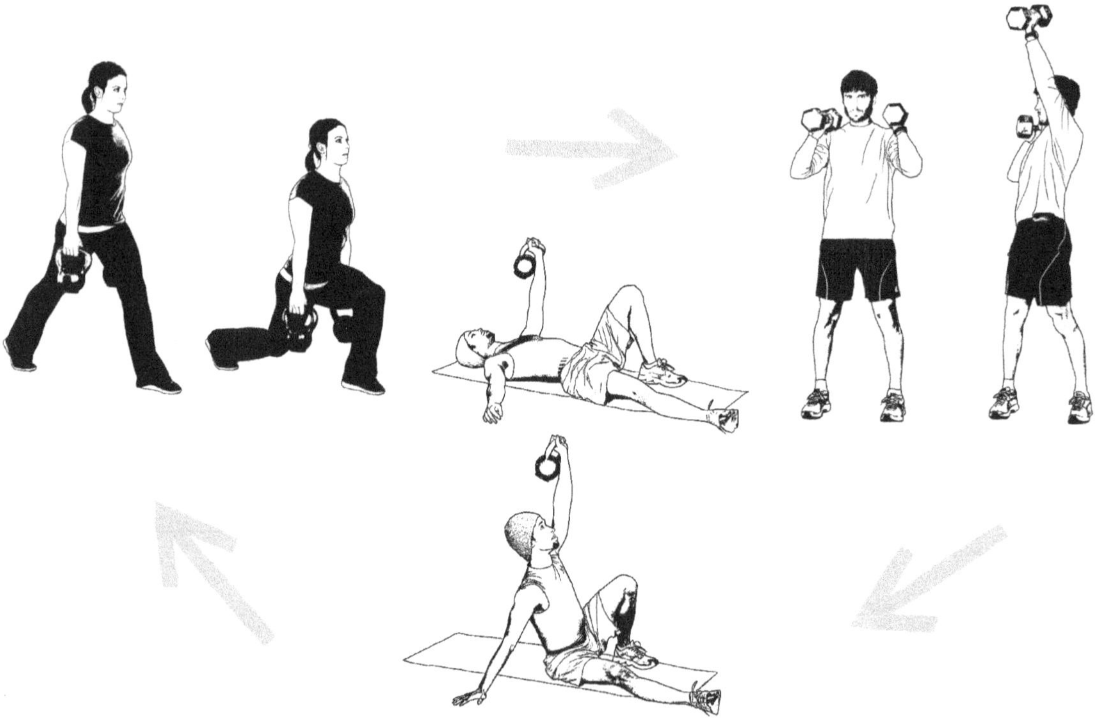

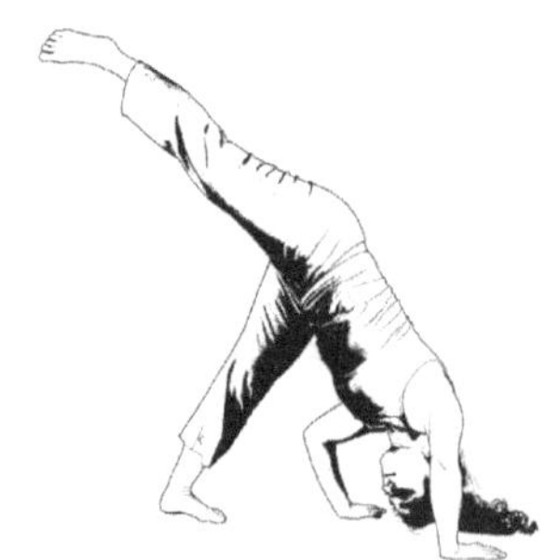

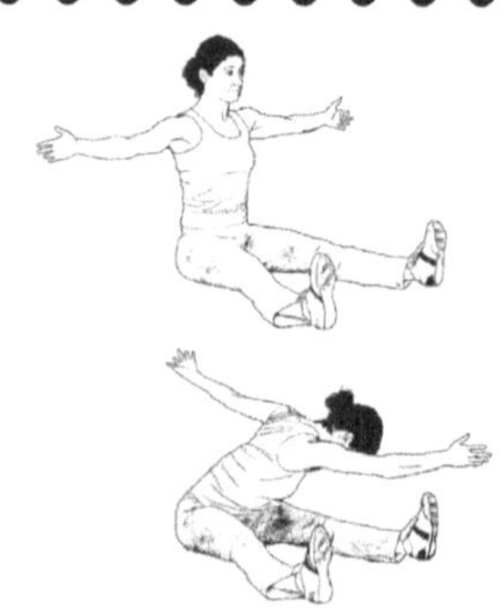

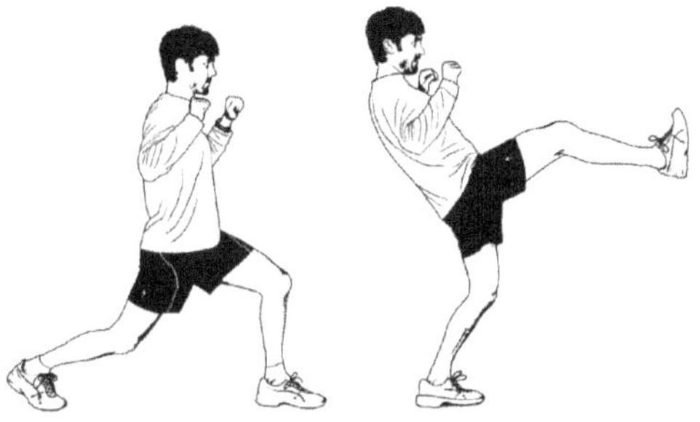

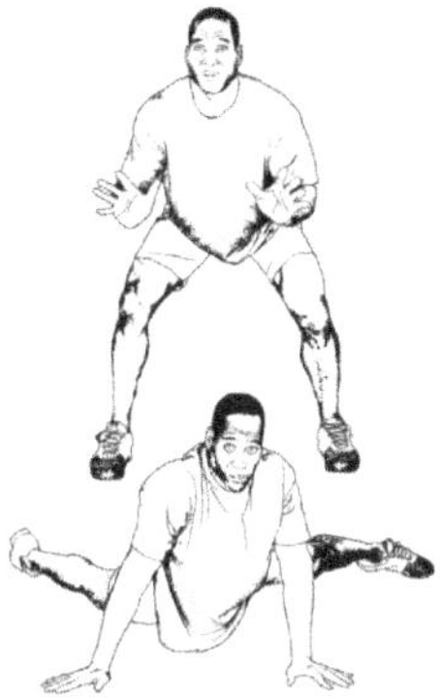

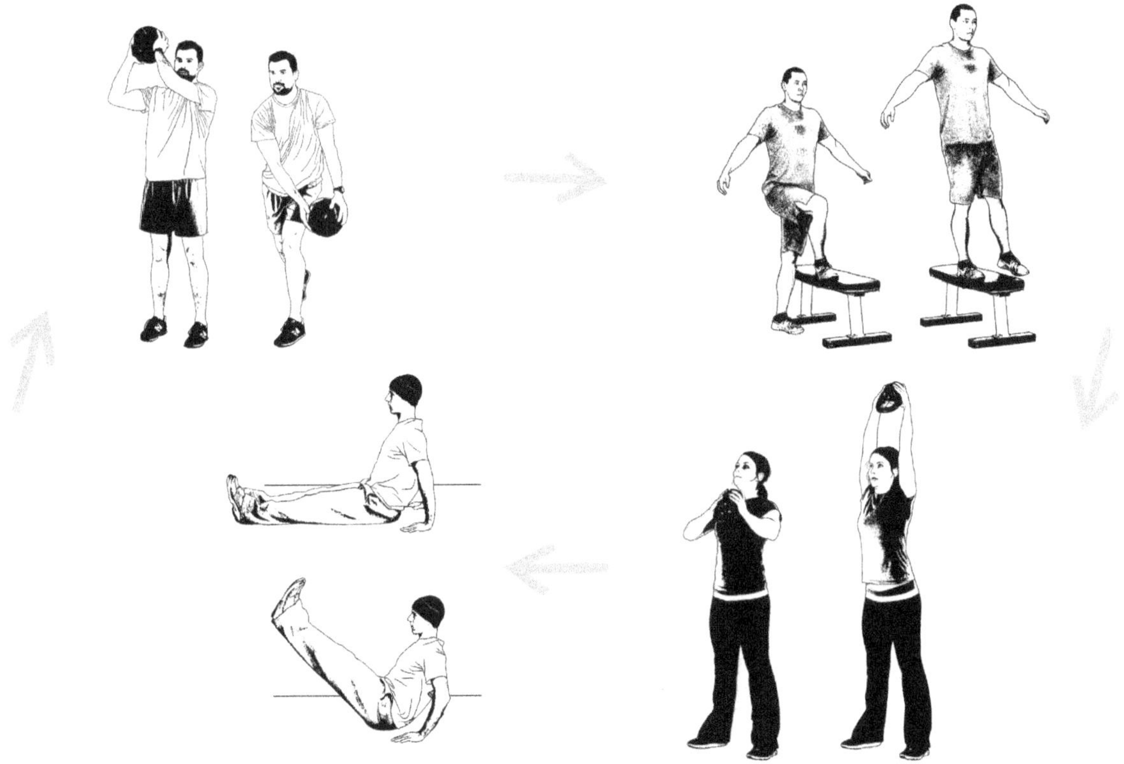

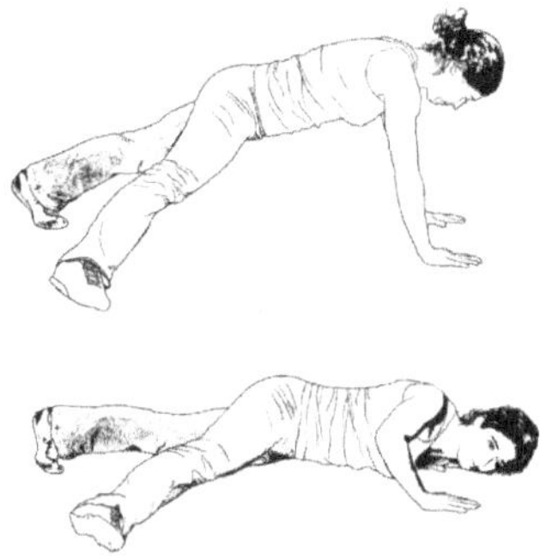

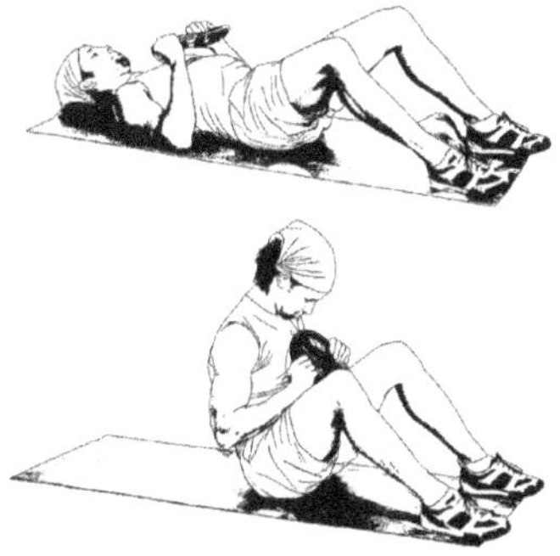

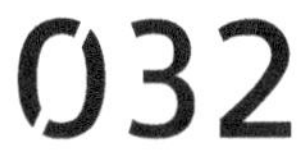

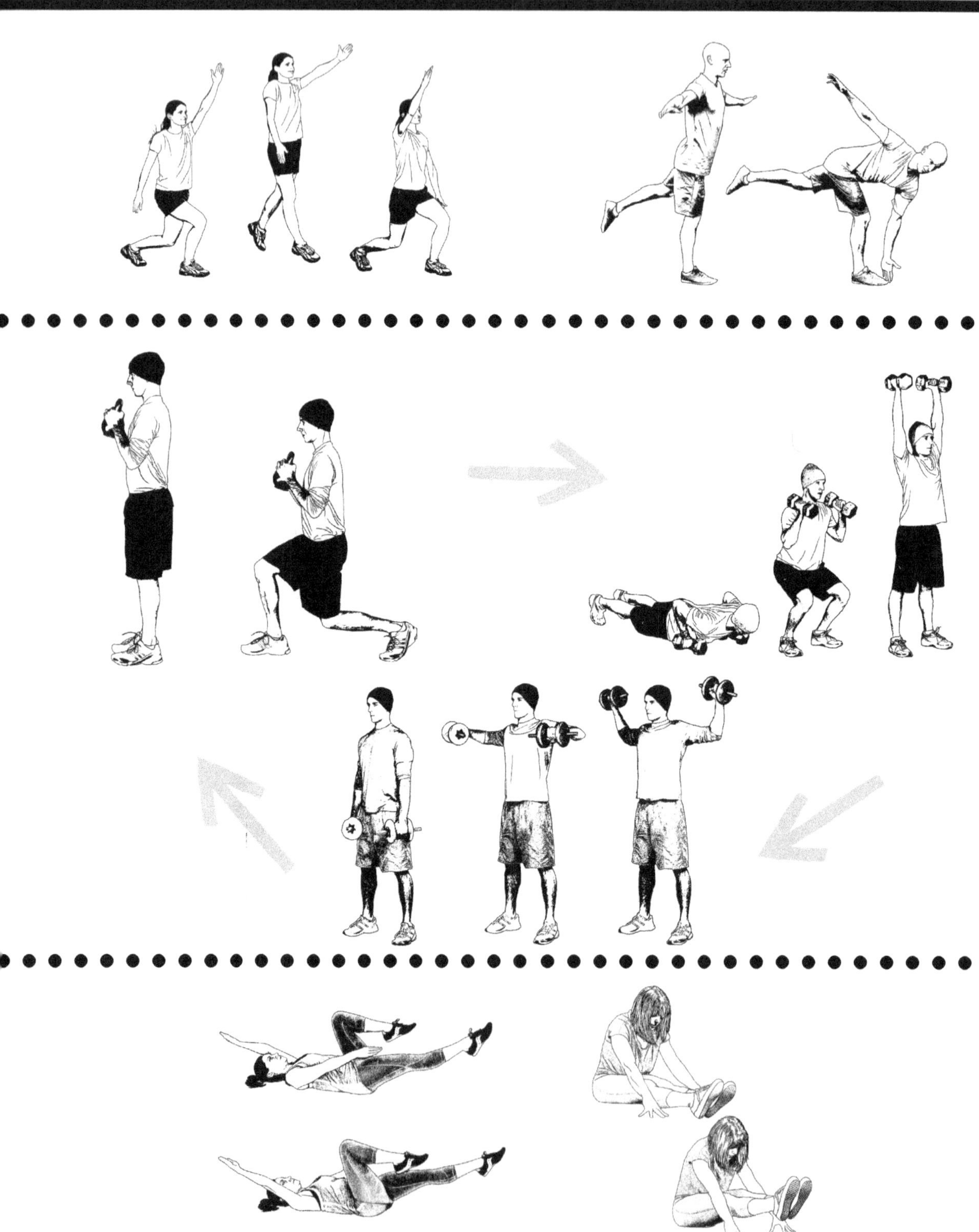

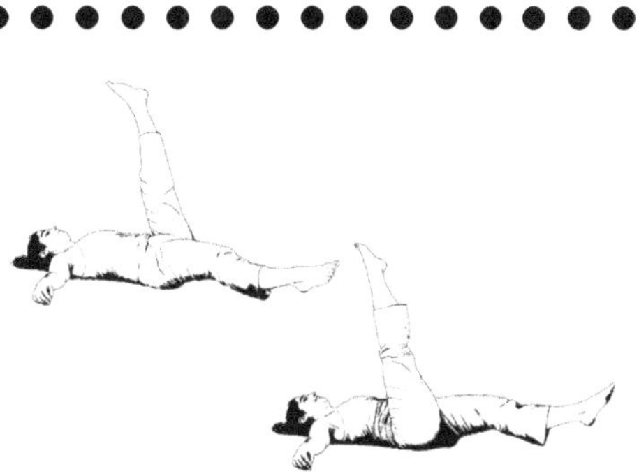

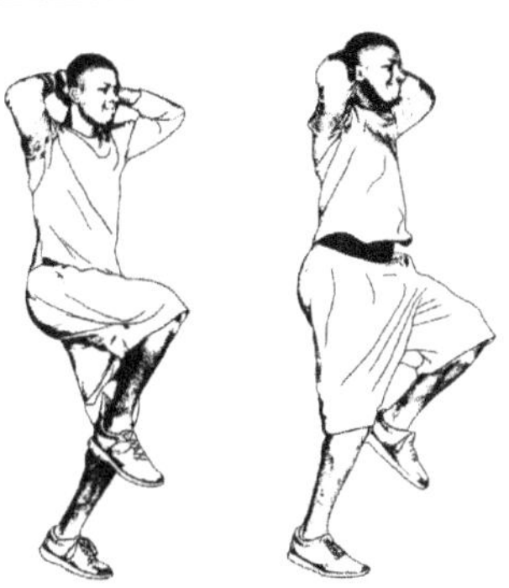

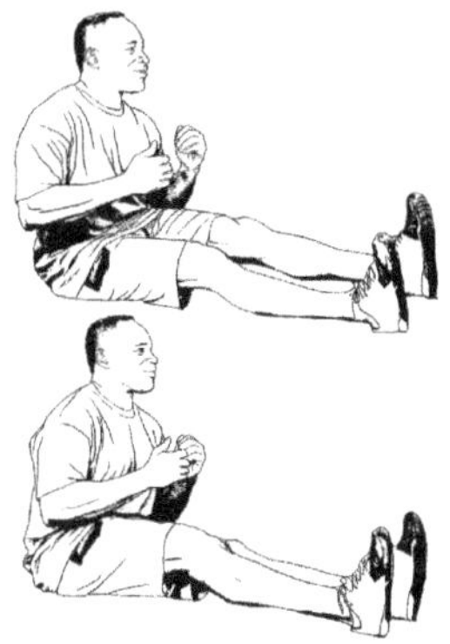

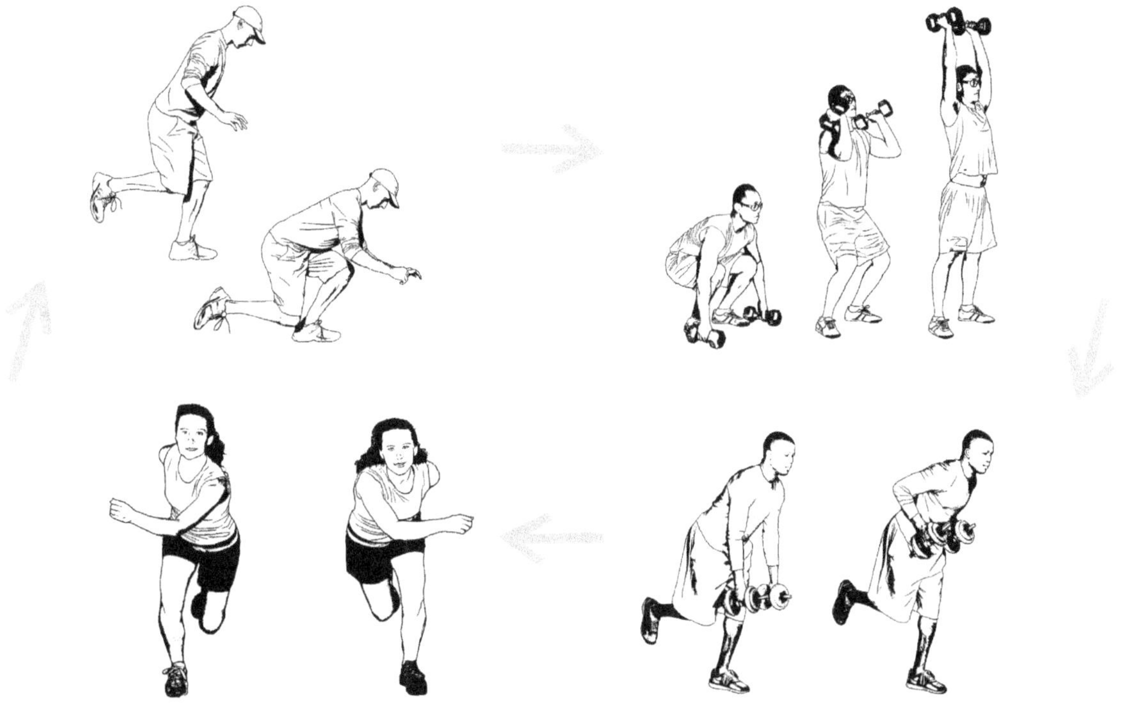

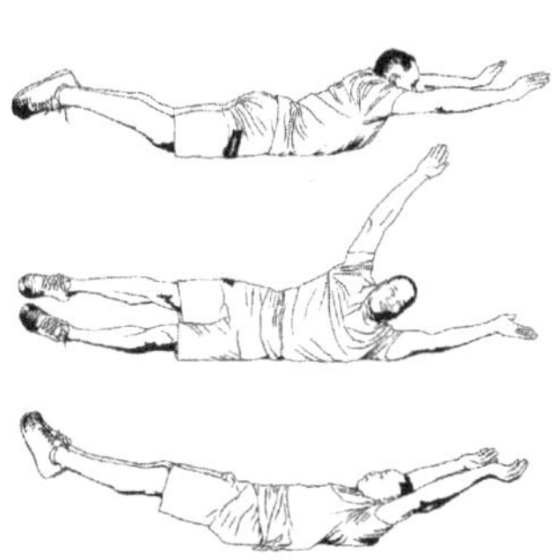

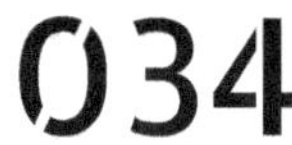

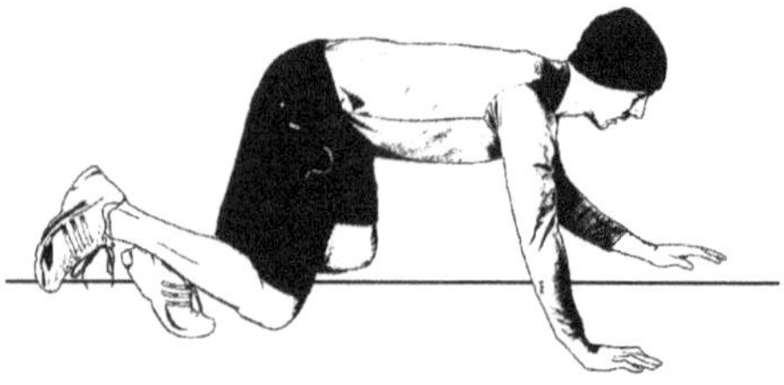

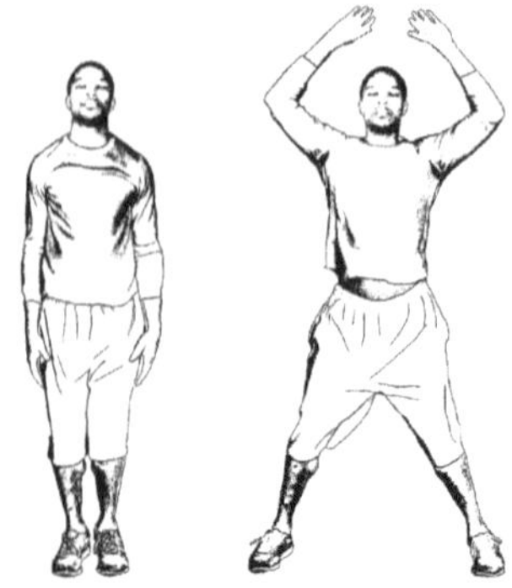

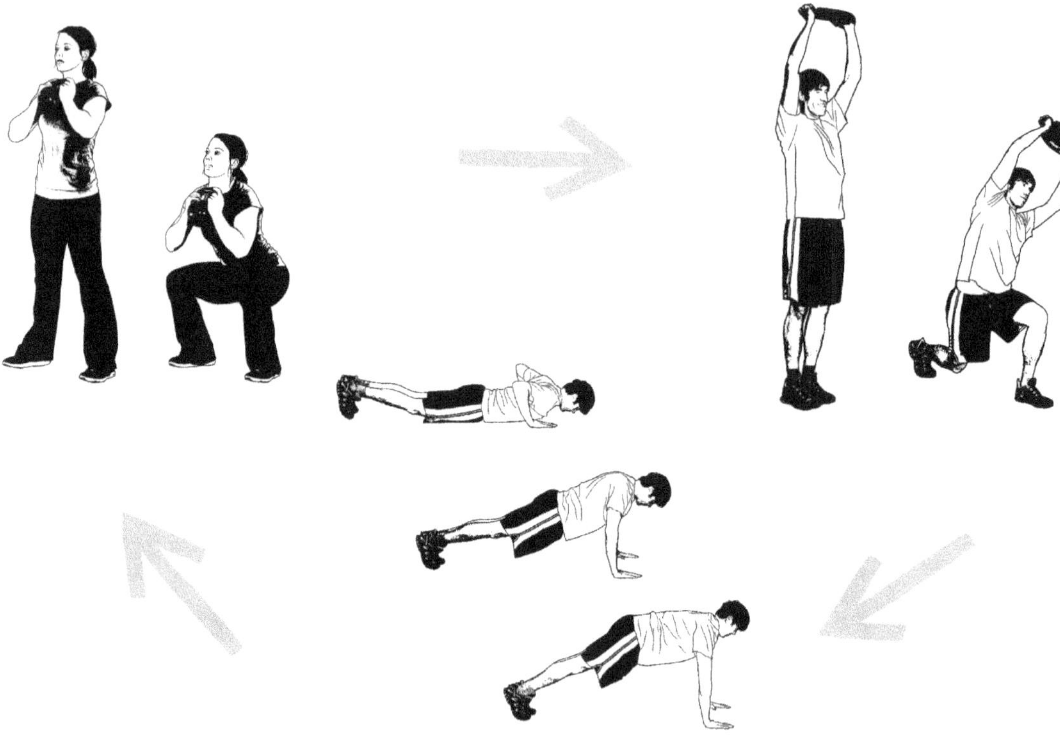

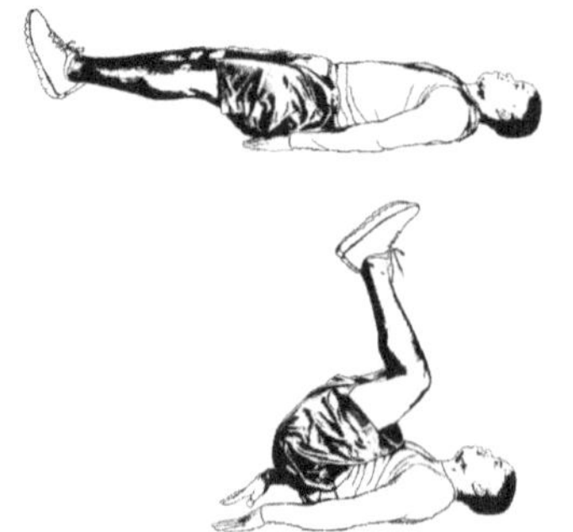
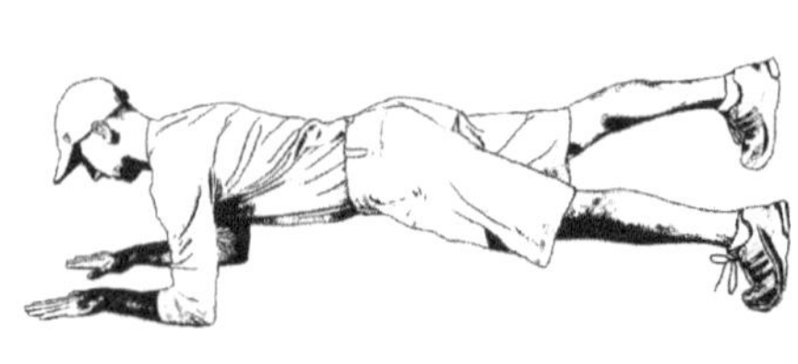

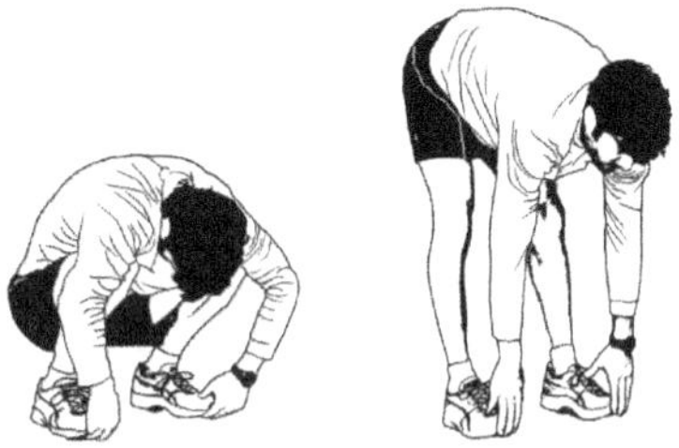

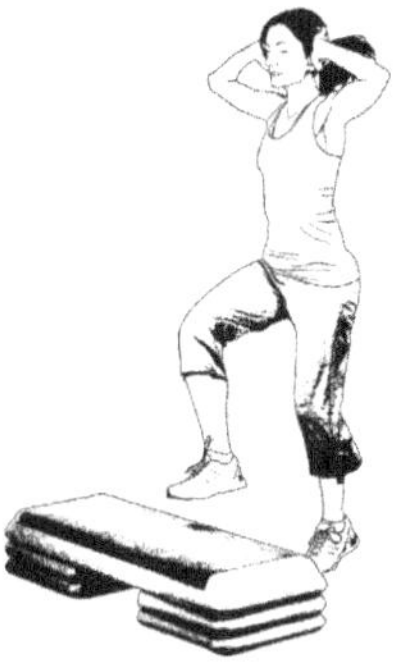

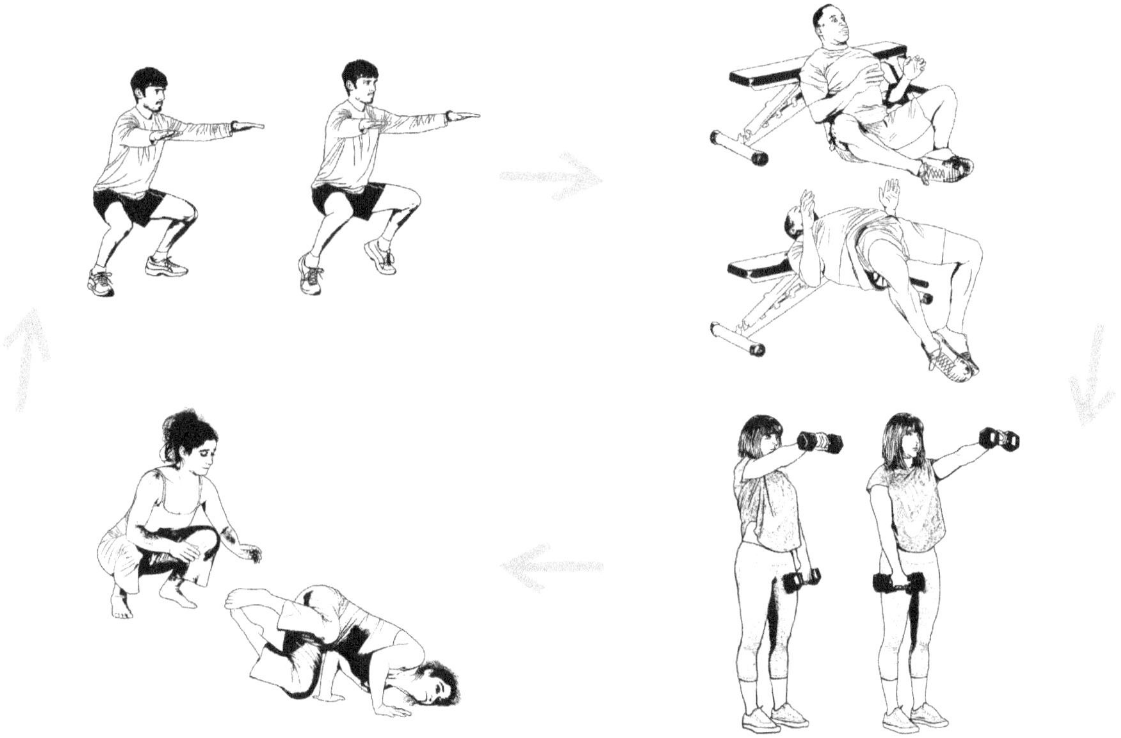

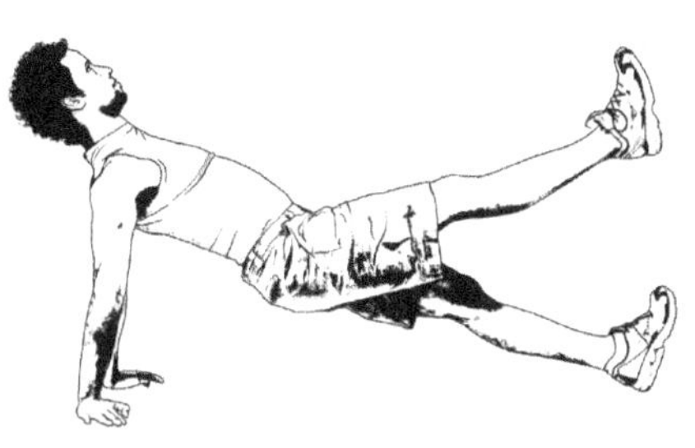
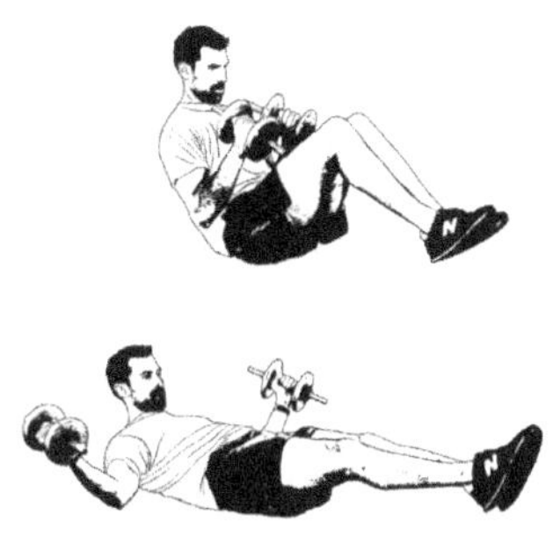

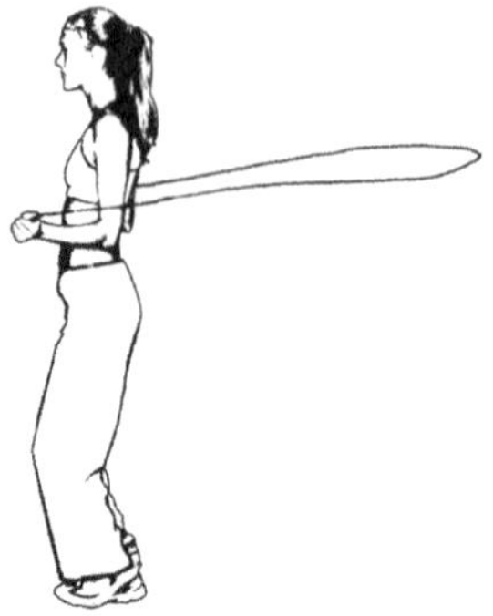

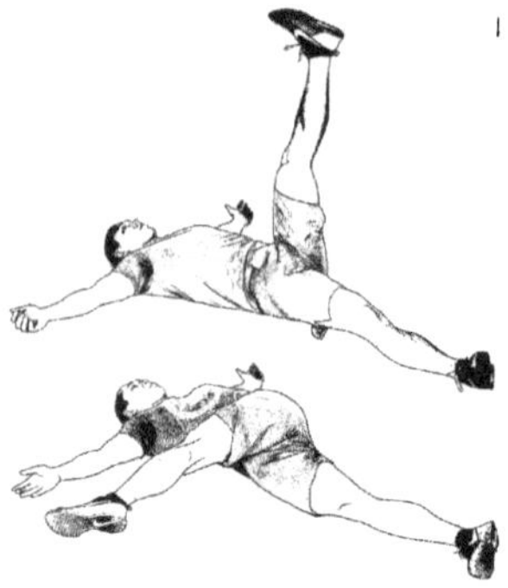

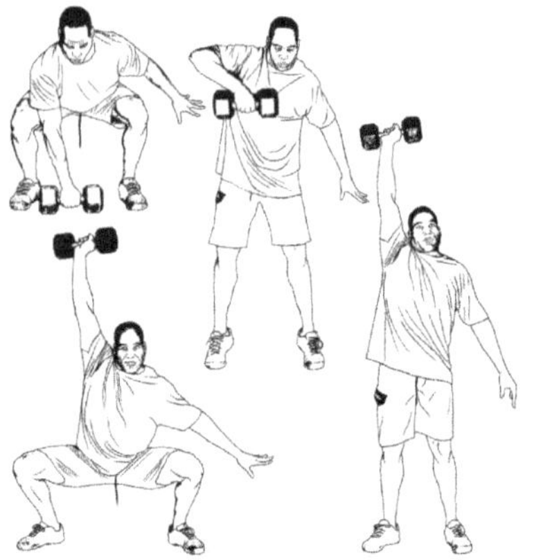

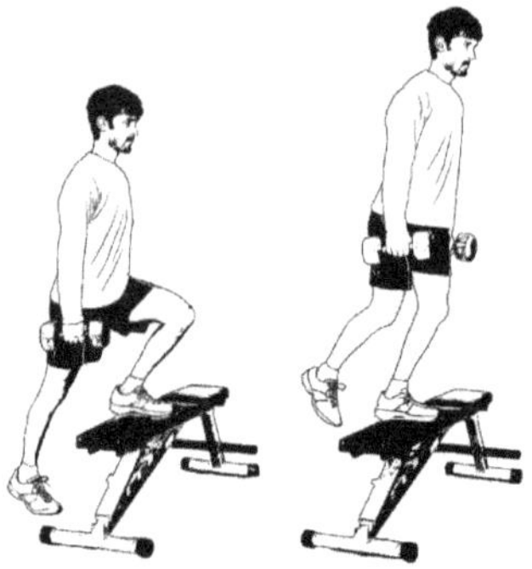

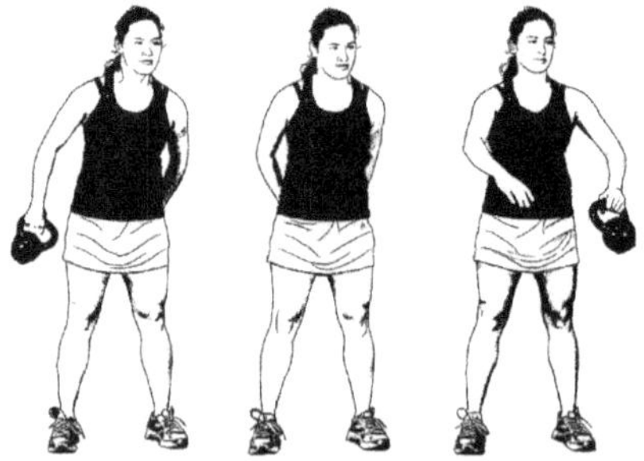

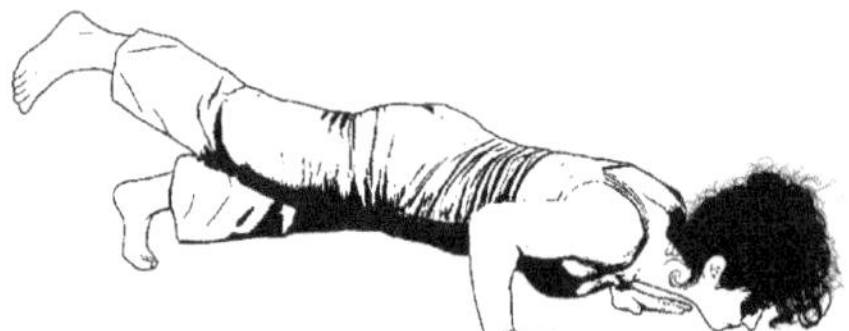

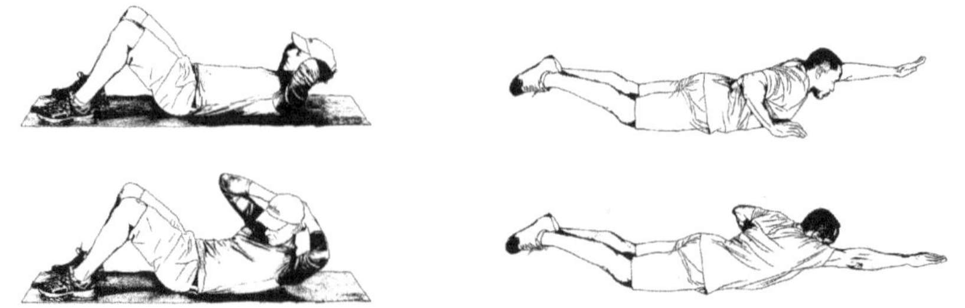

SIDE A

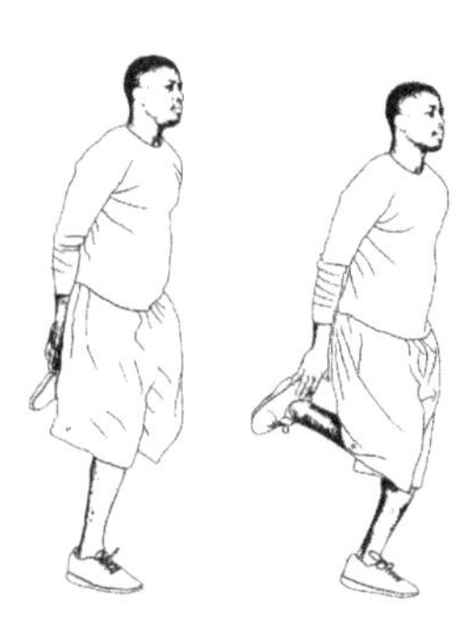
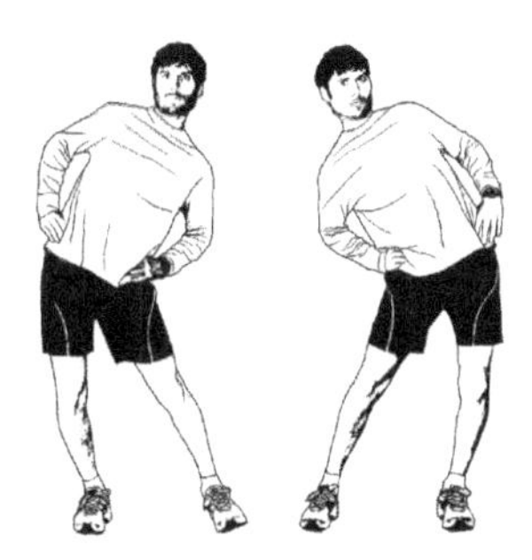
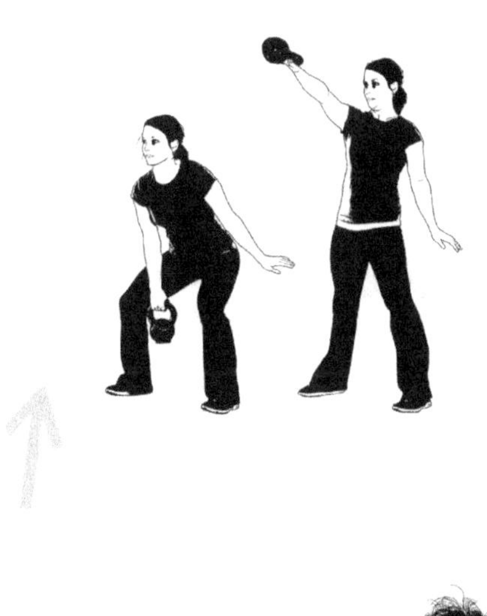
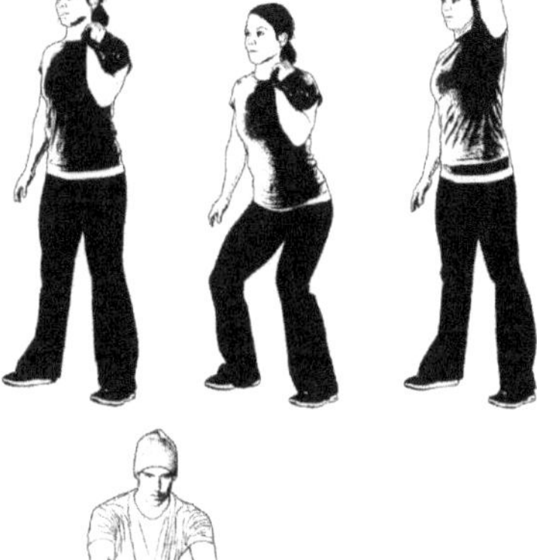
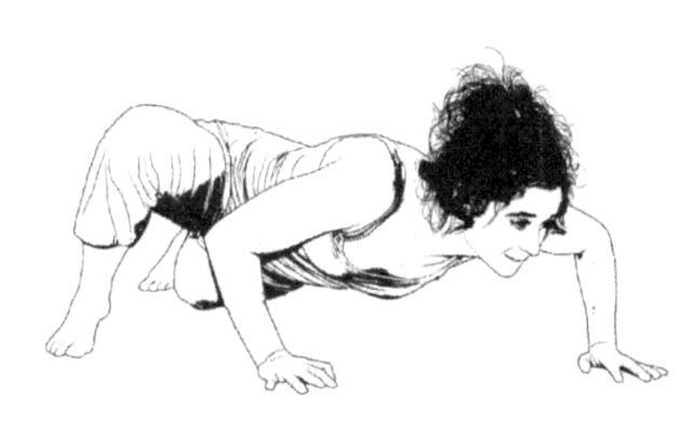
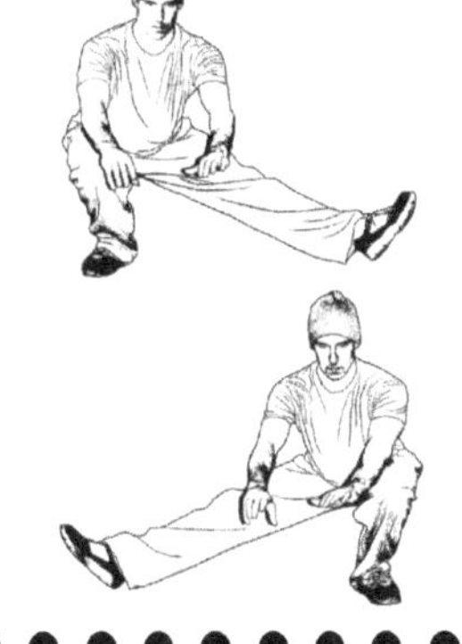
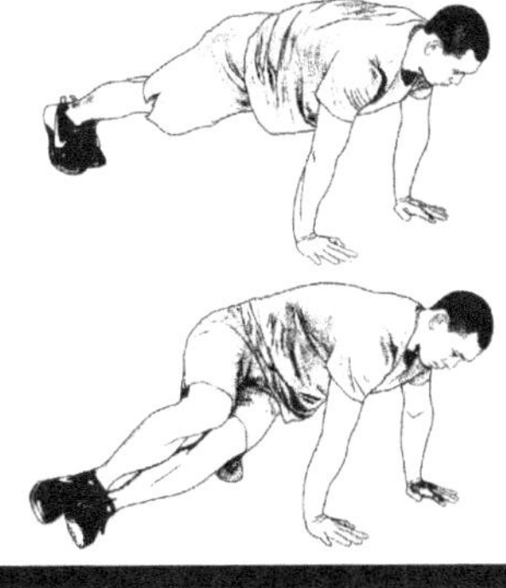
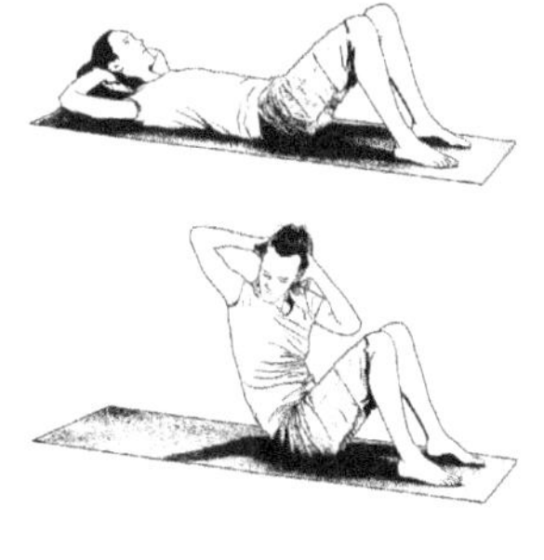

SIDE A

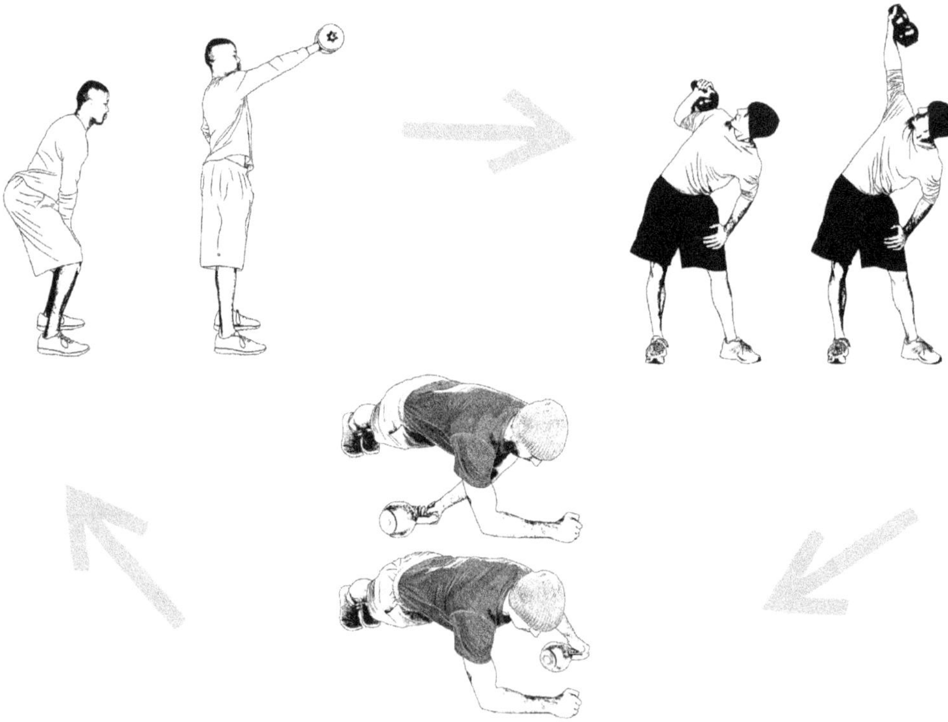

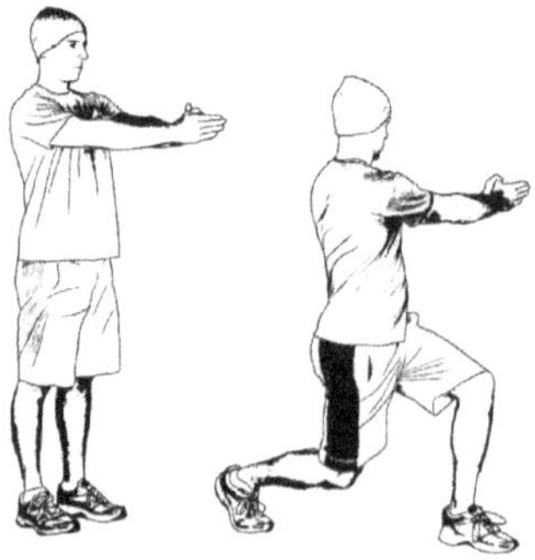

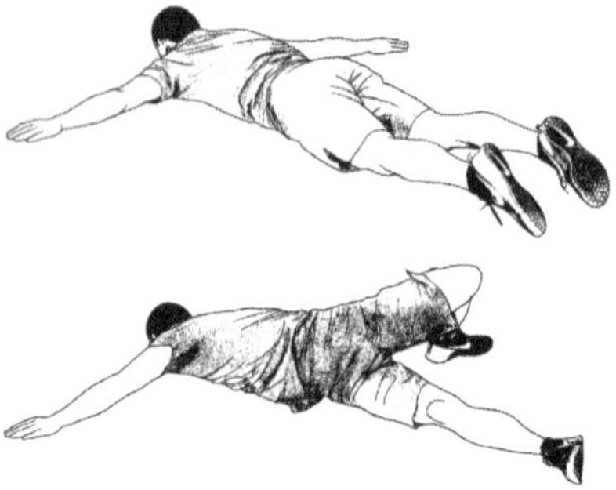

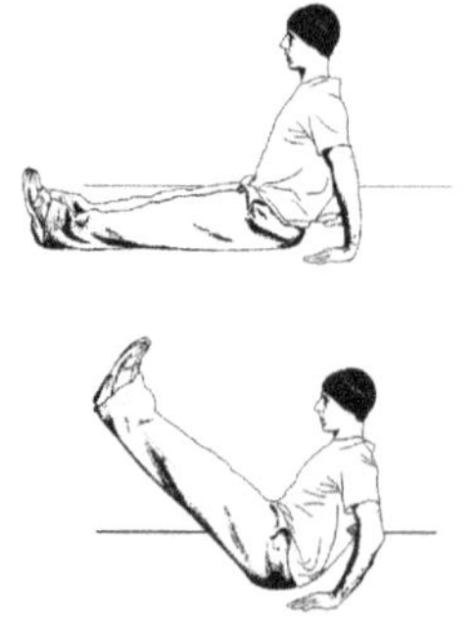

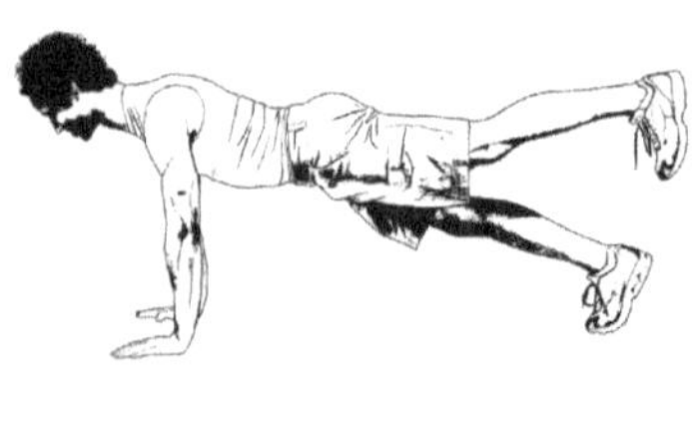

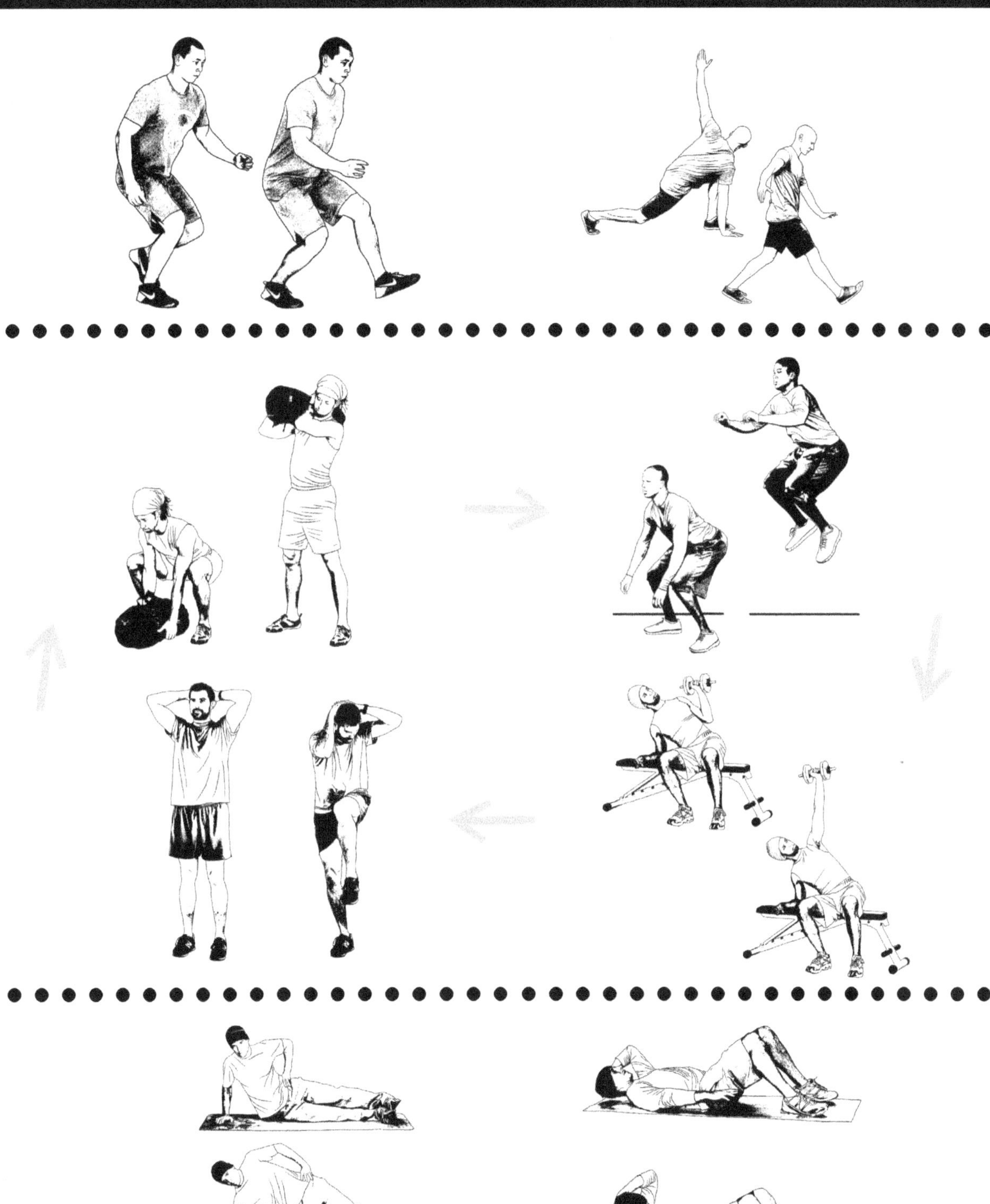

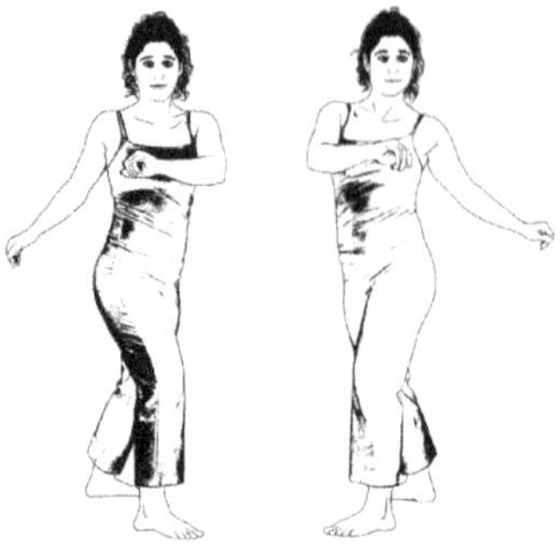

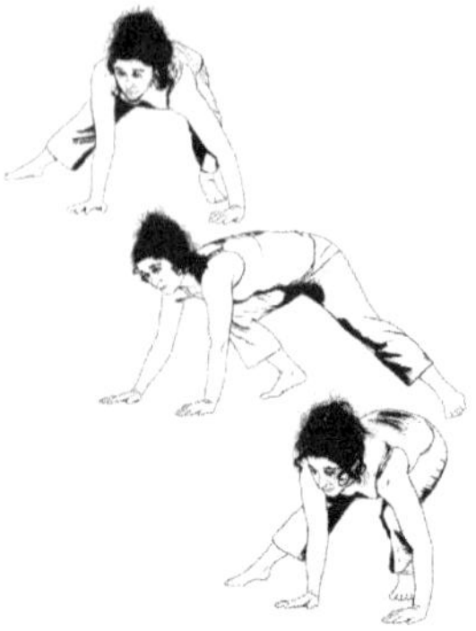

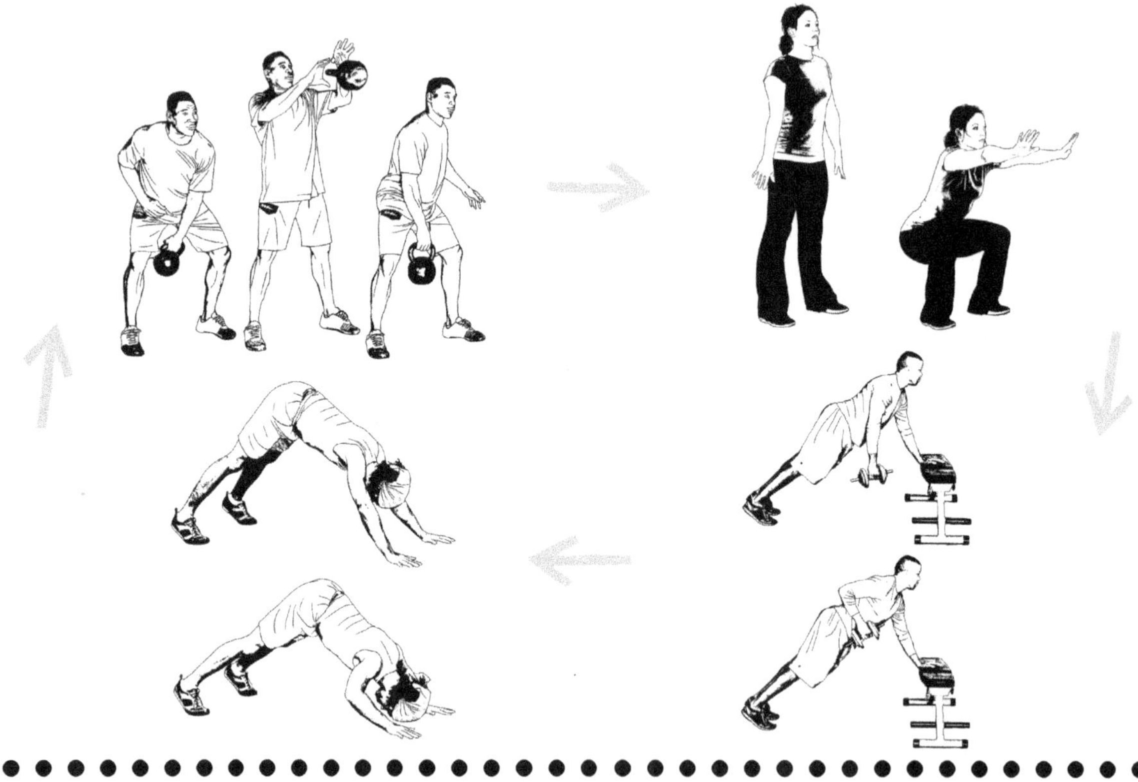

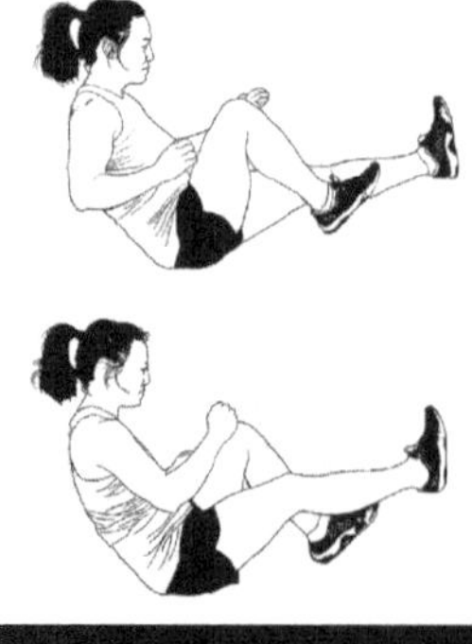

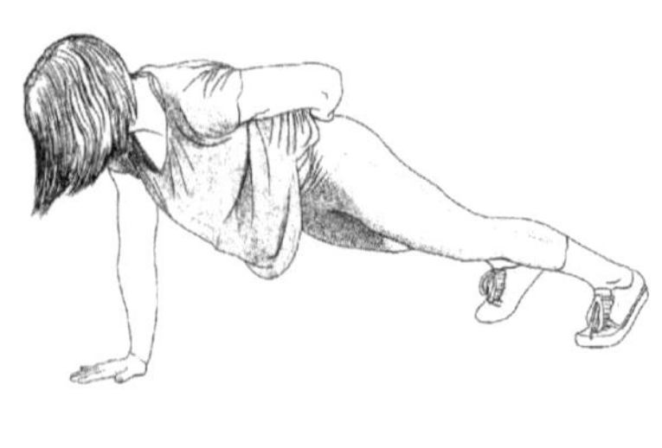

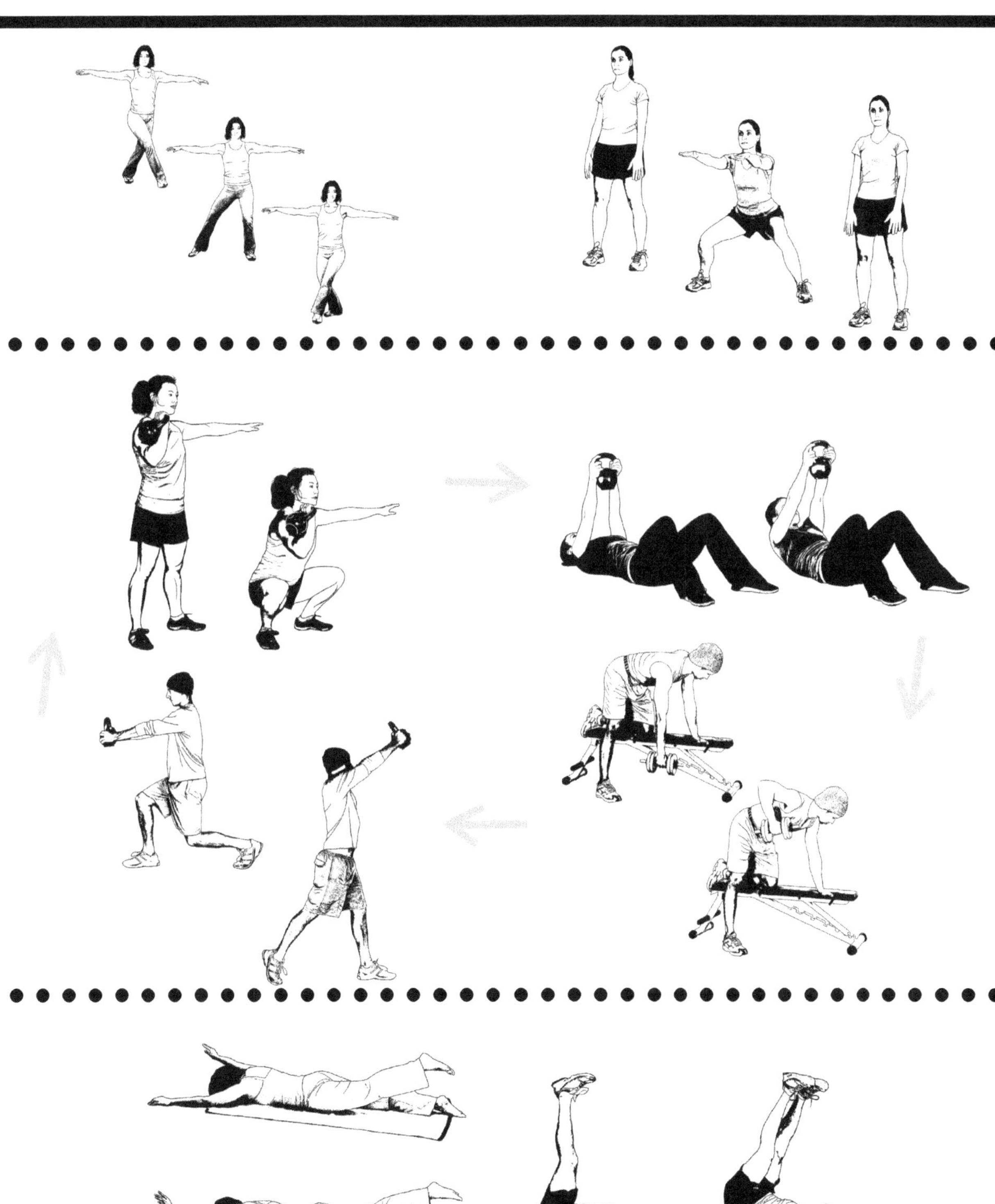

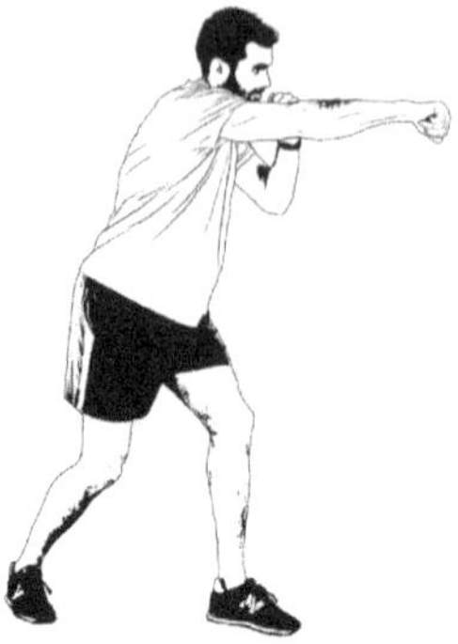

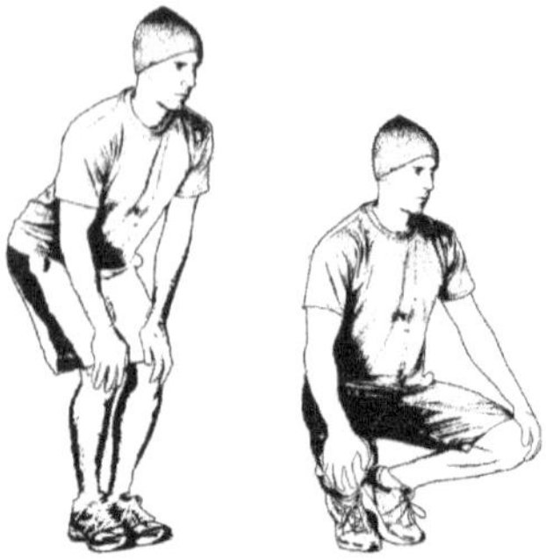

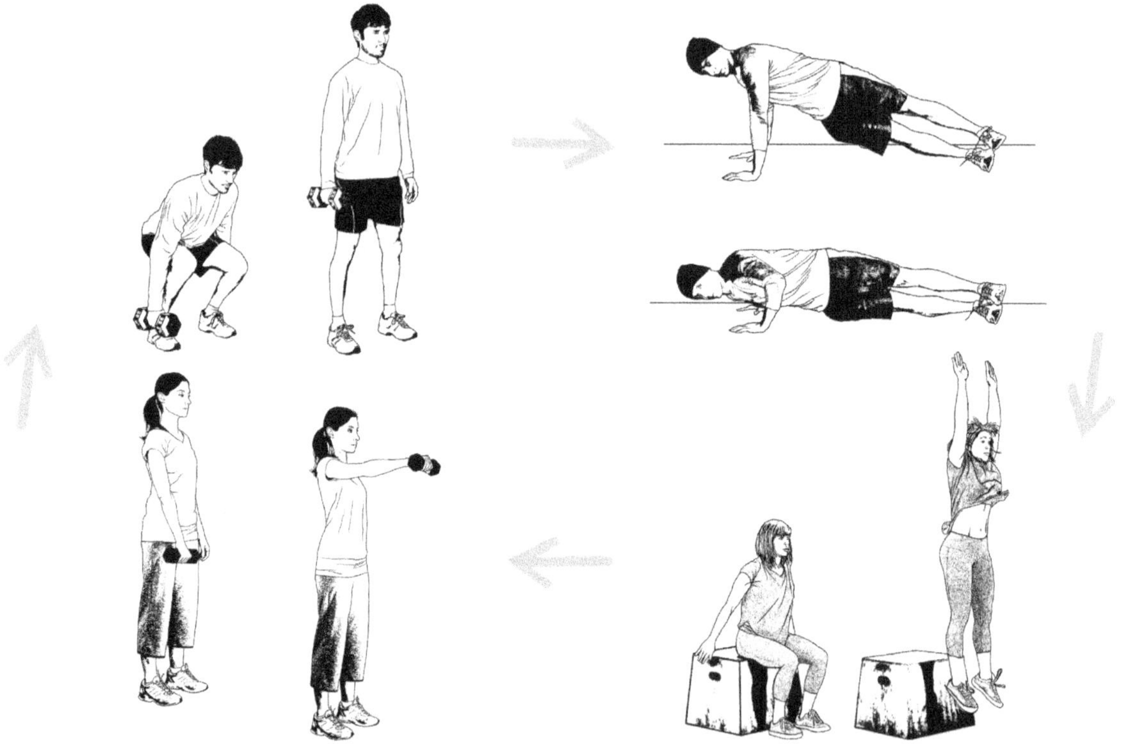

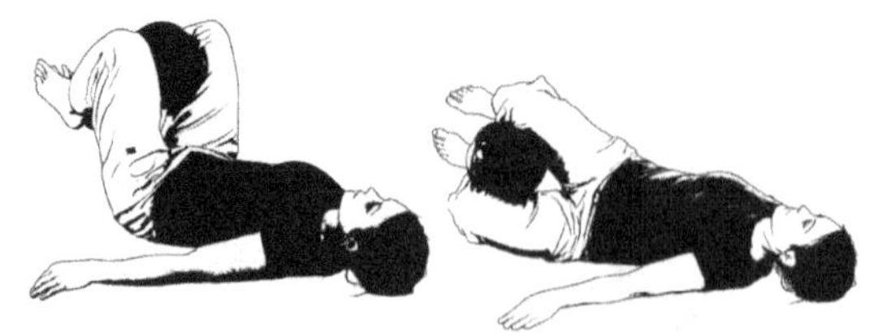

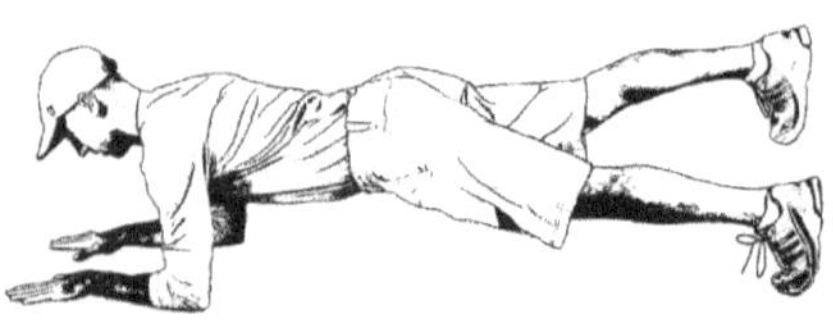

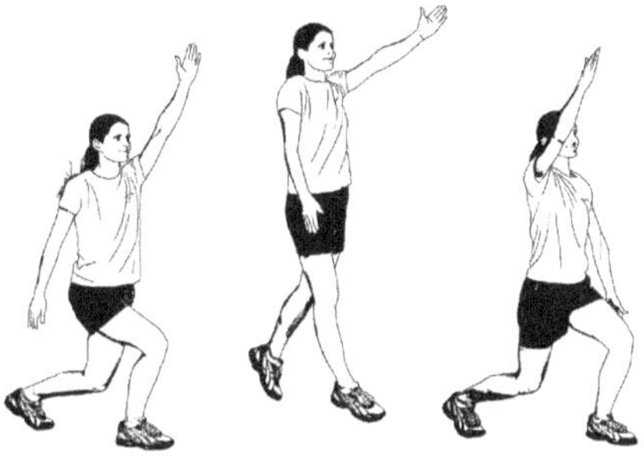

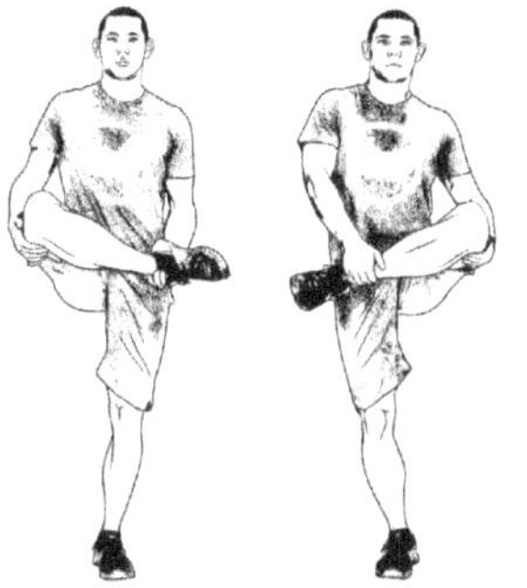

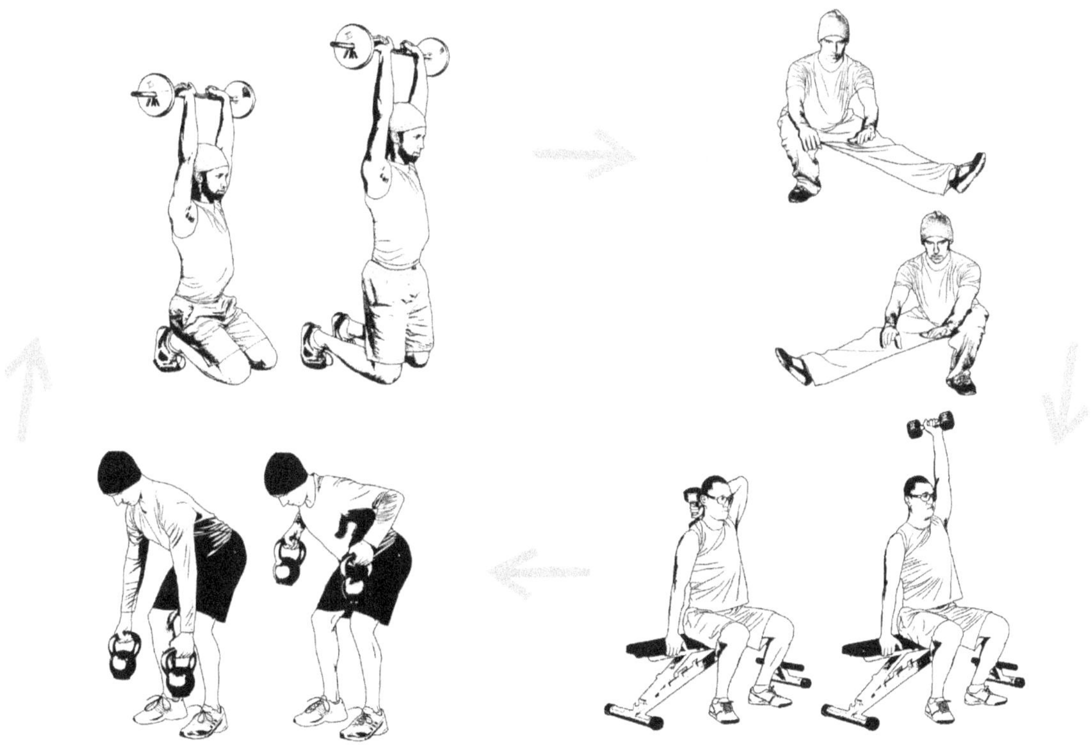

SIDE A

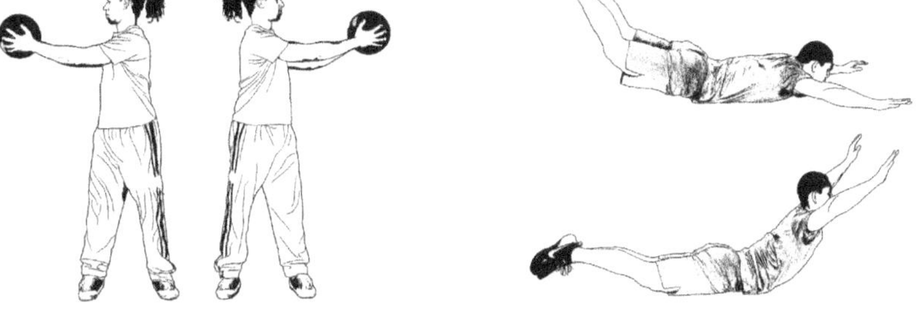

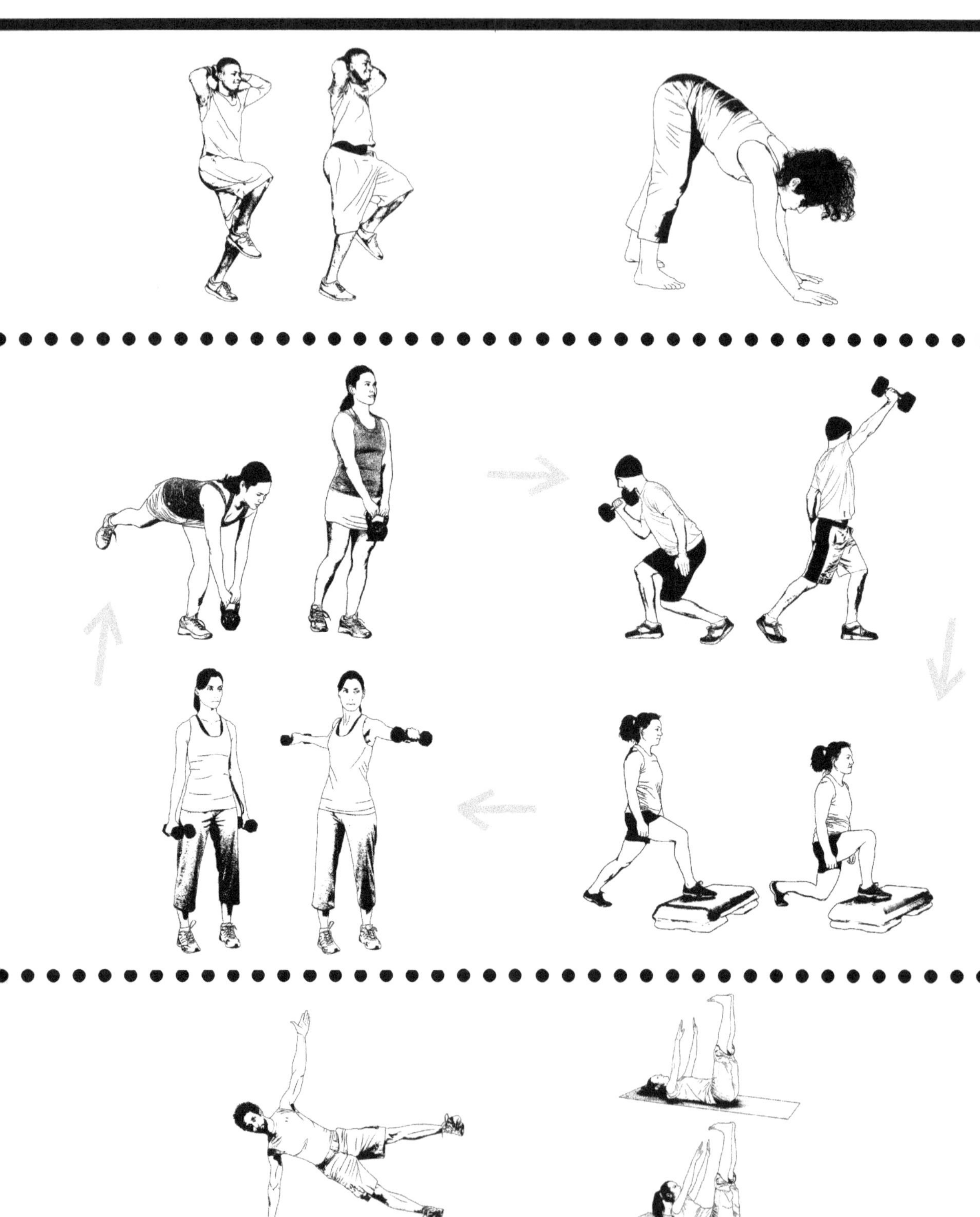

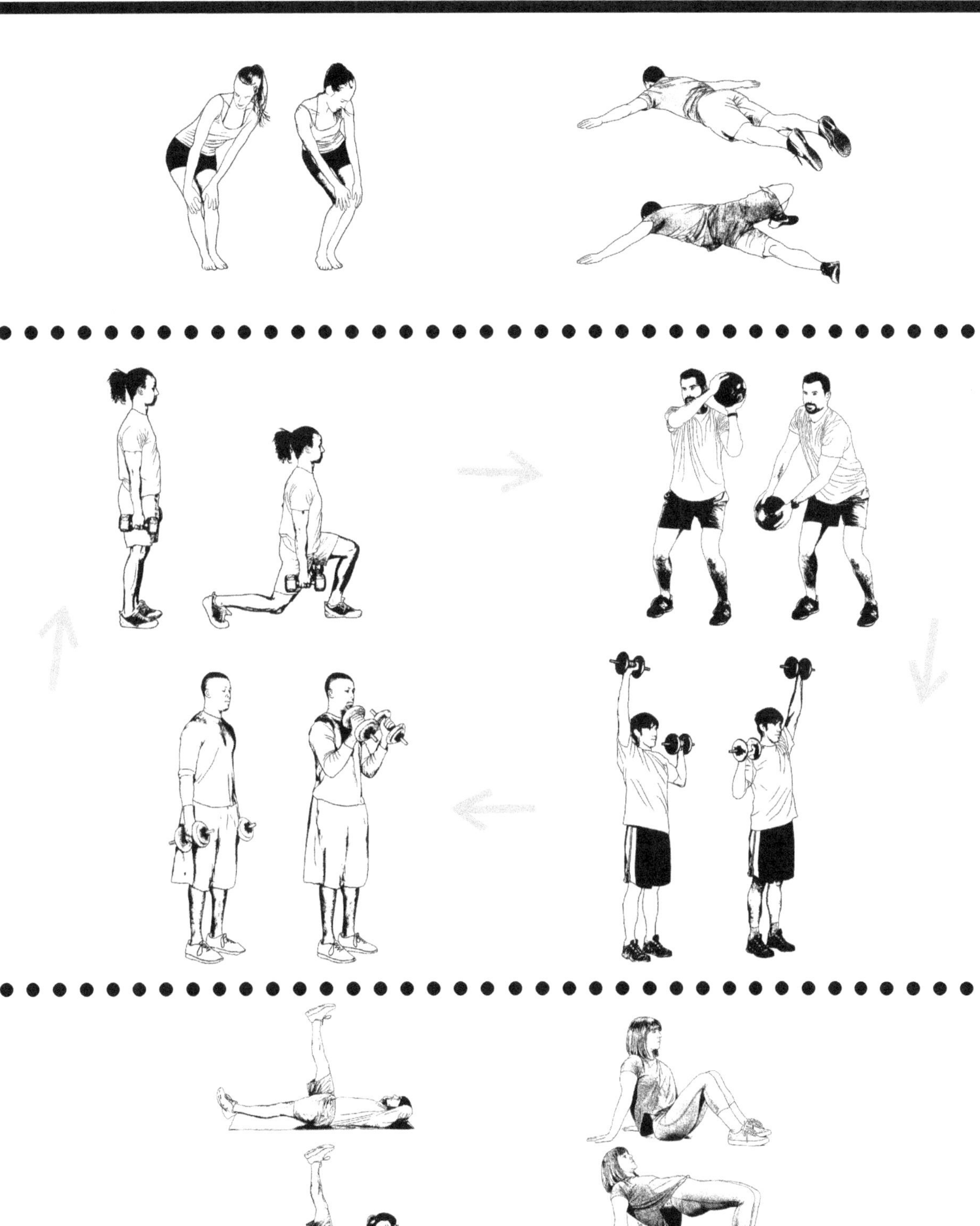

SIDE A

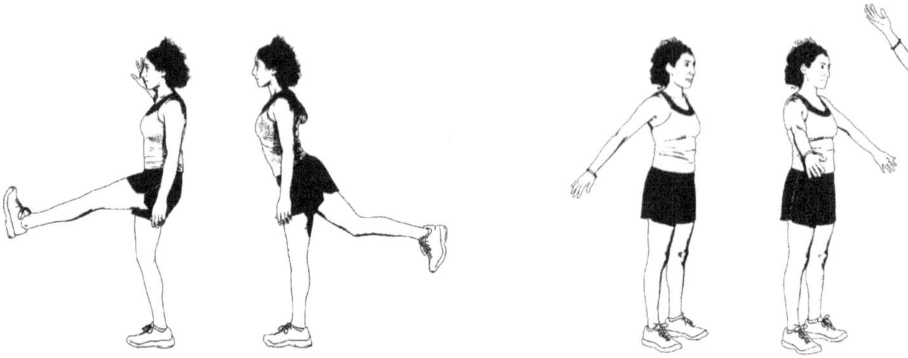

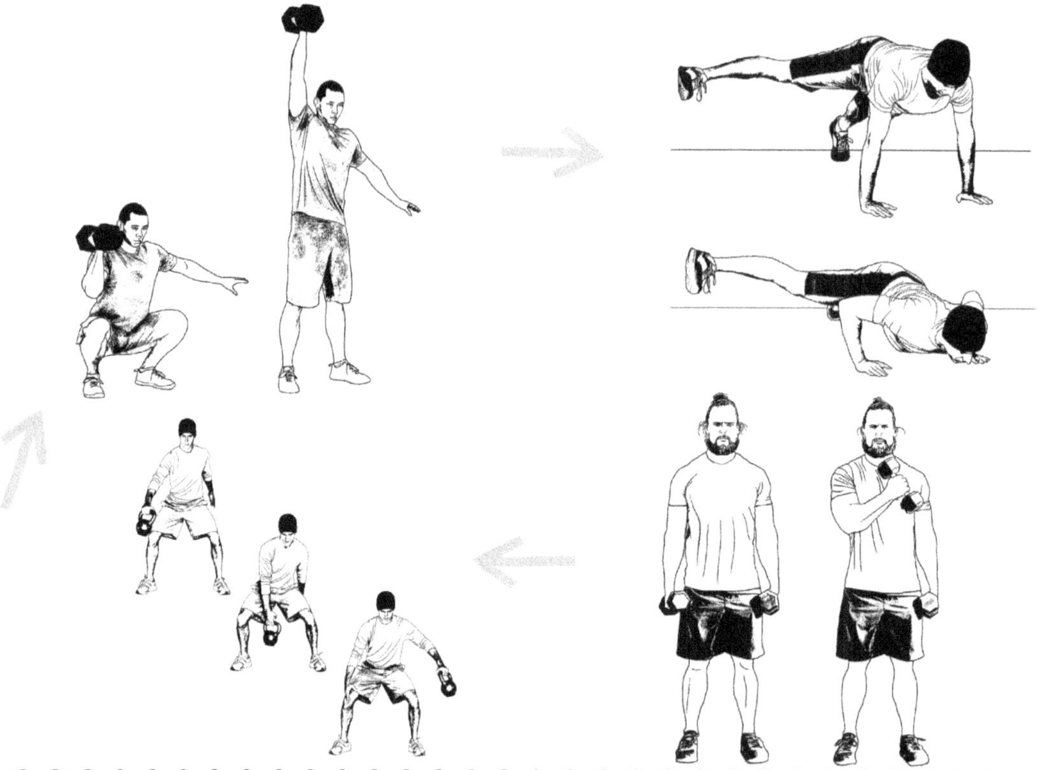

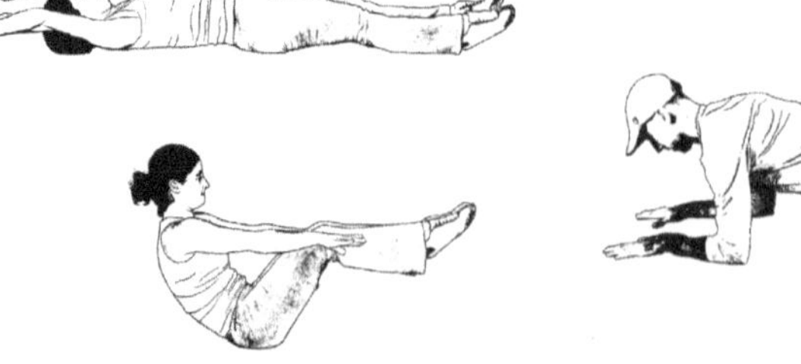

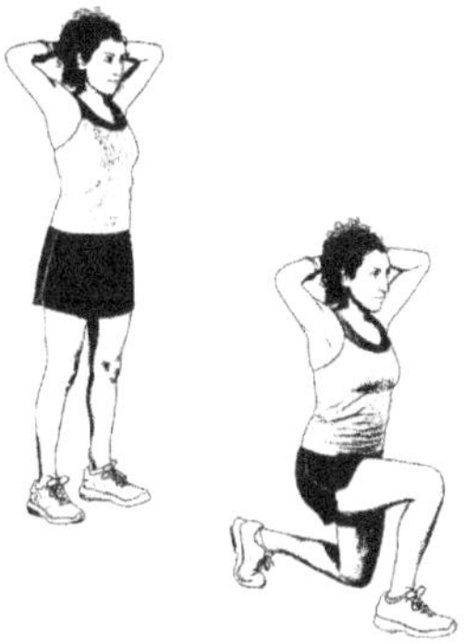

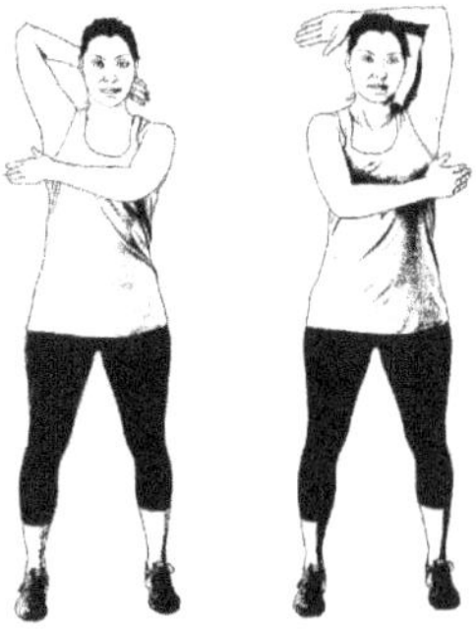

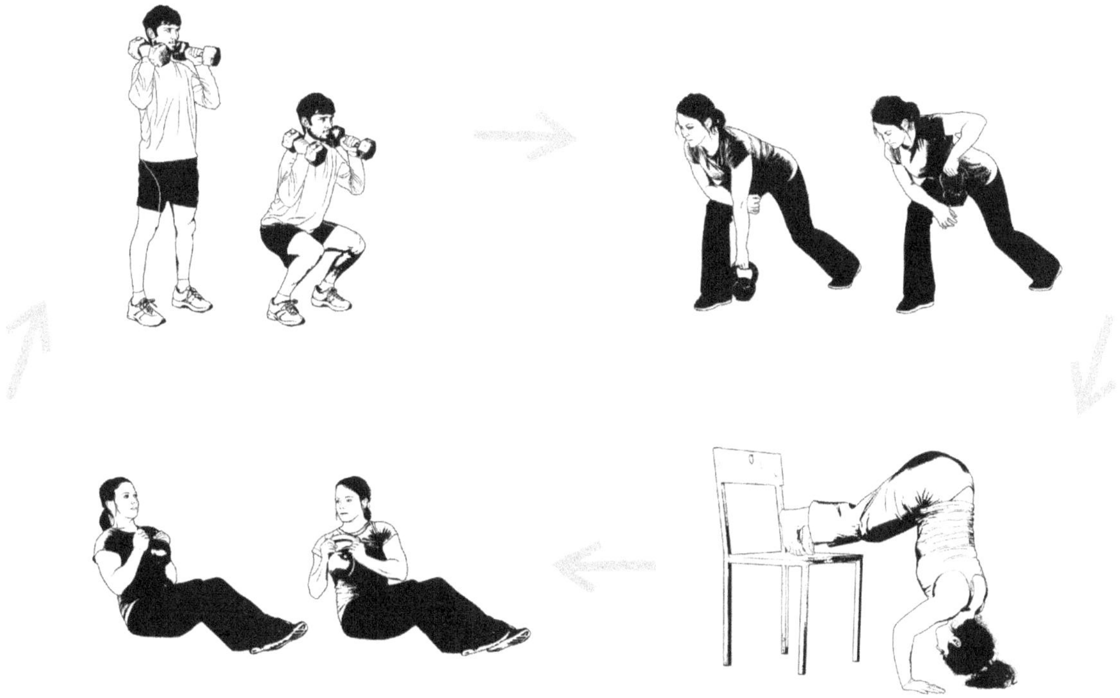

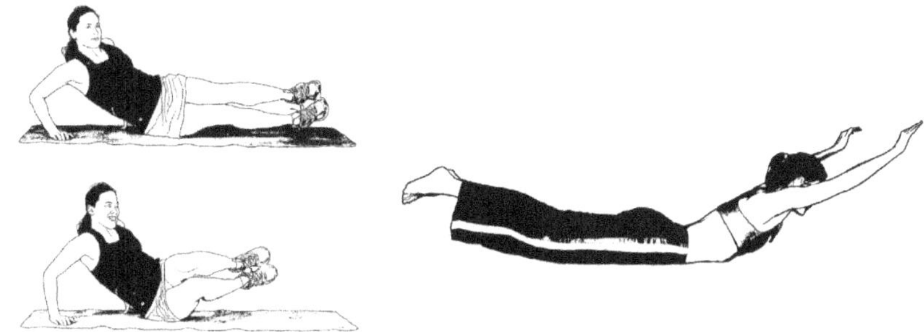

SIDE A

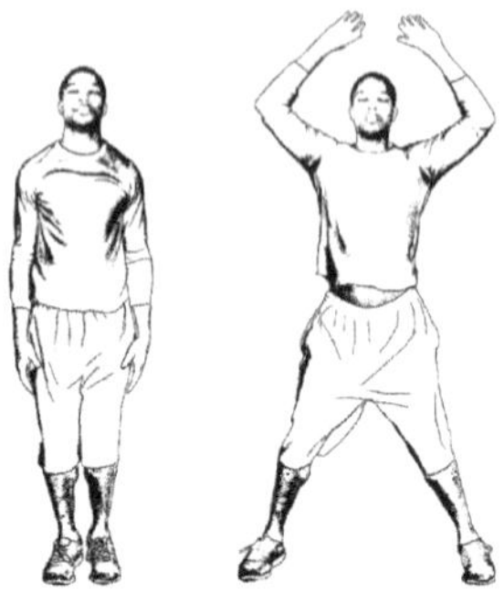

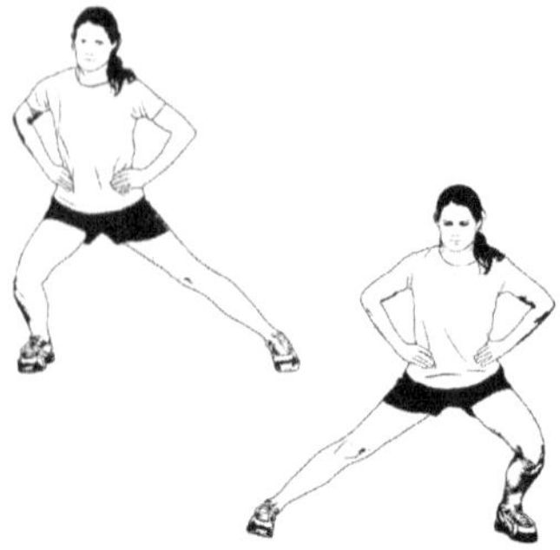

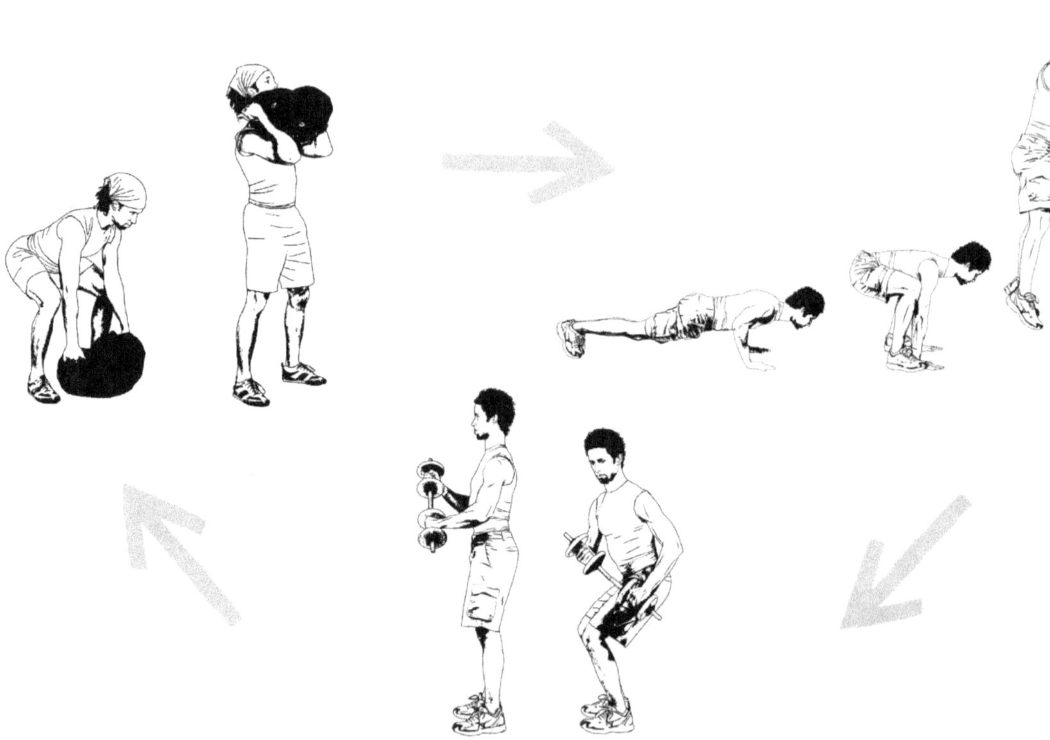

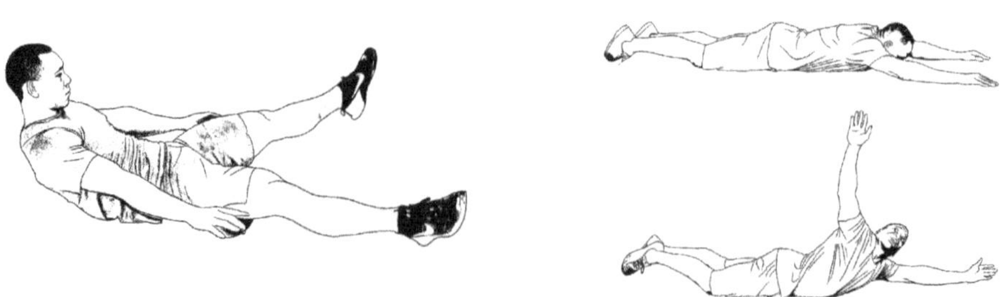

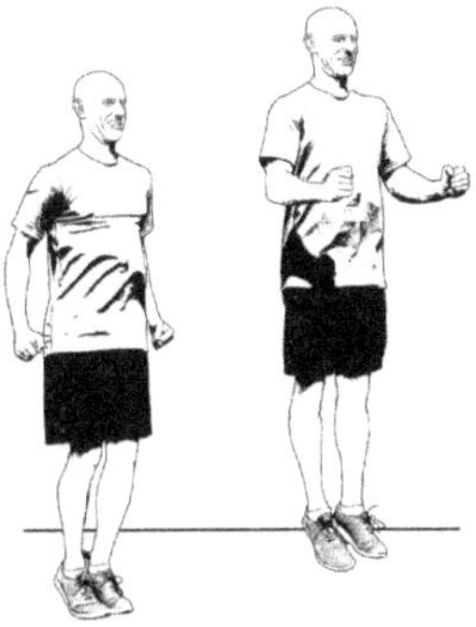

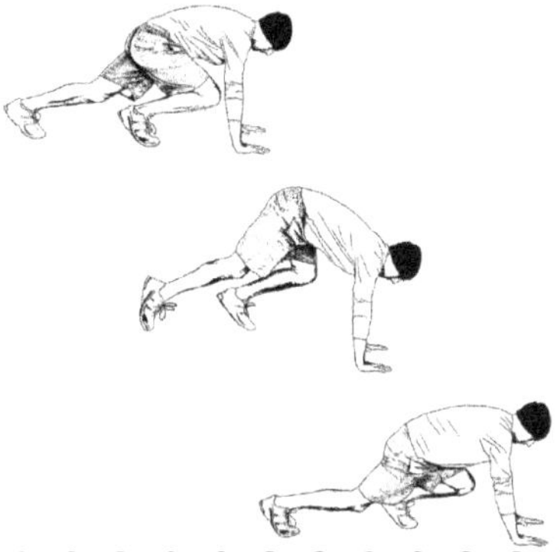

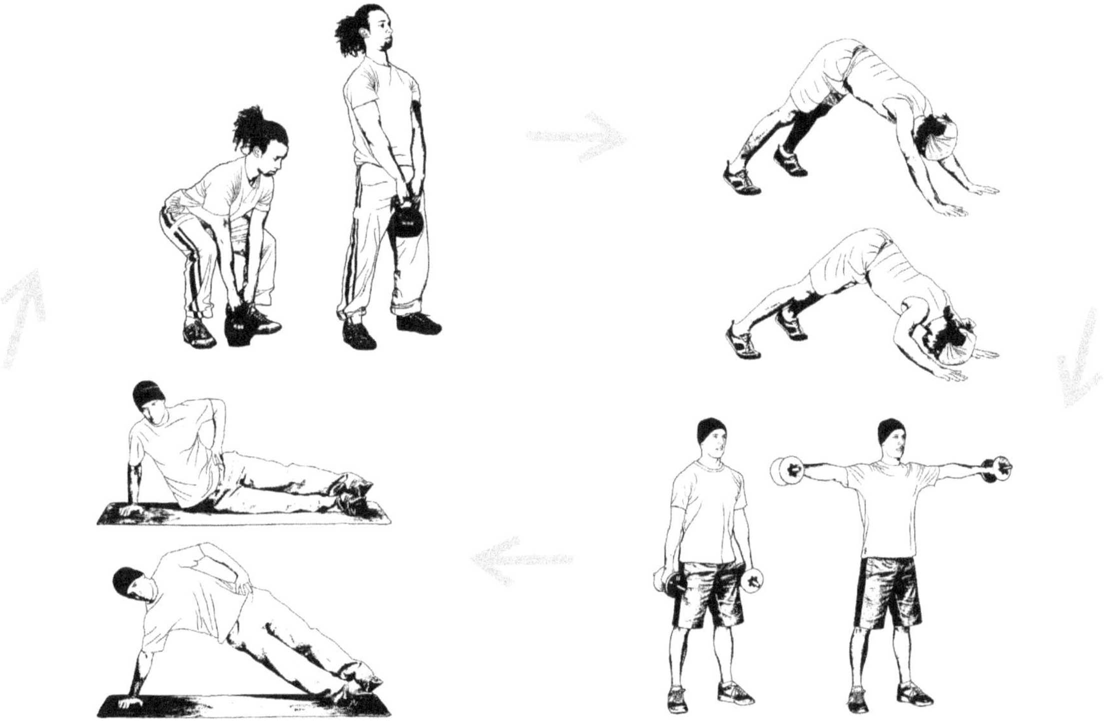

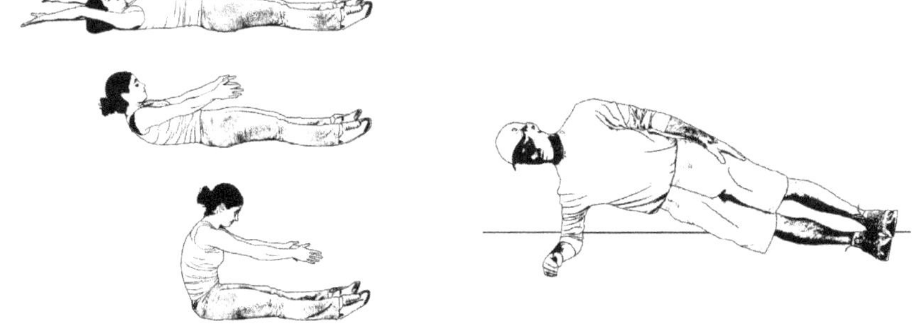

SIDE A

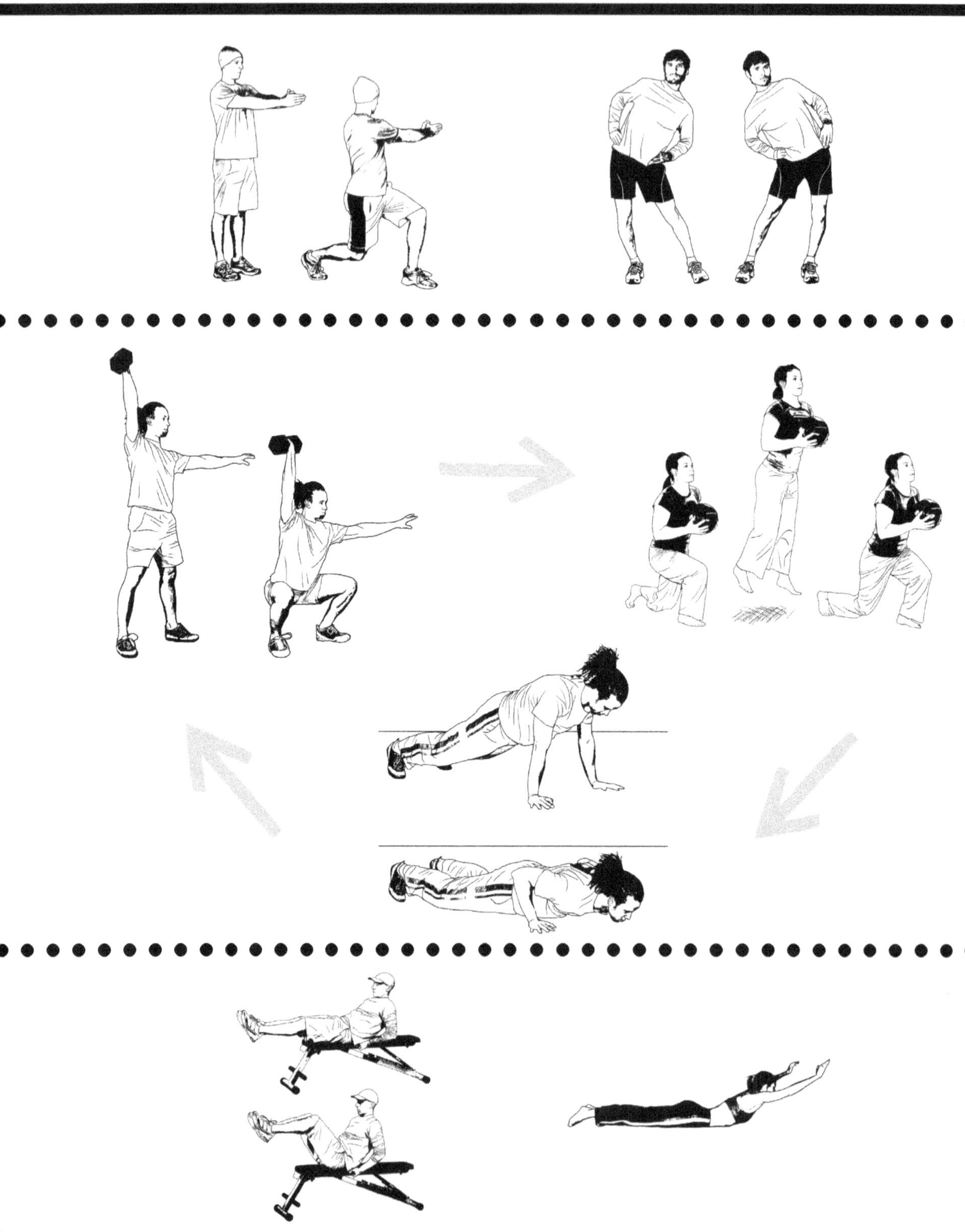

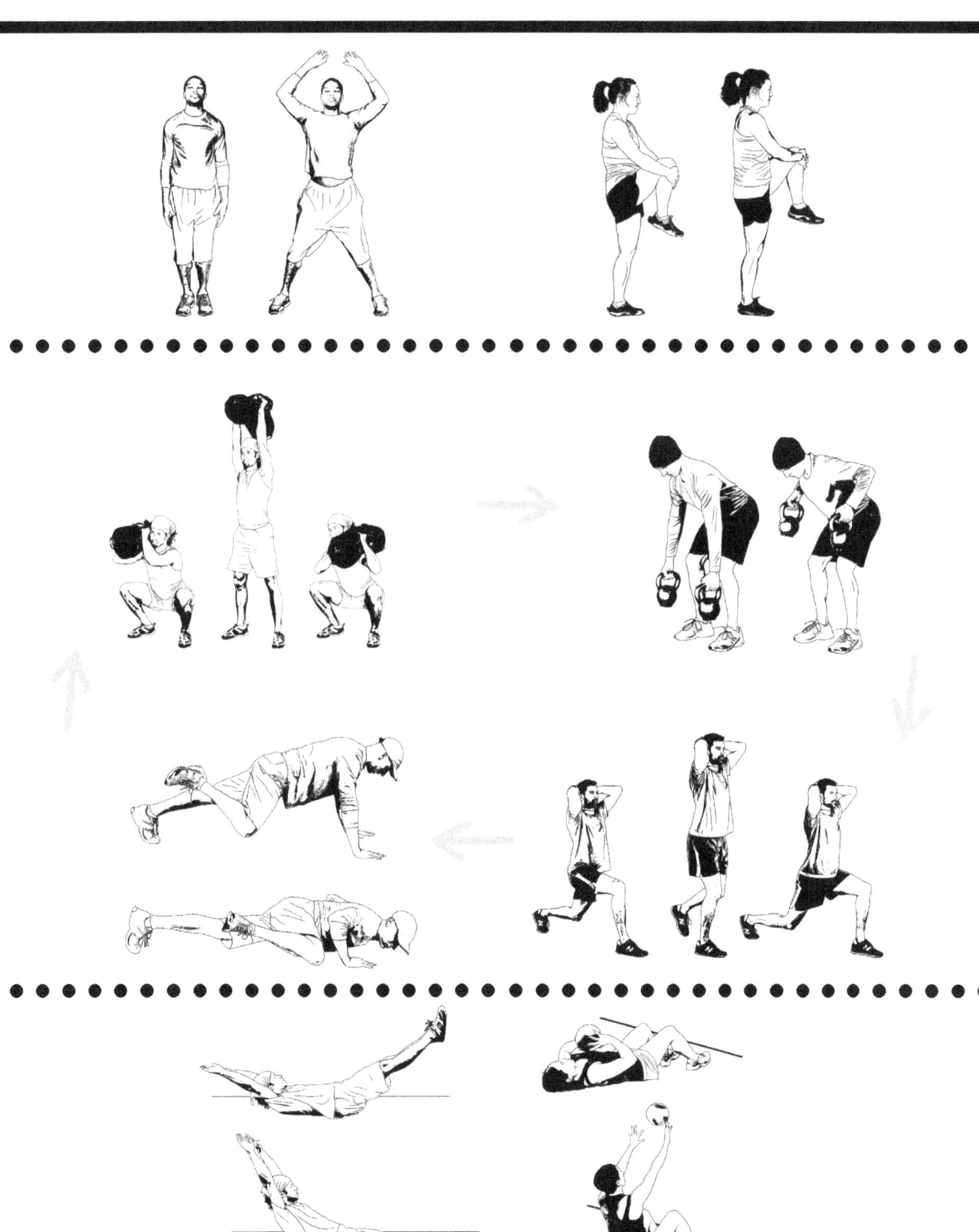

SIDE A

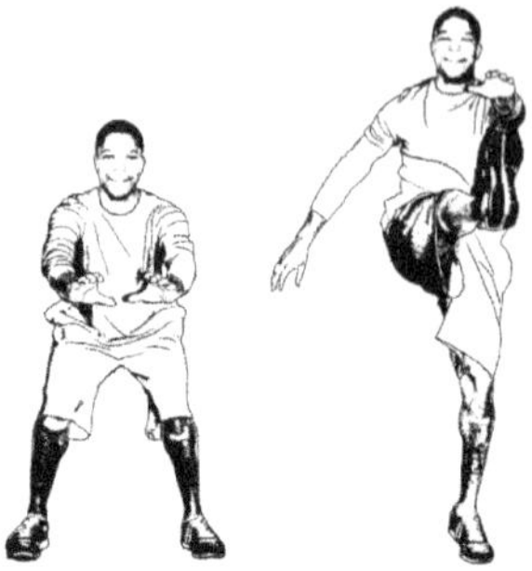

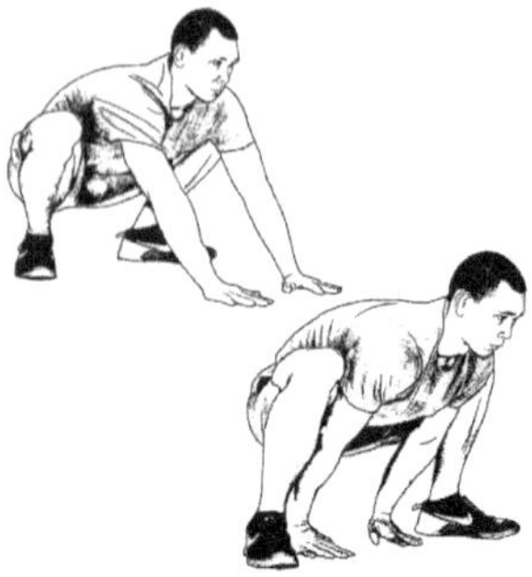

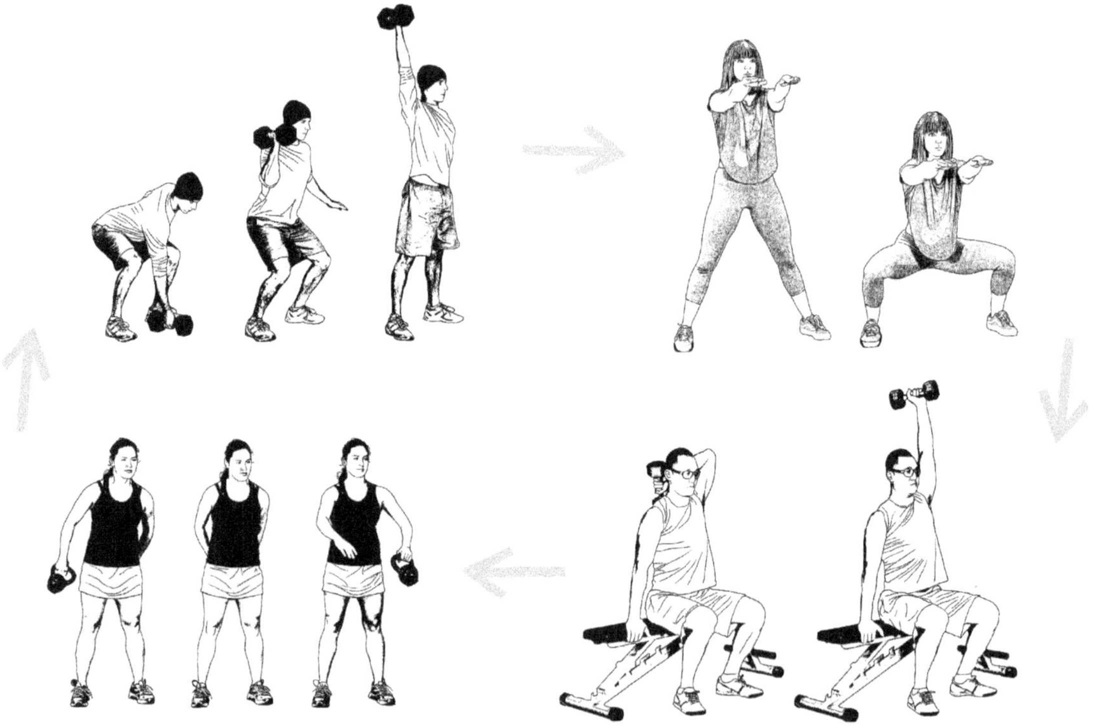

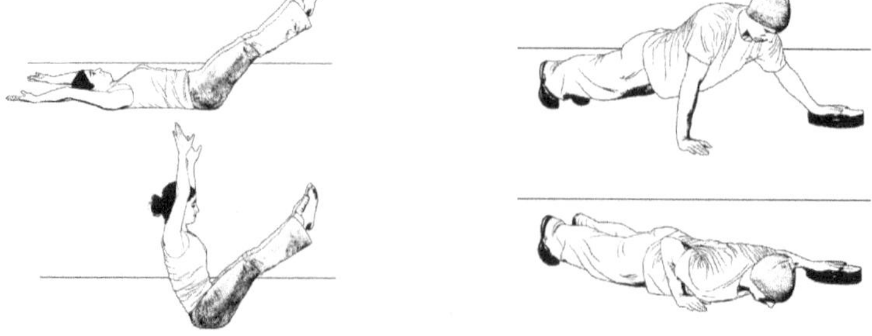

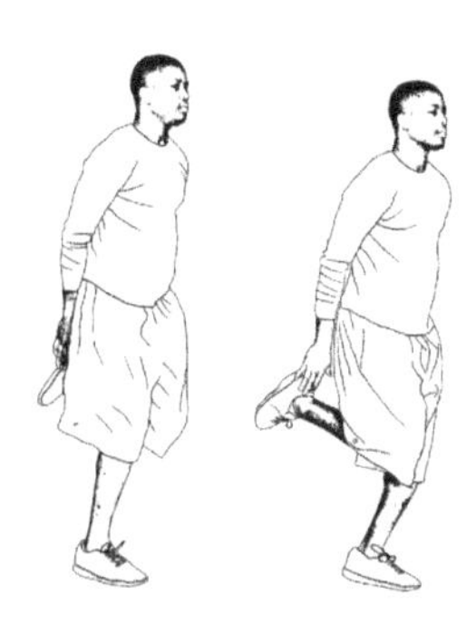
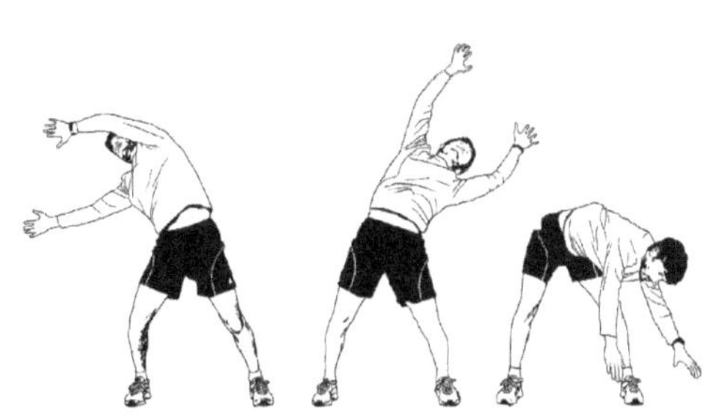
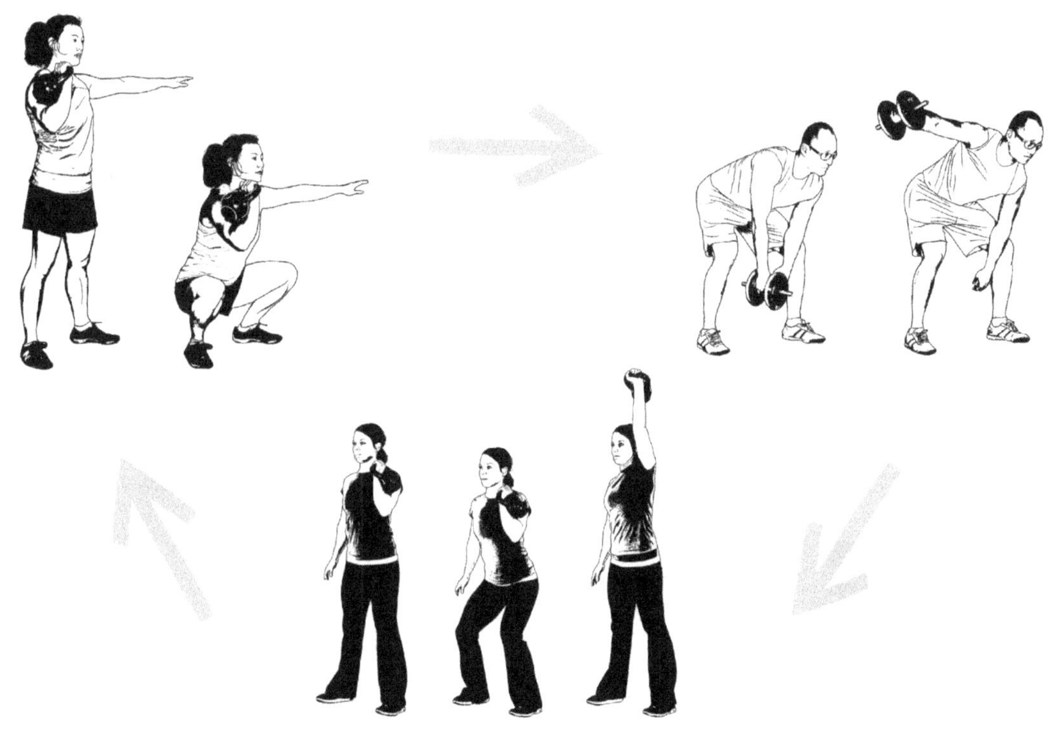
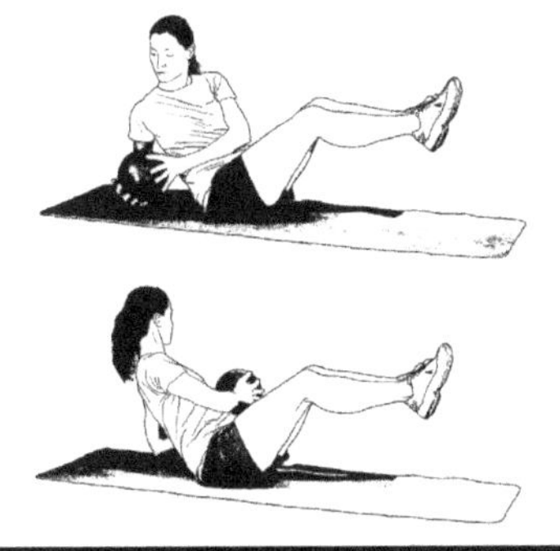
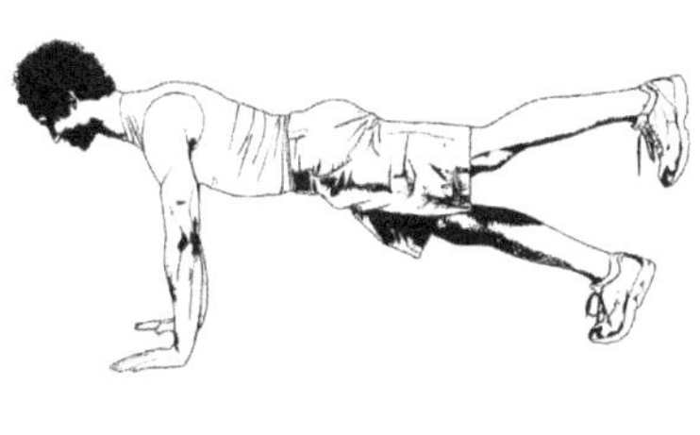

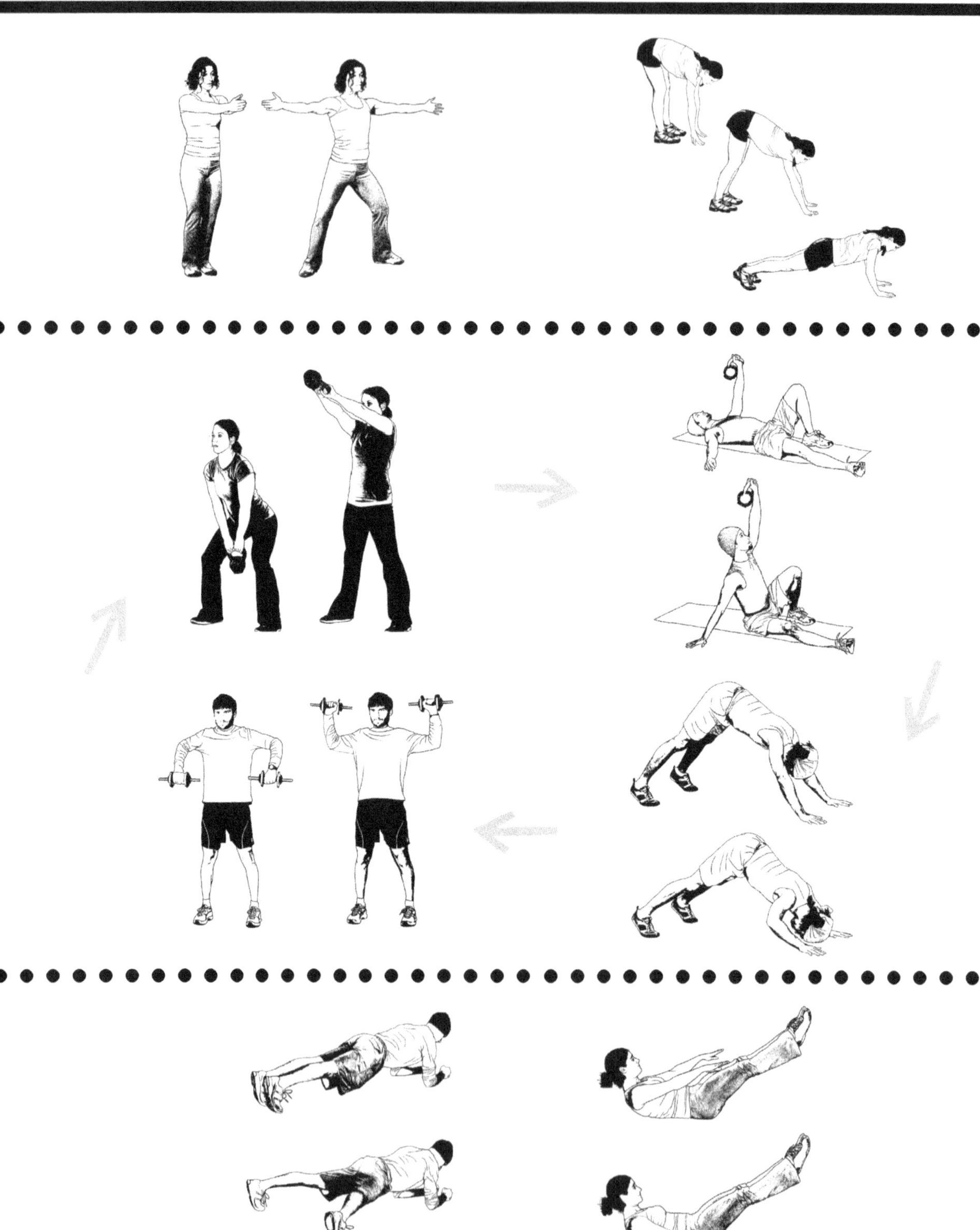

SIDE A

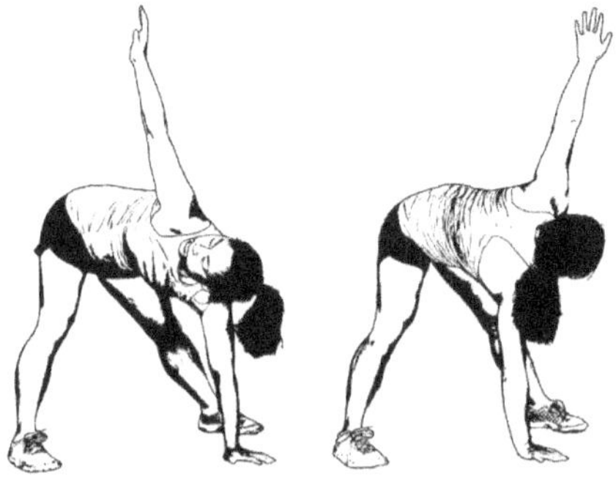

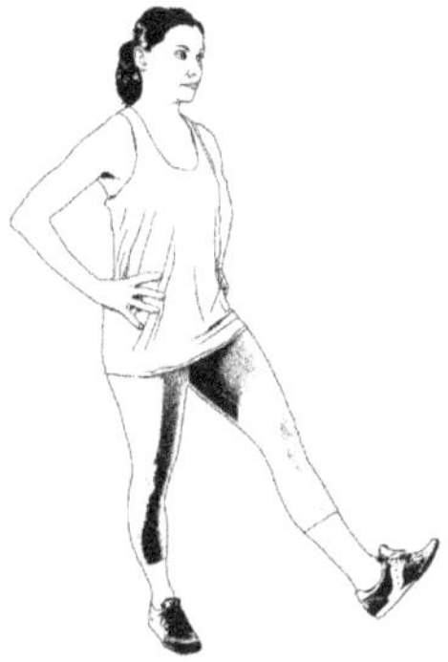

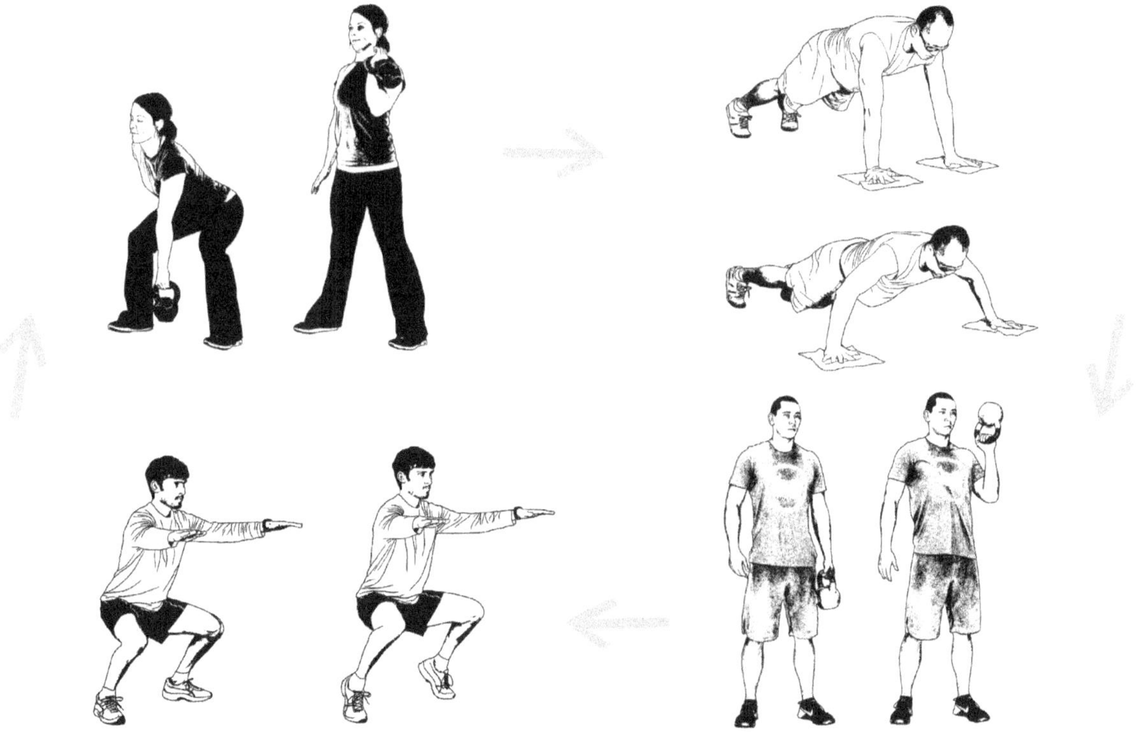

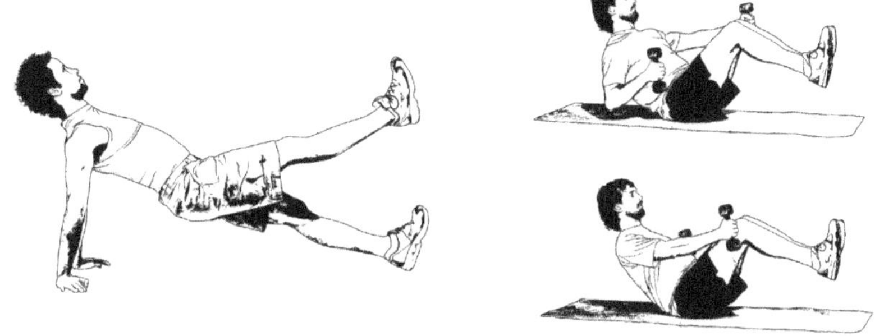

SIDE A

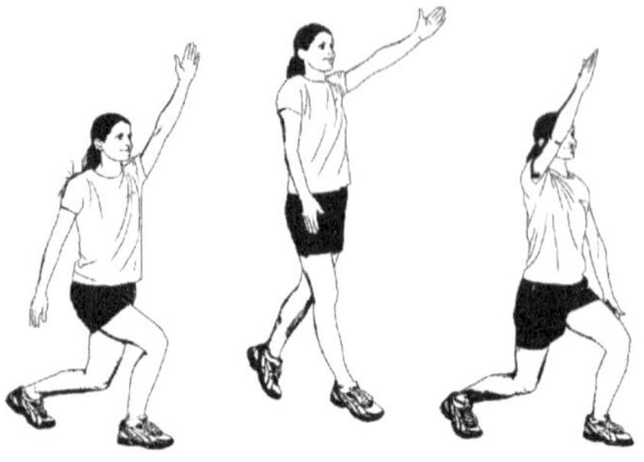

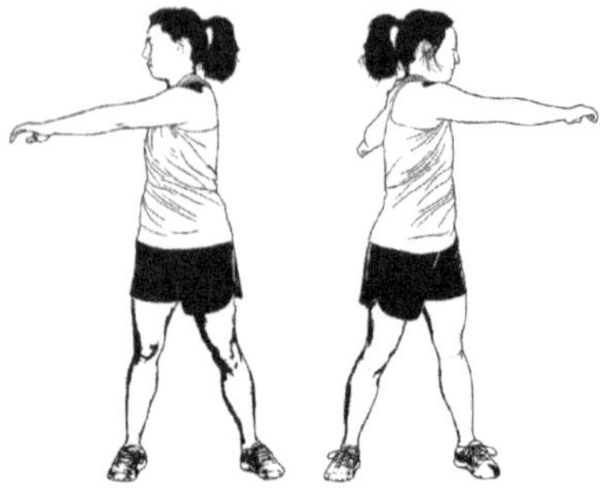

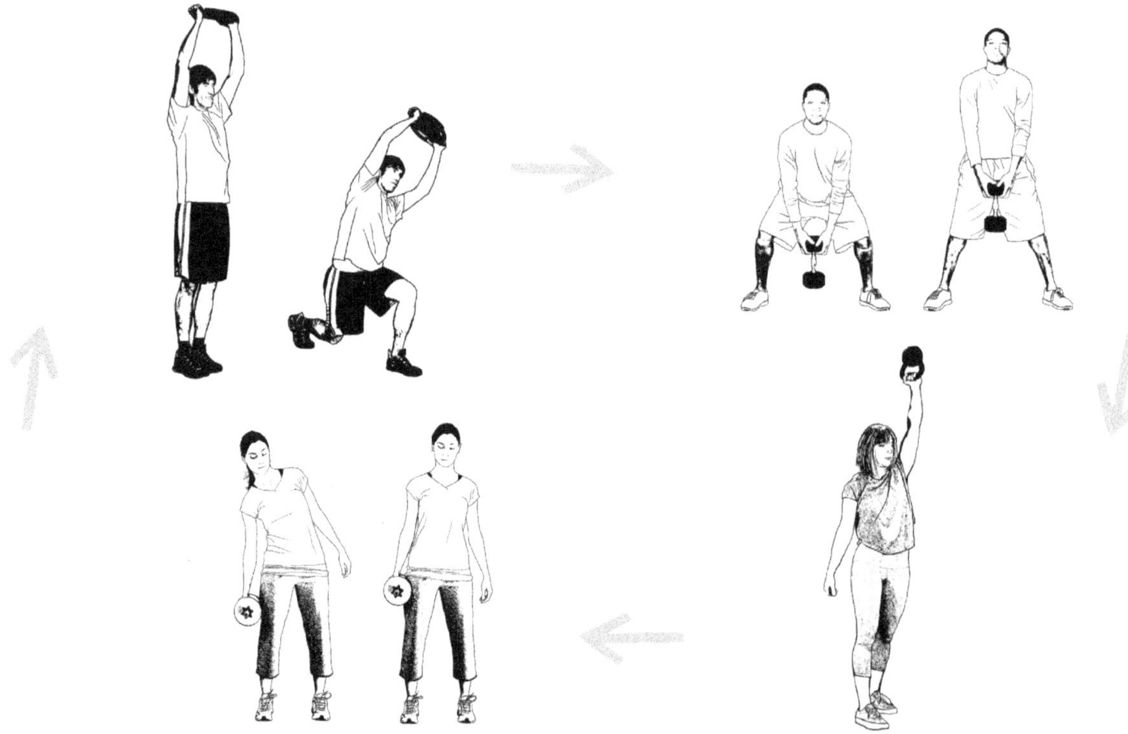

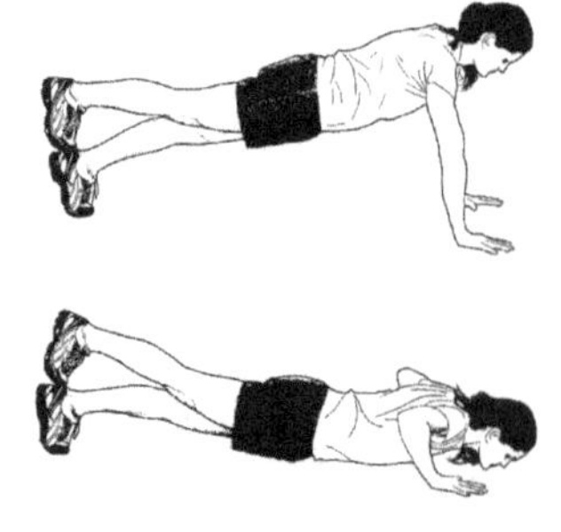

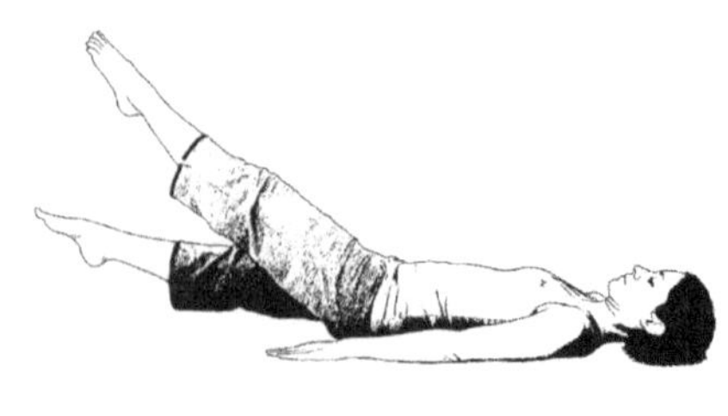

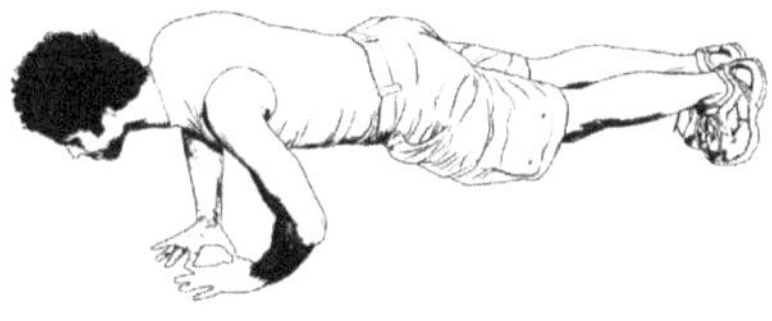

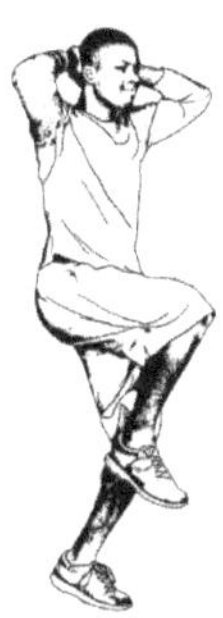

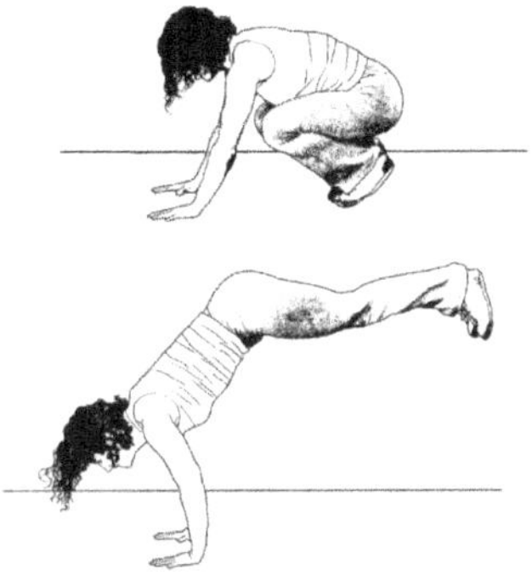

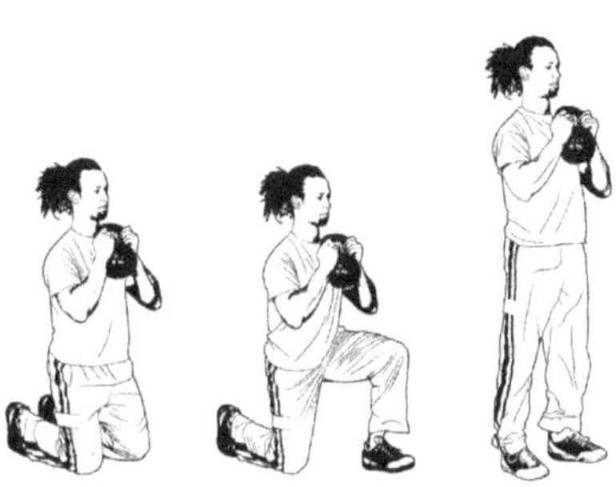

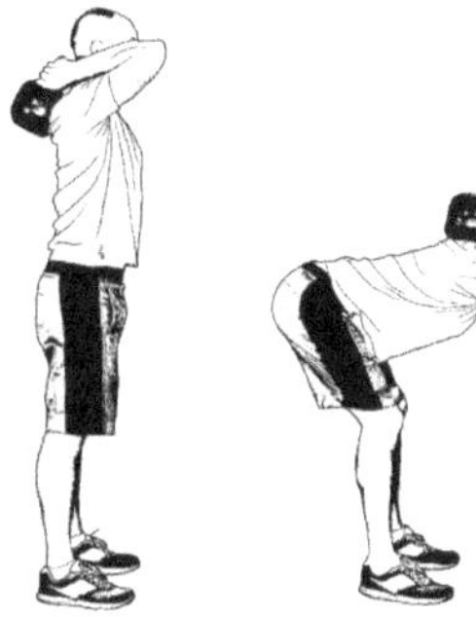

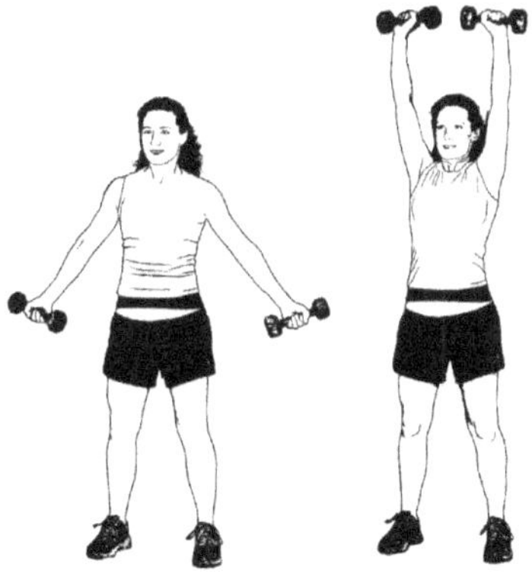

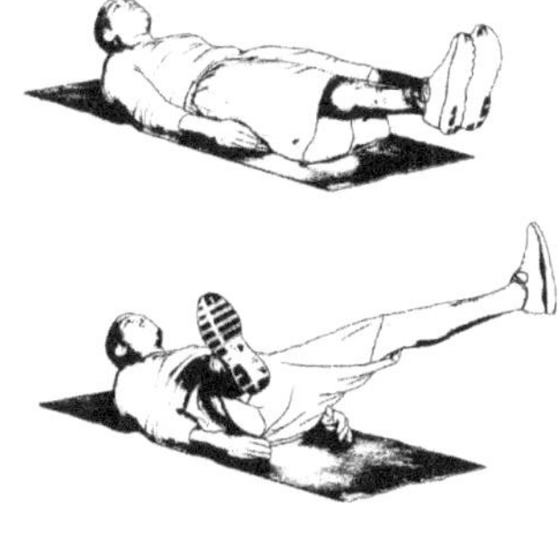

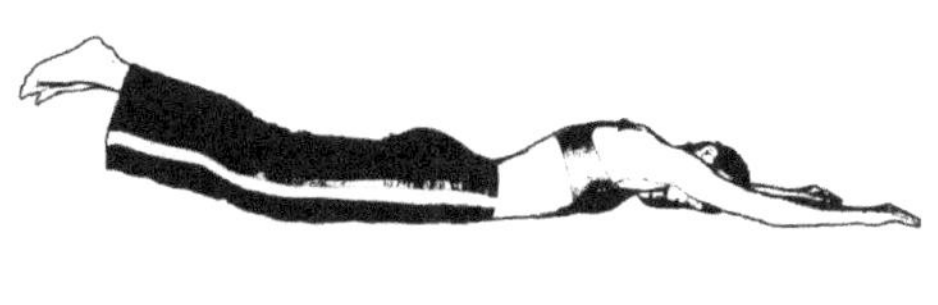

SIDE A

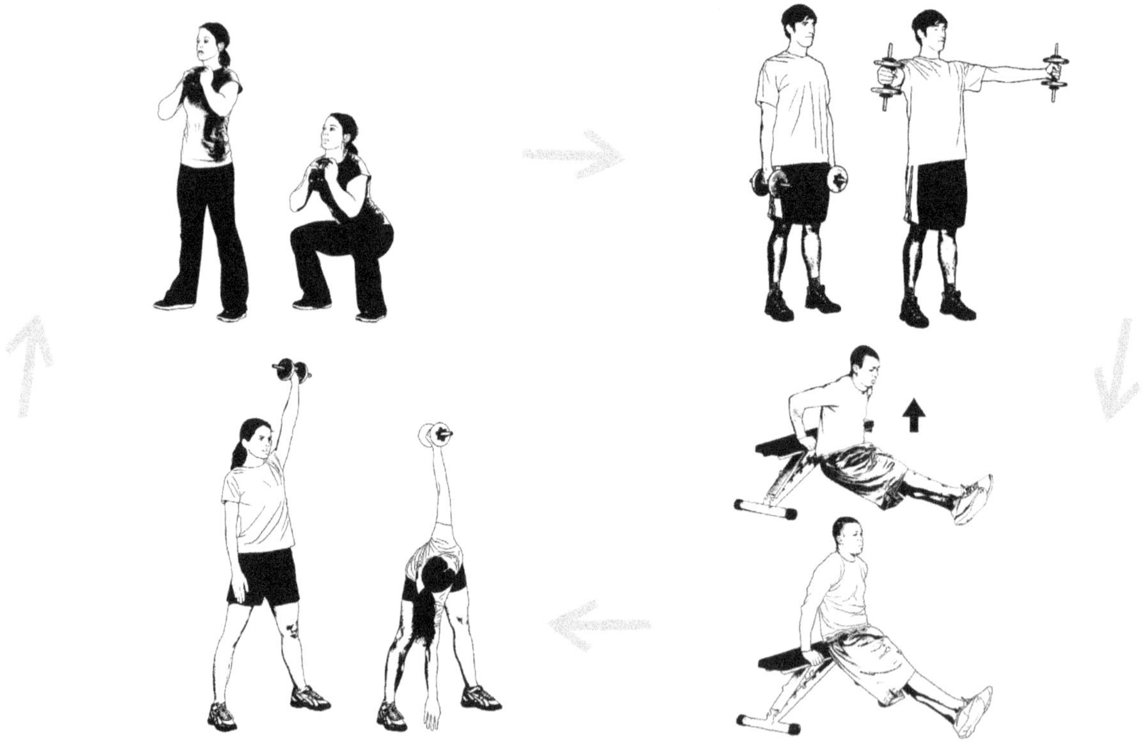

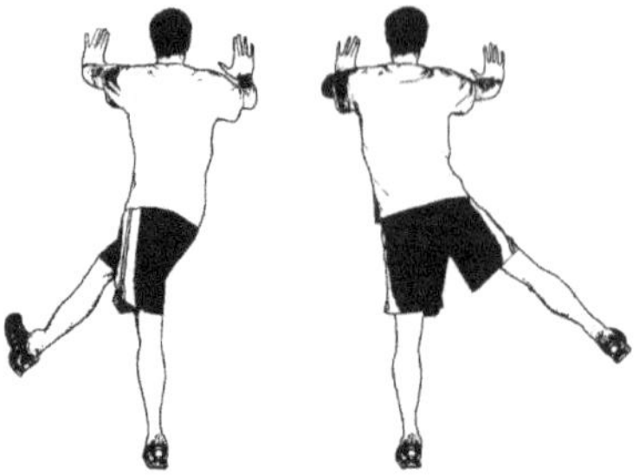

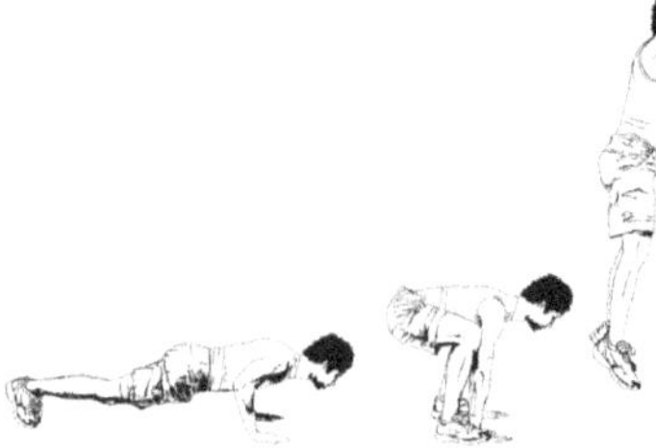

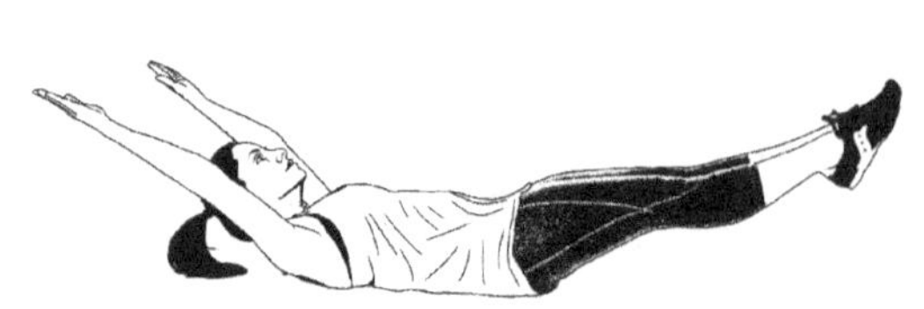

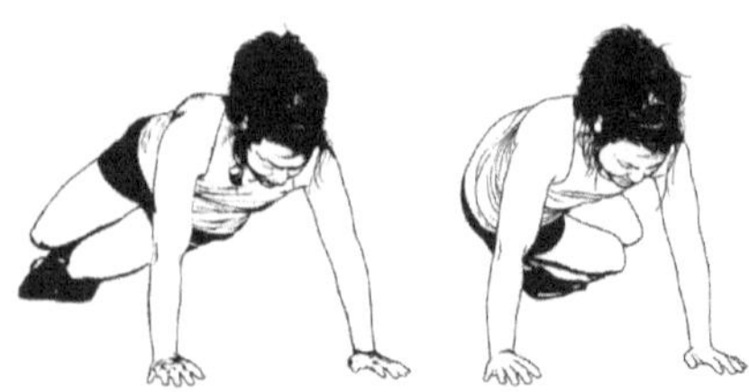

SIDE A

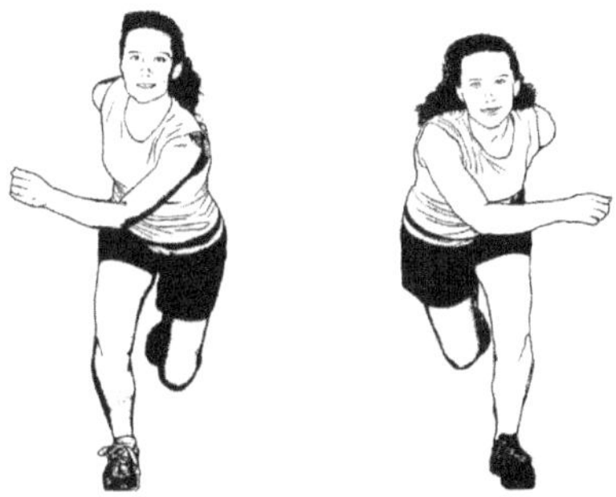

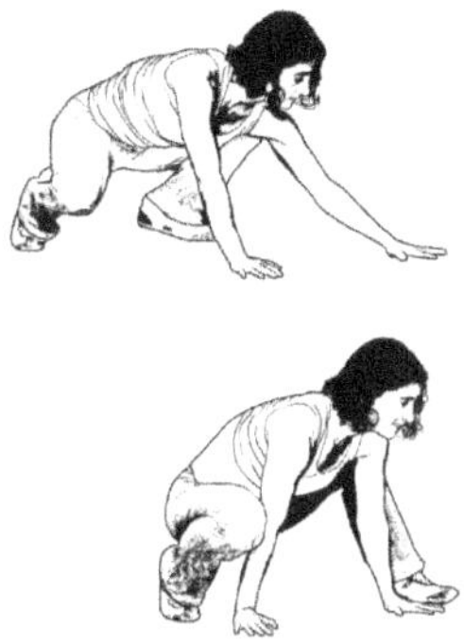

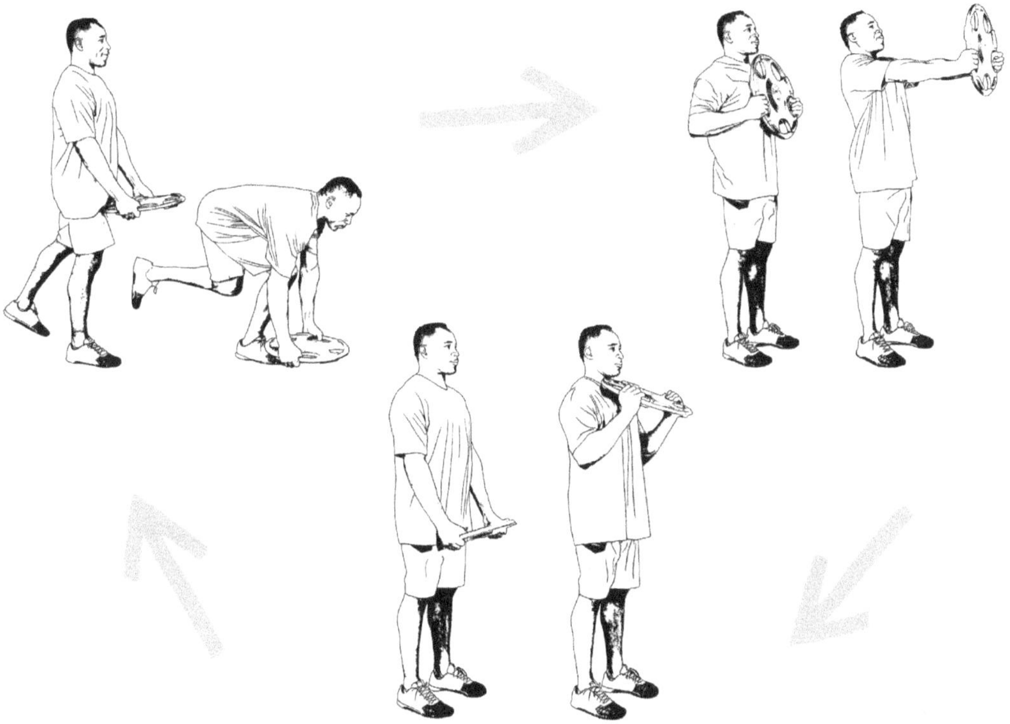

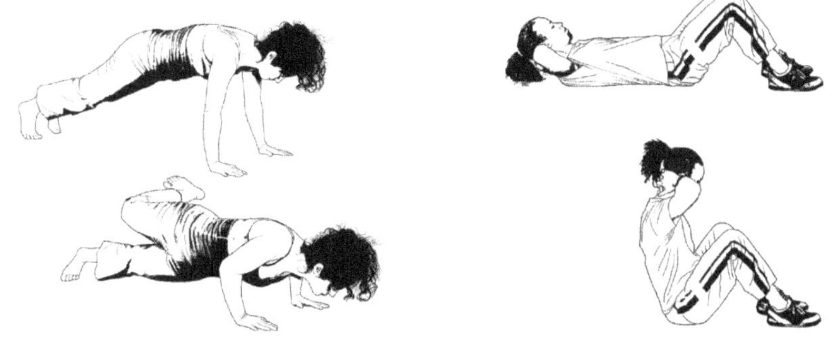

Side B

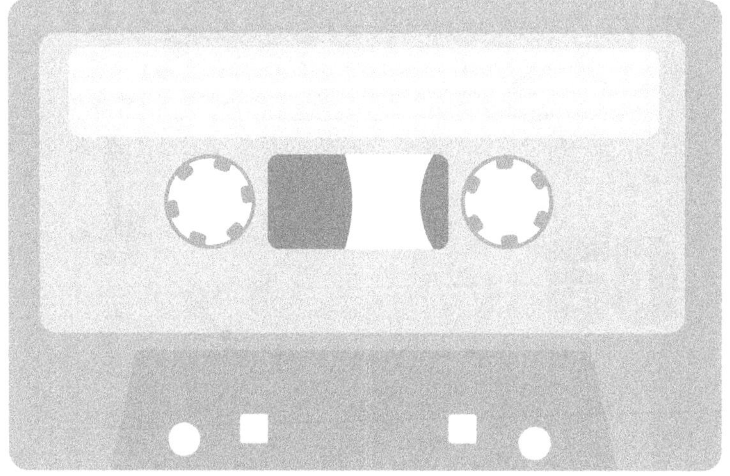

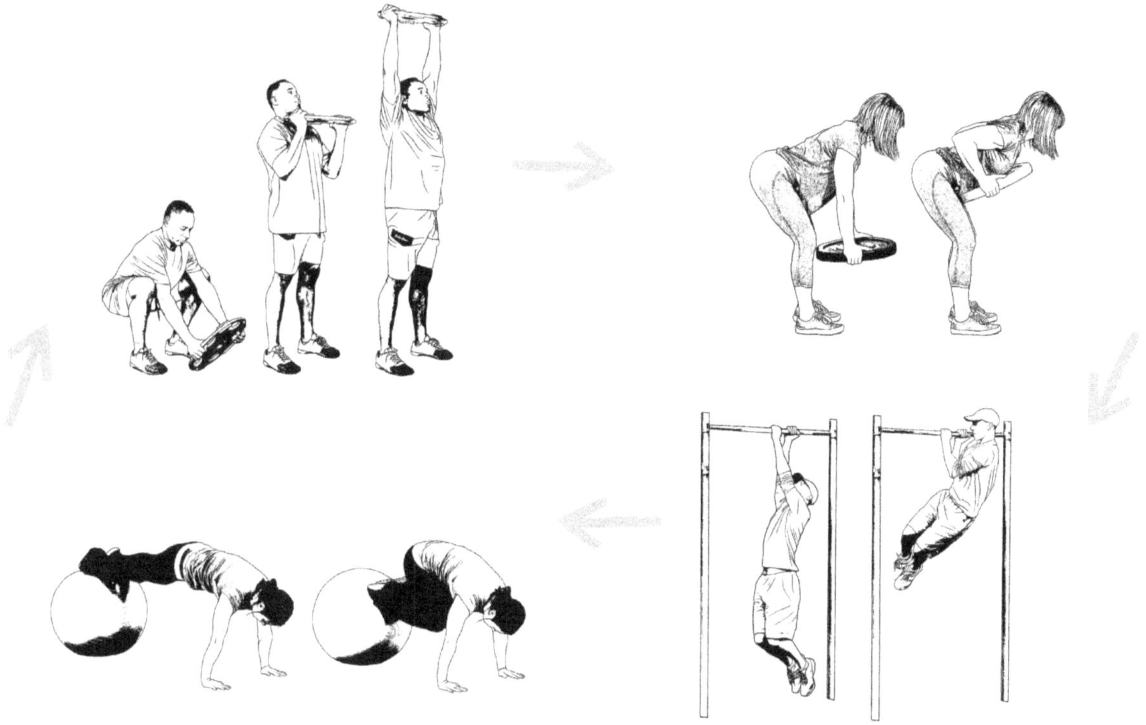

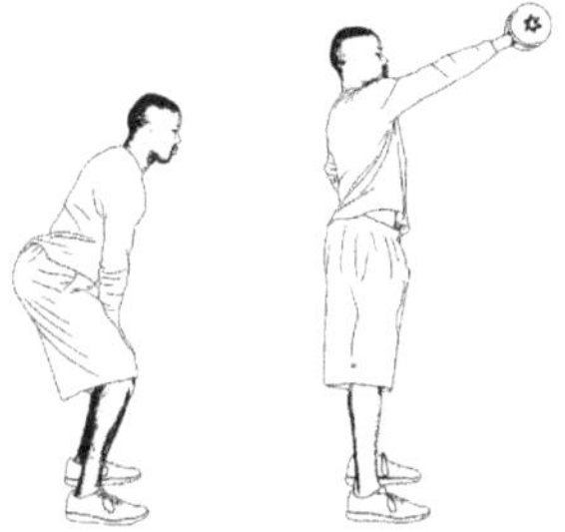

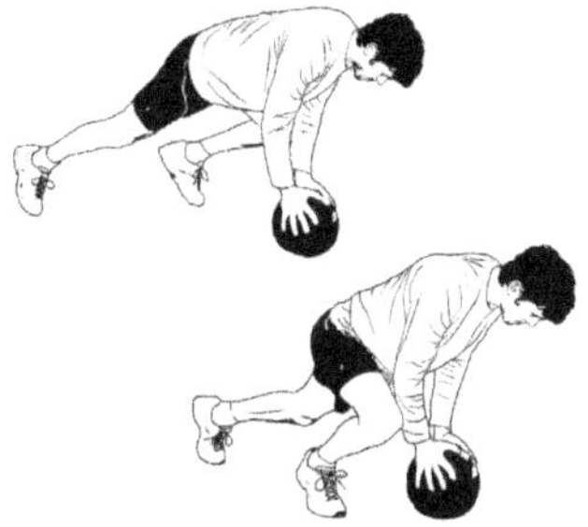

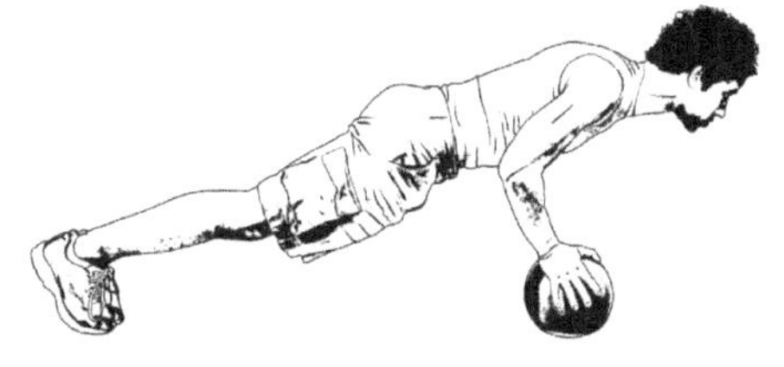
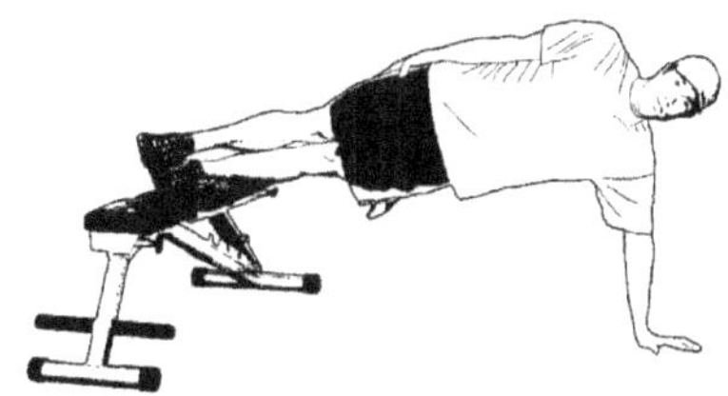

Side B

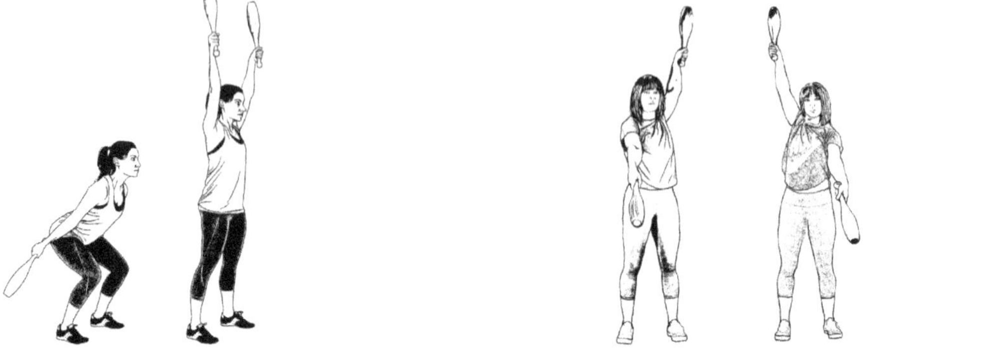

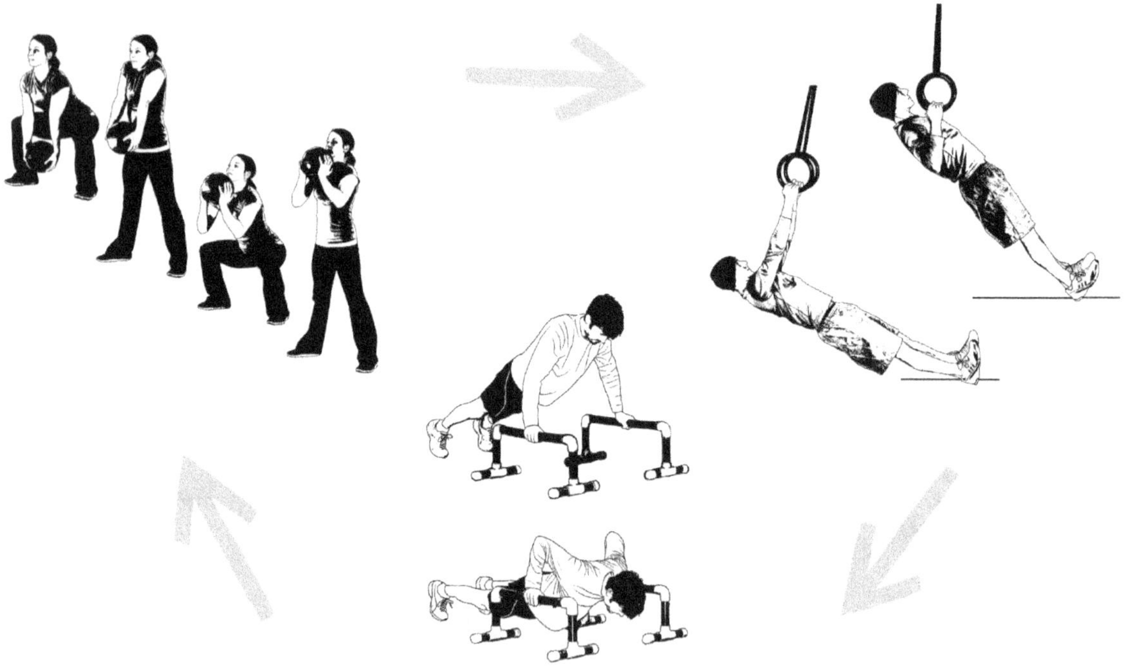

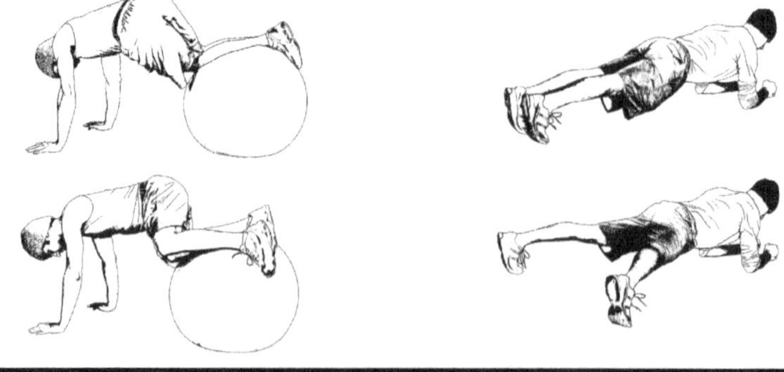

Side B

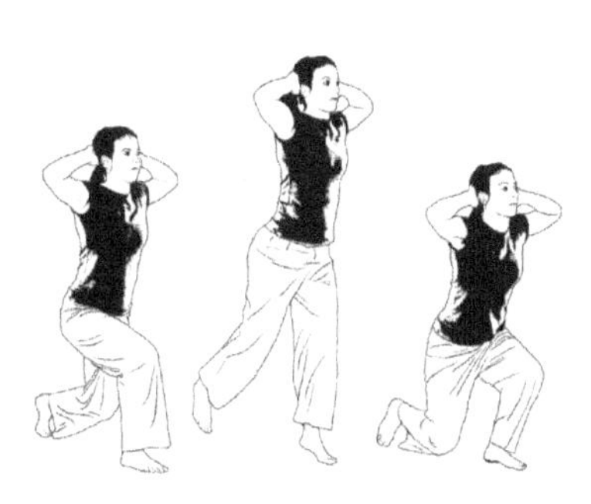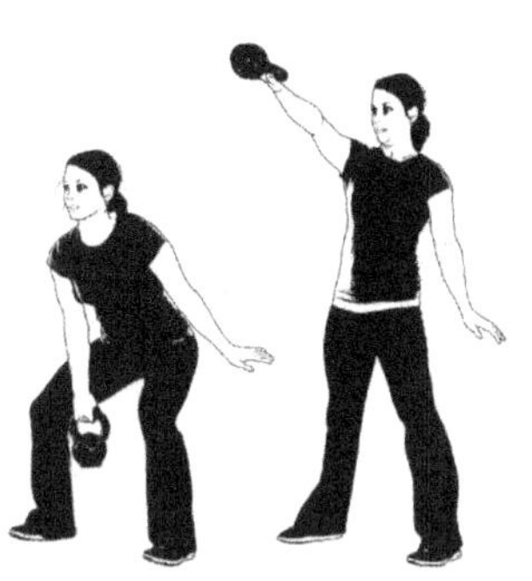

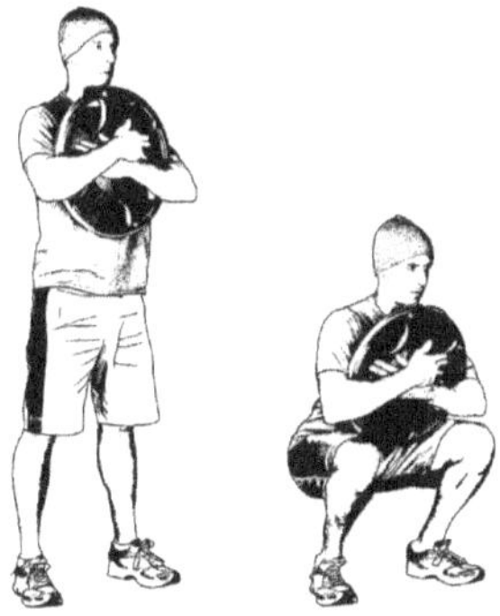

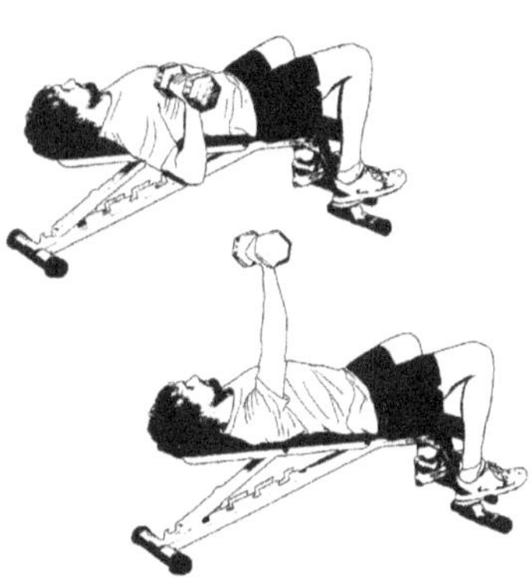

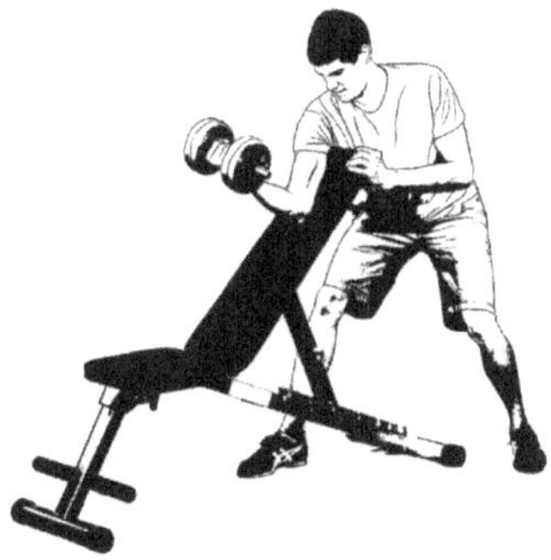

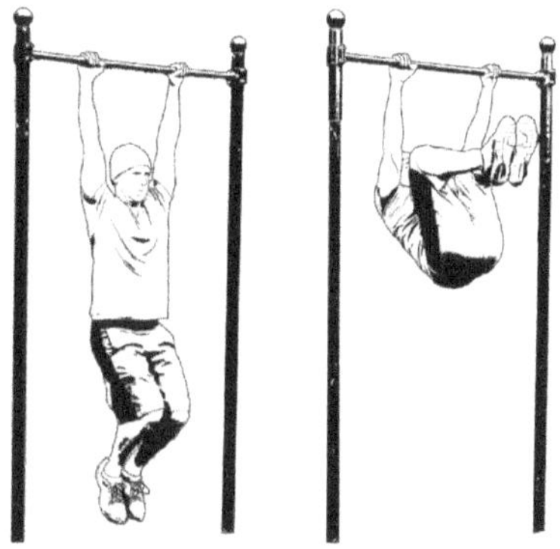

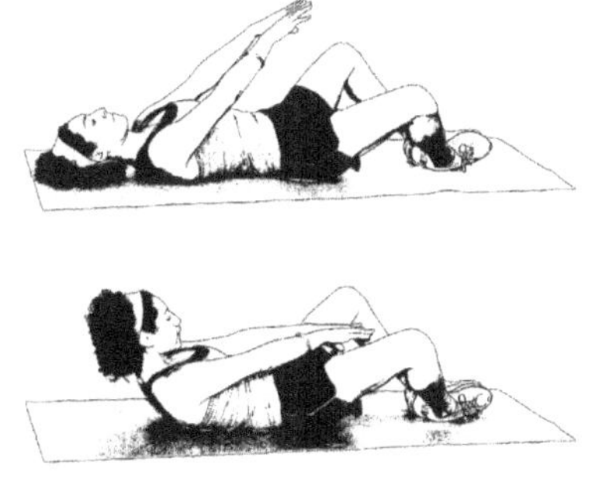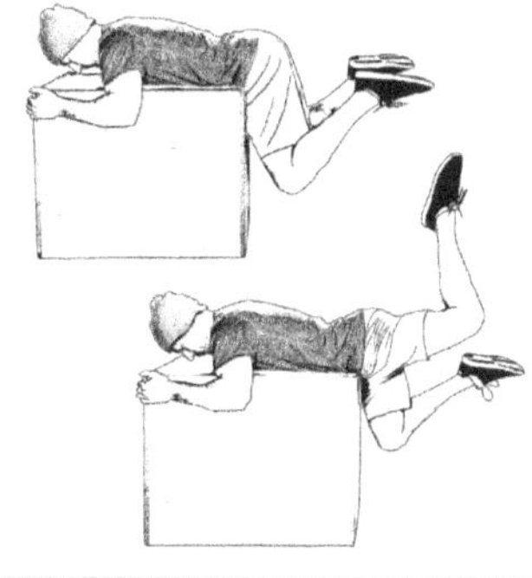

SIDE B

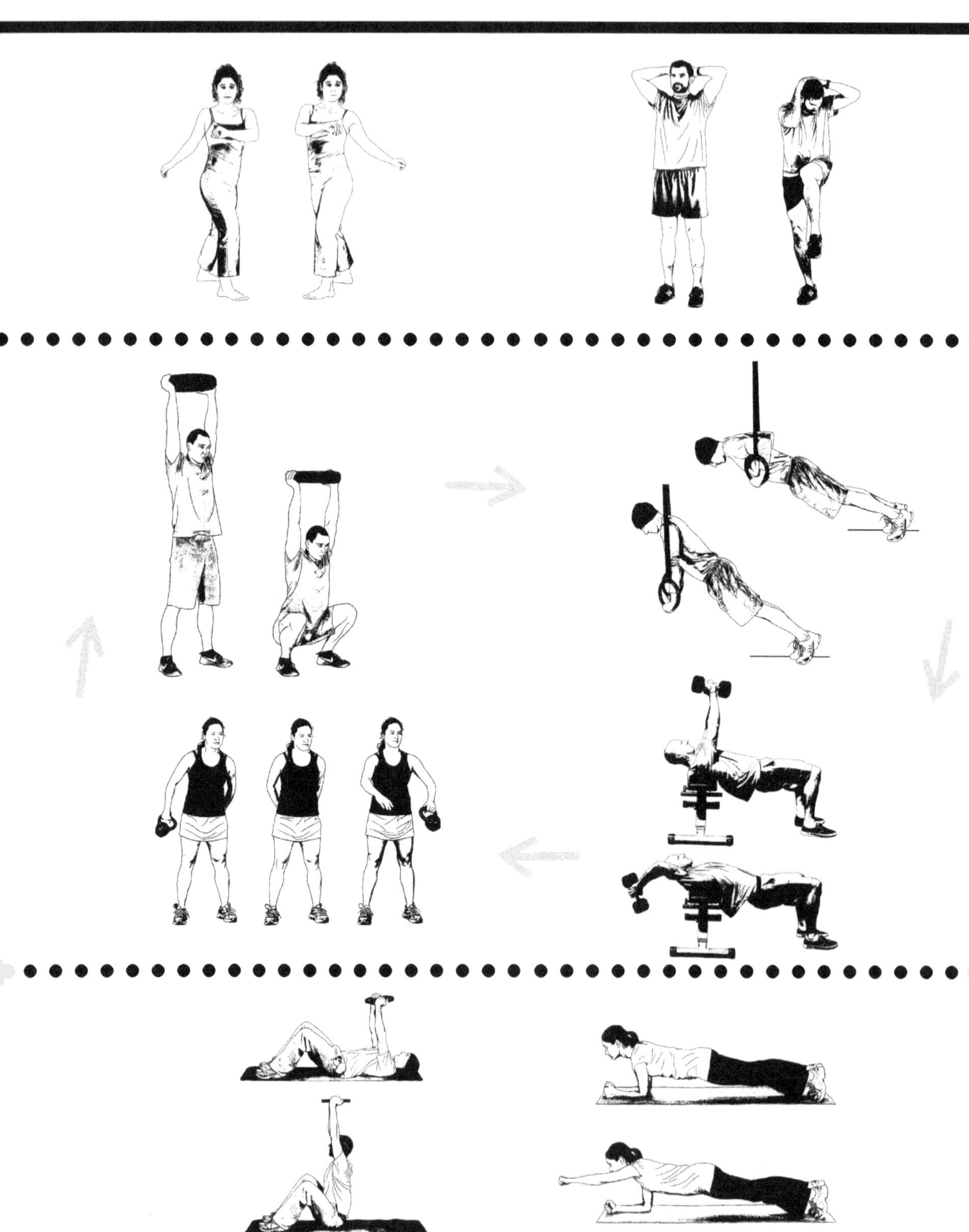

SIDE B

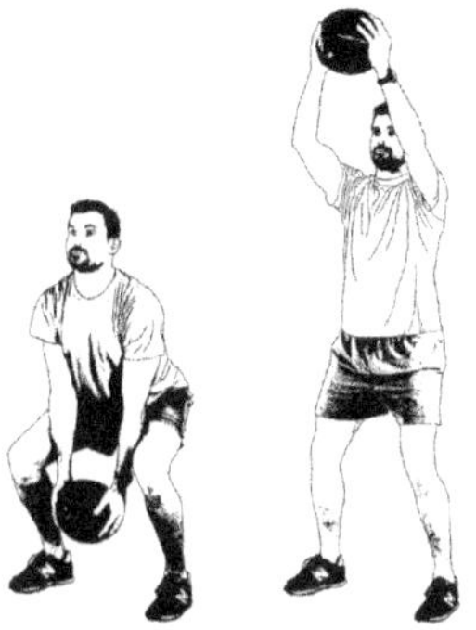

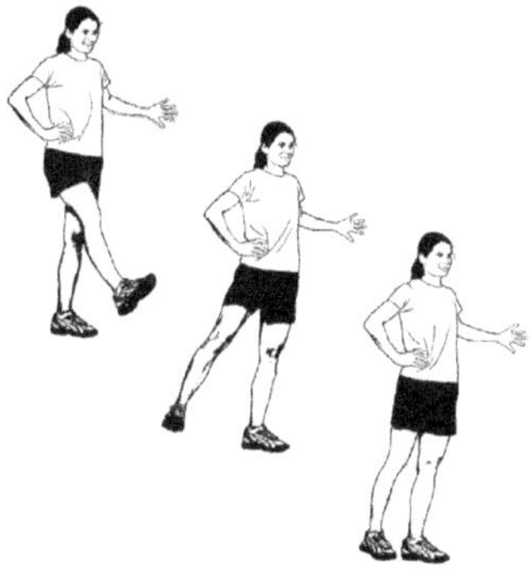

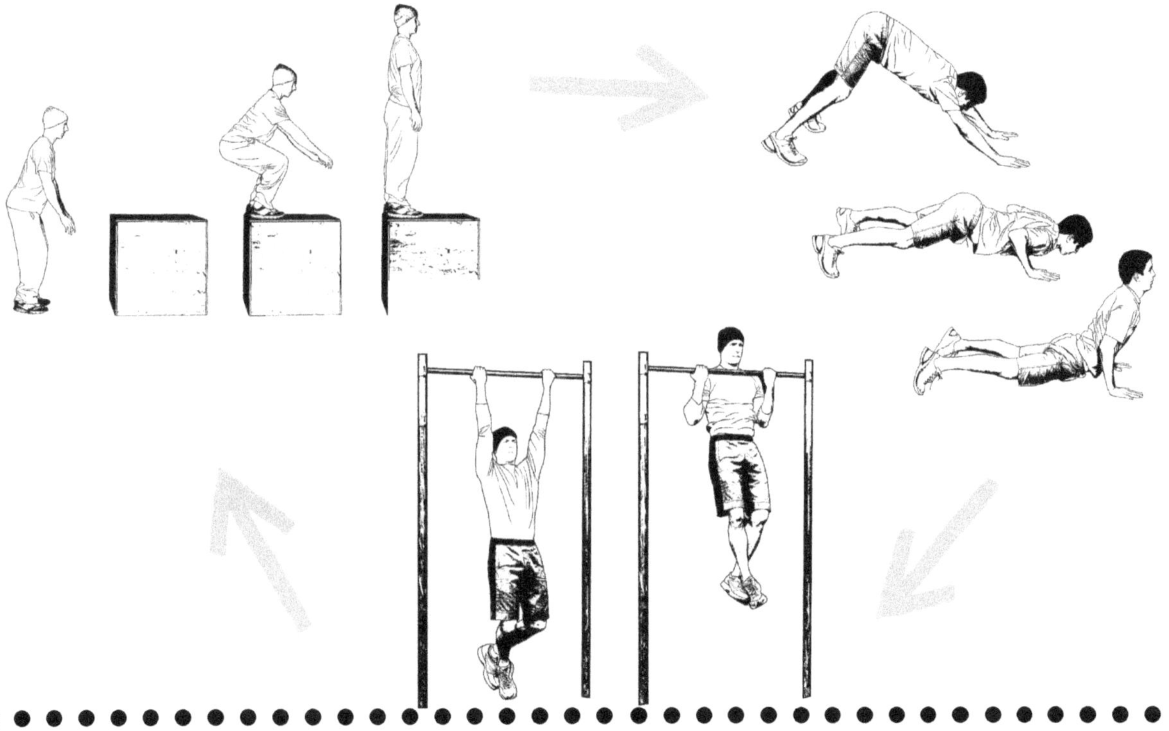

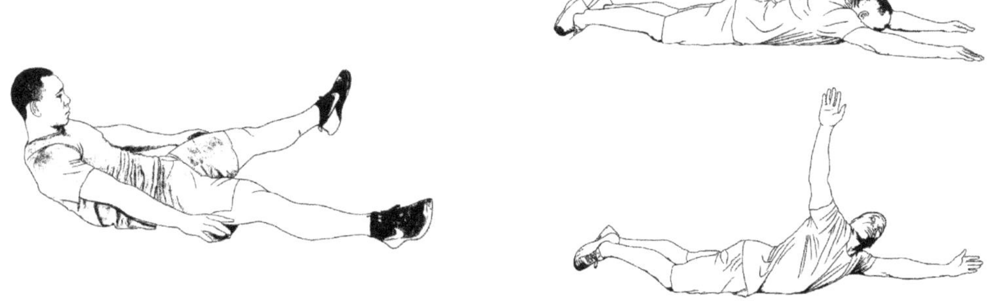

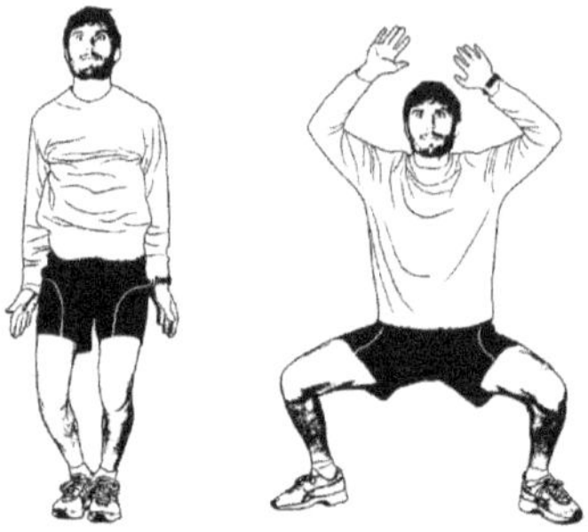

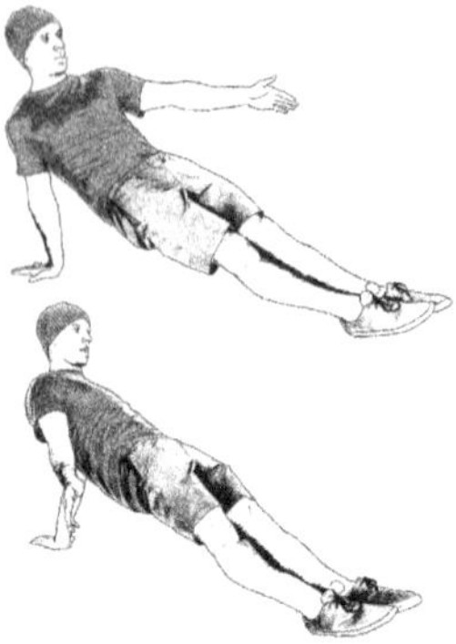

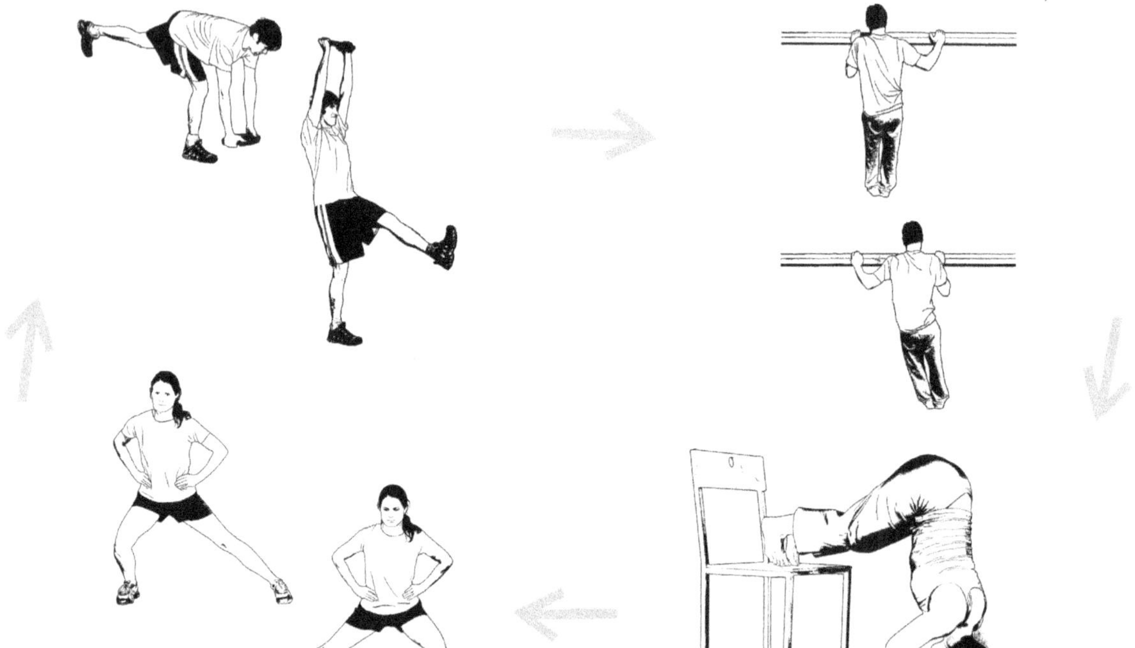

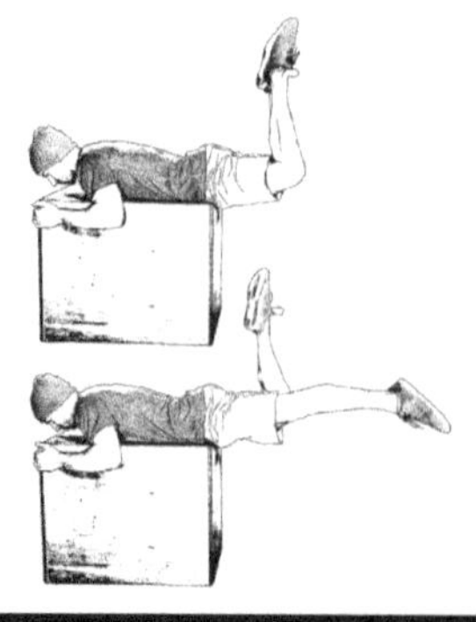
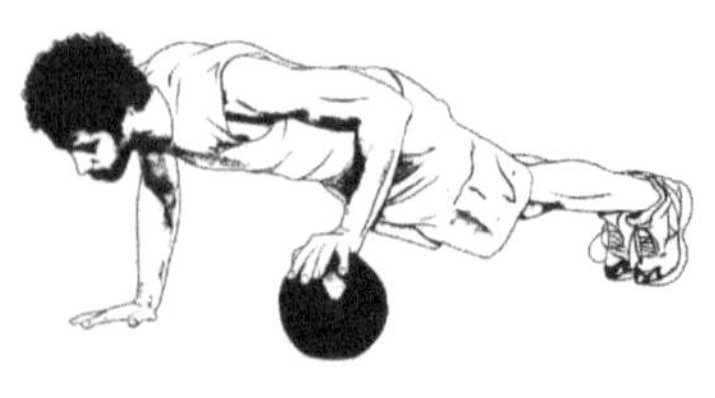

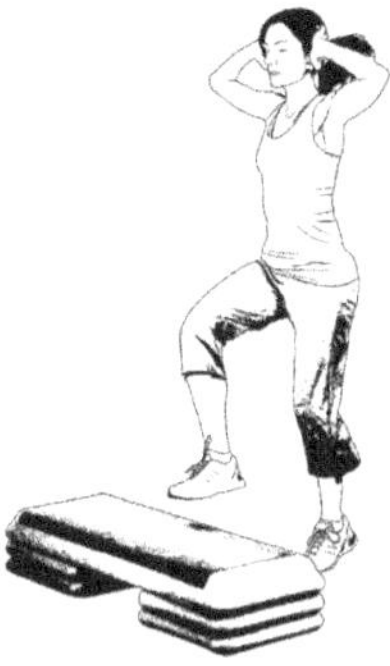

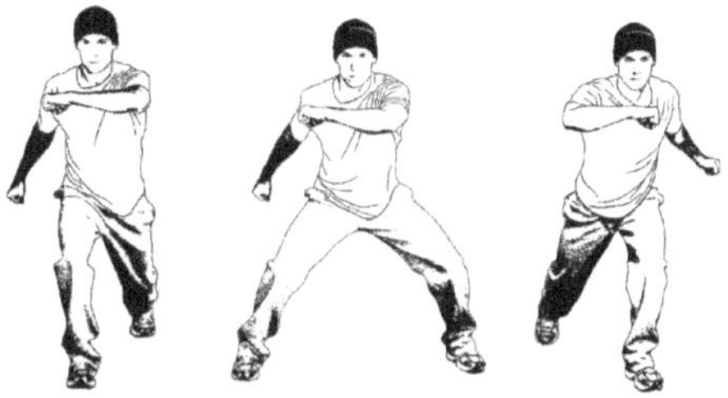

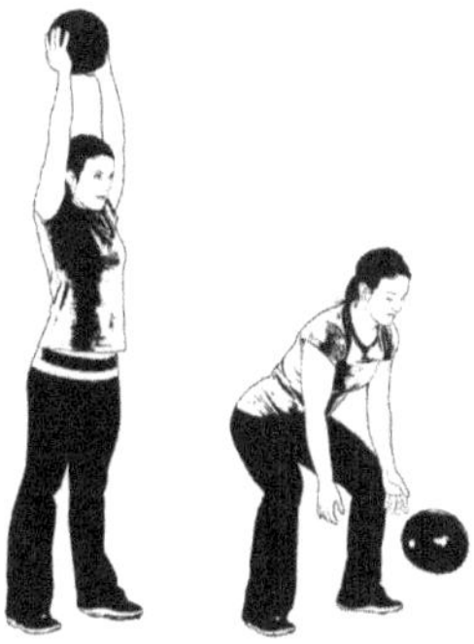

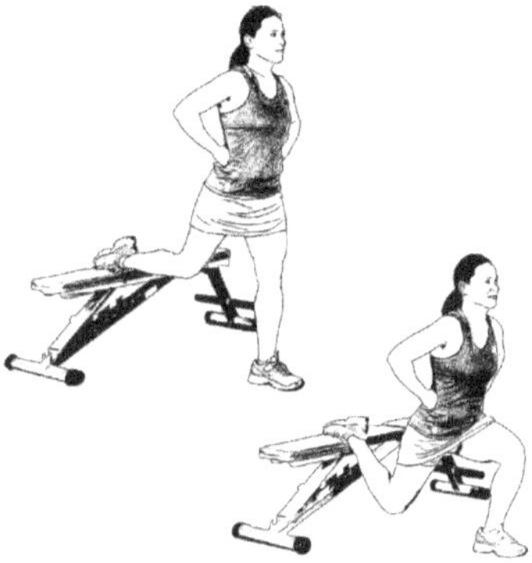

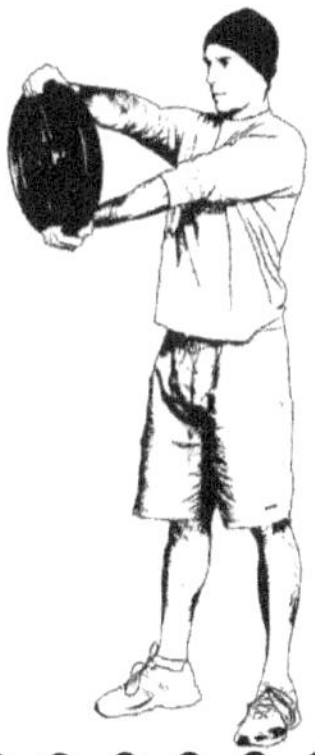

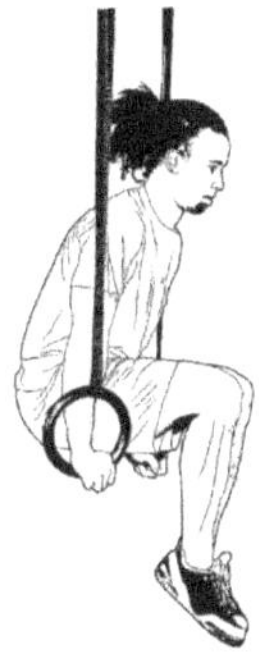

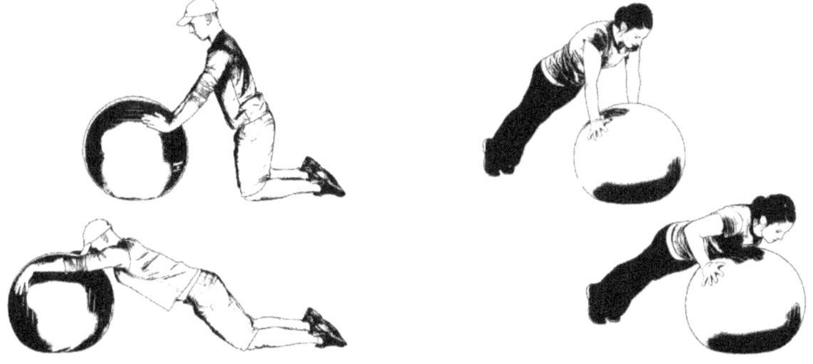

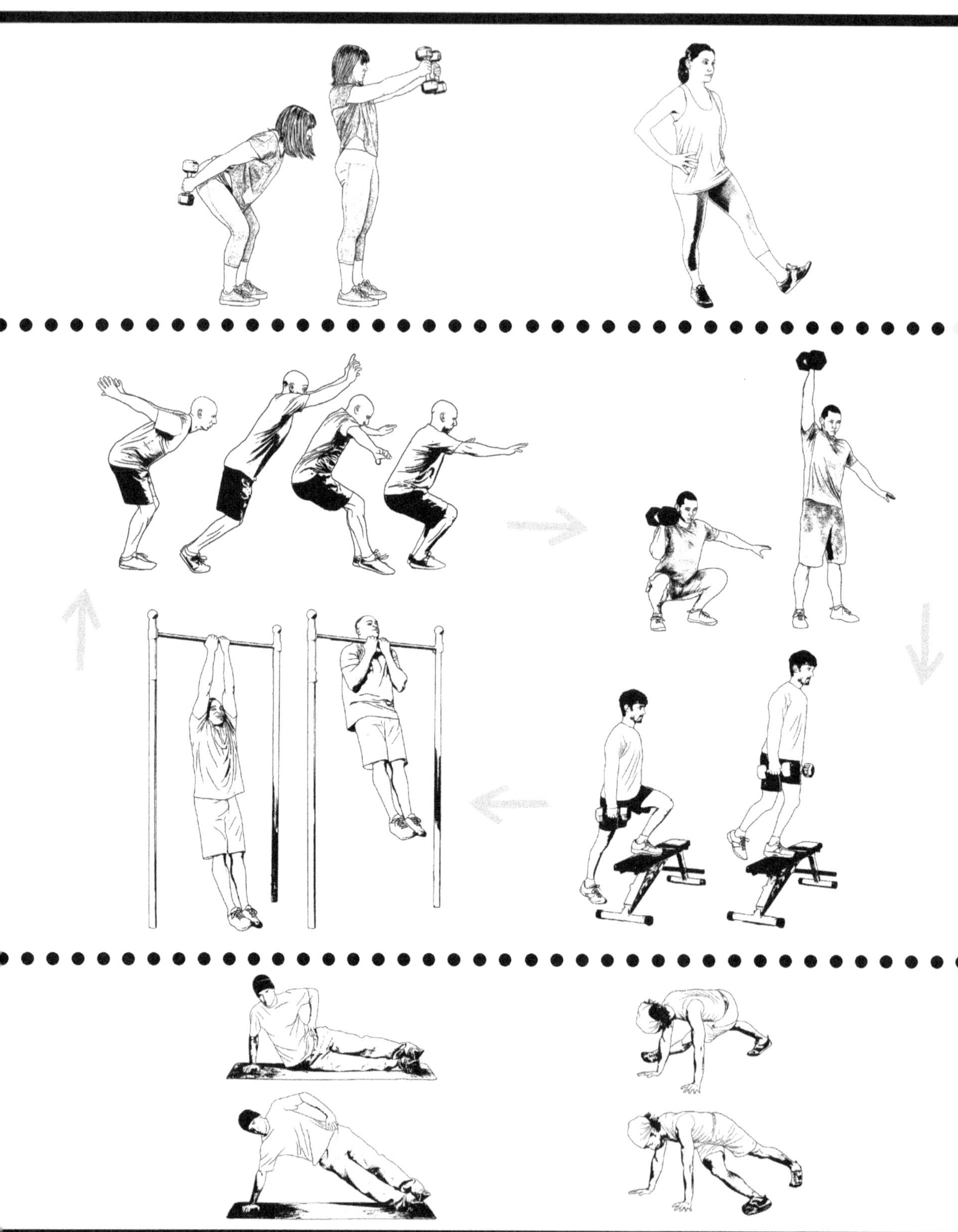

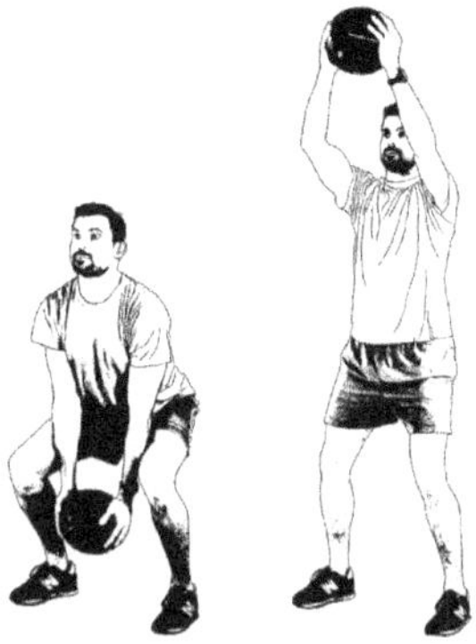

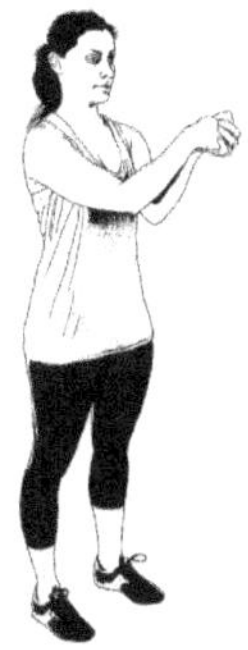

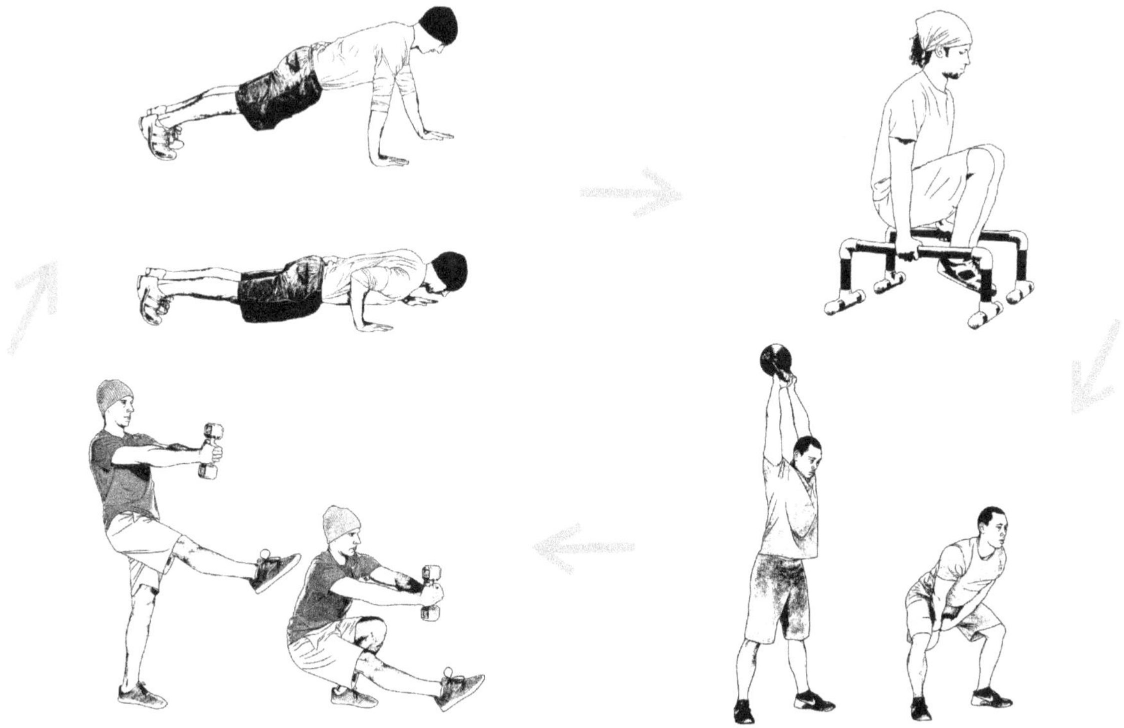

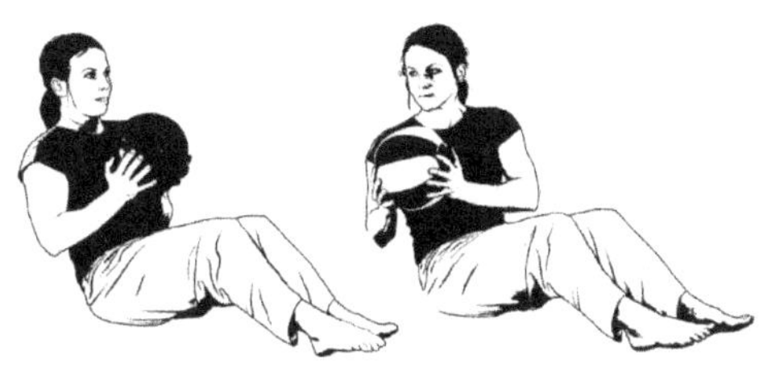

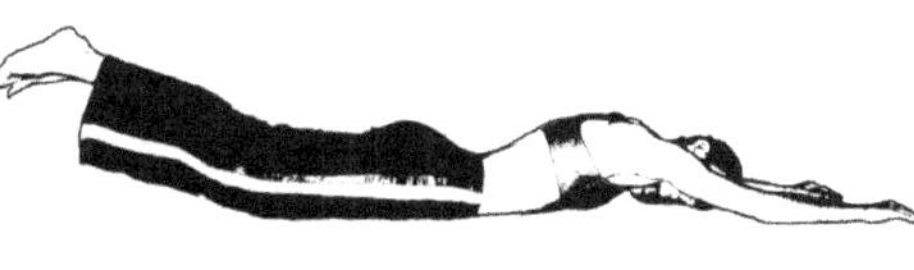

SIDE B

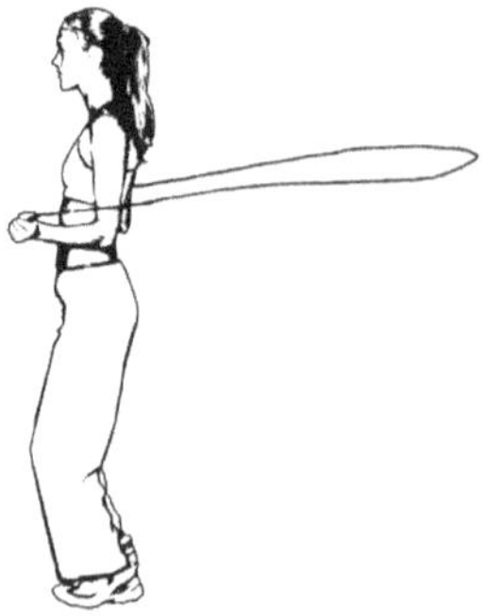

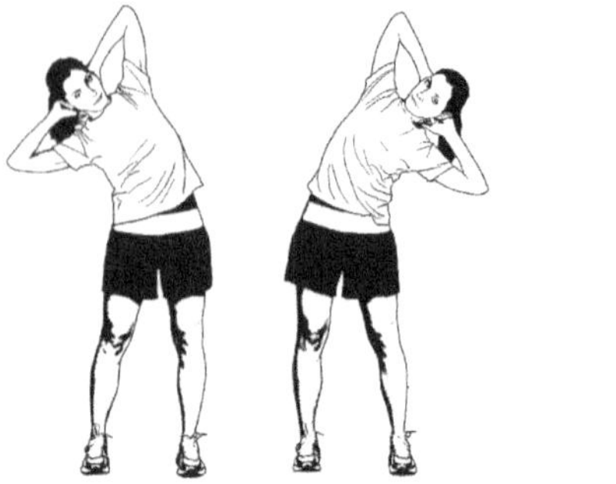

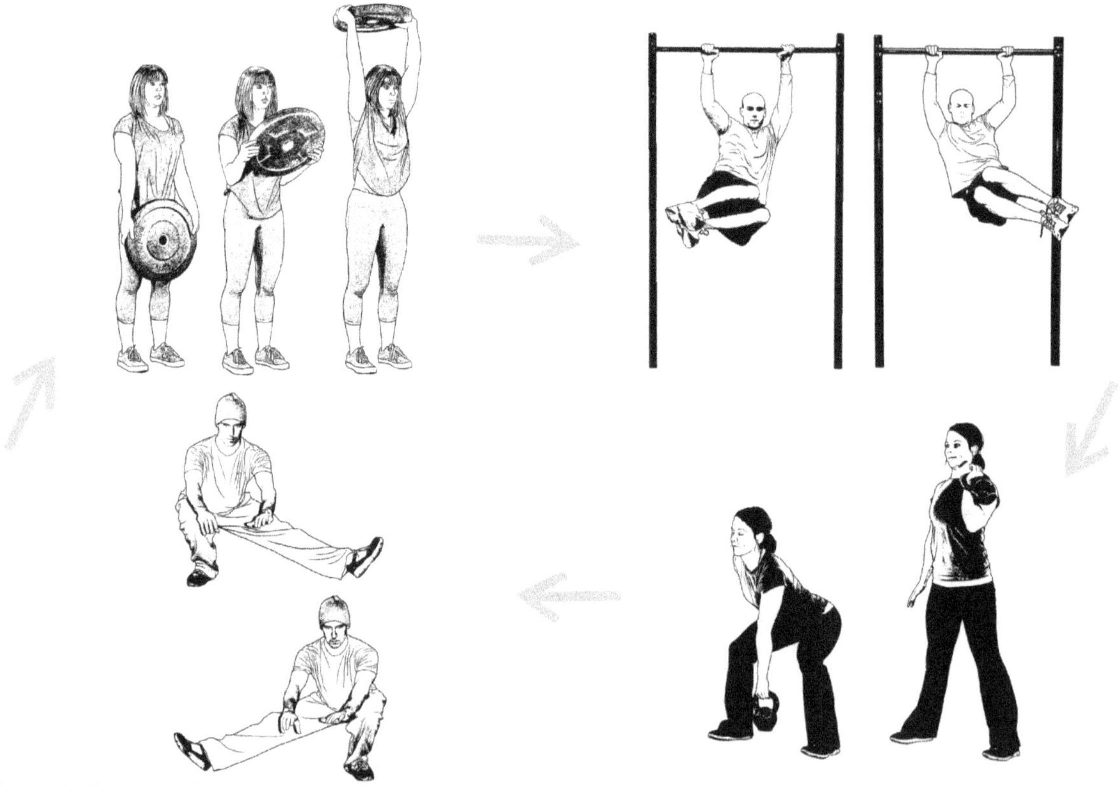

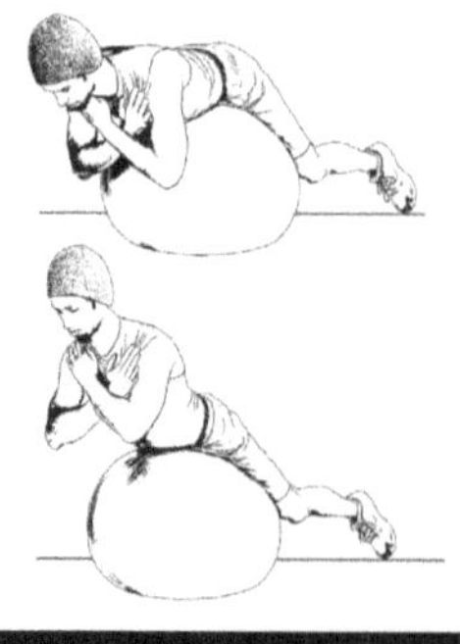

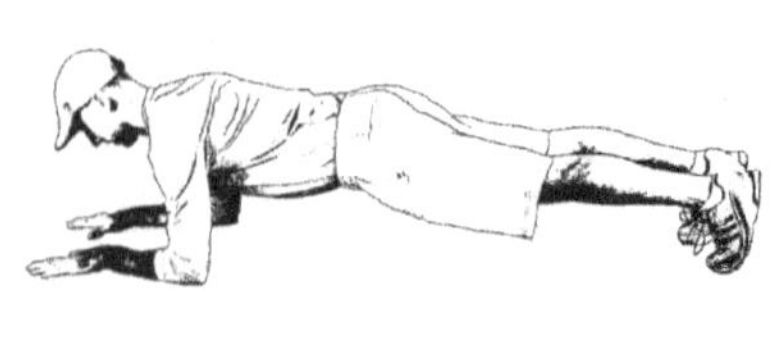

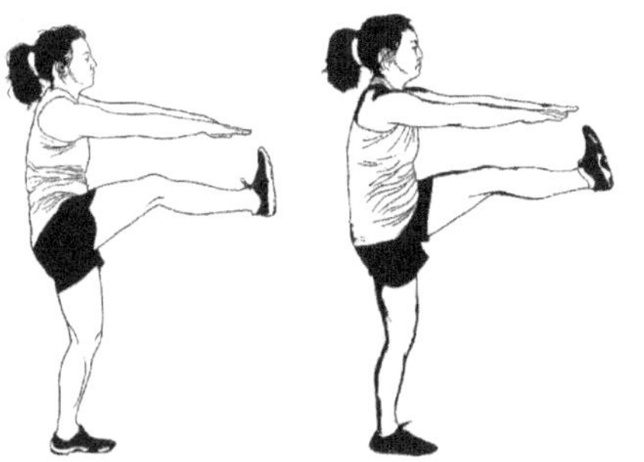

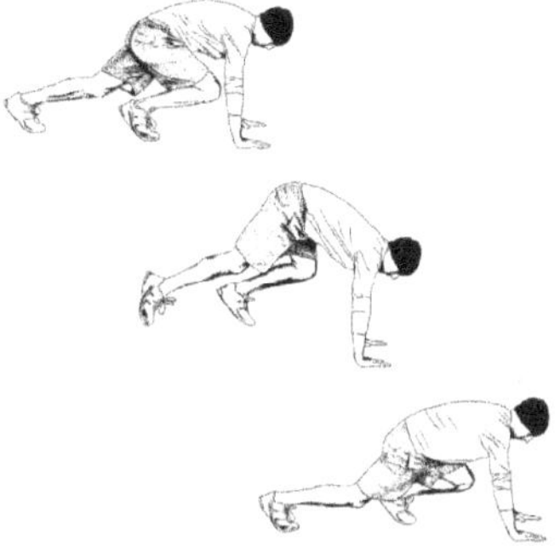

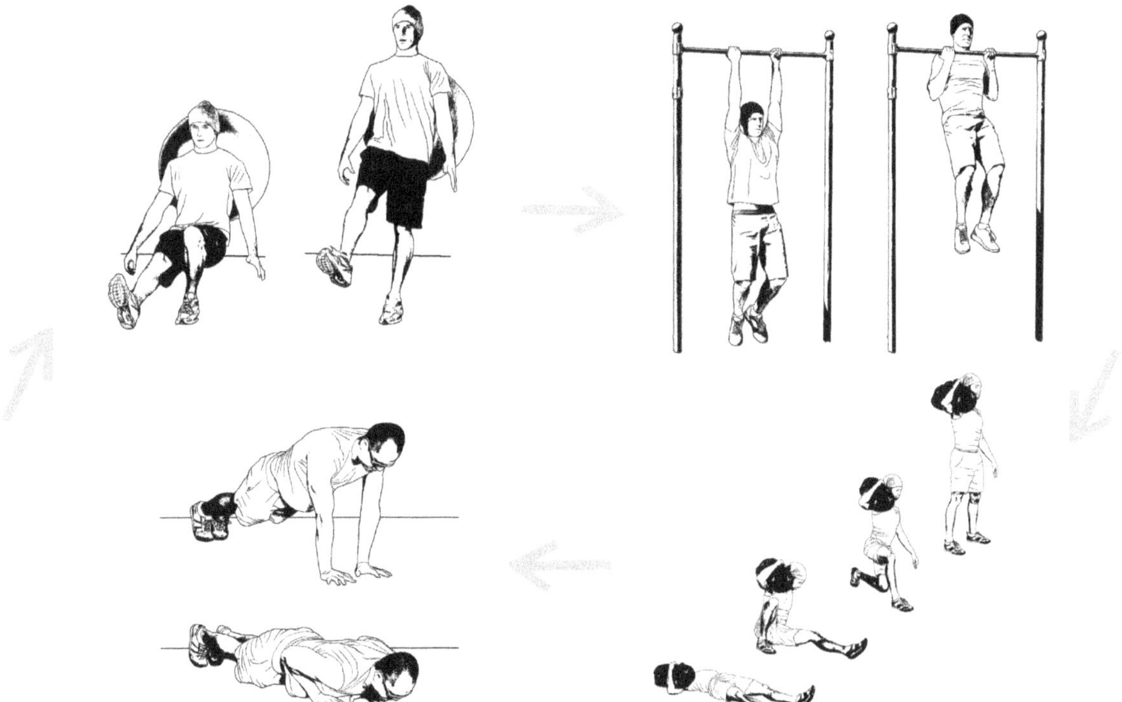

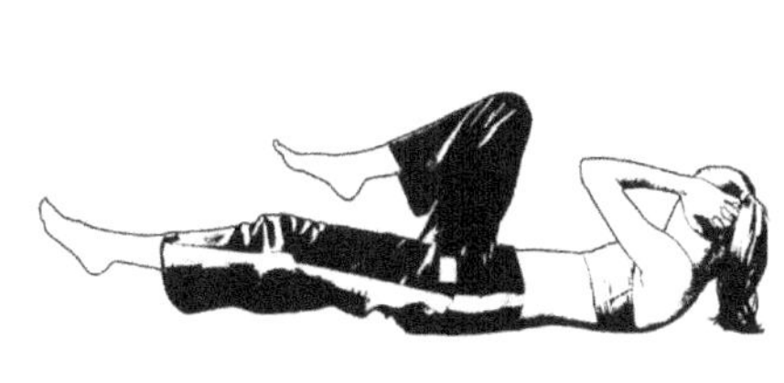

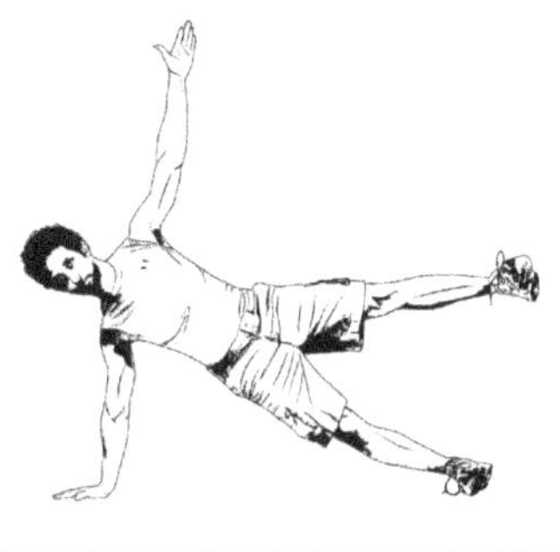

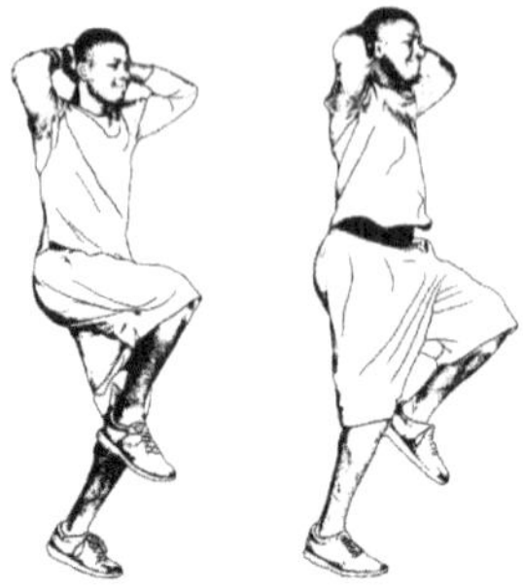

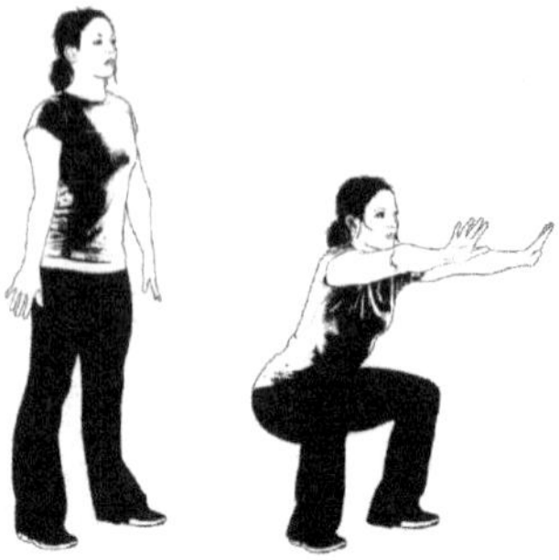

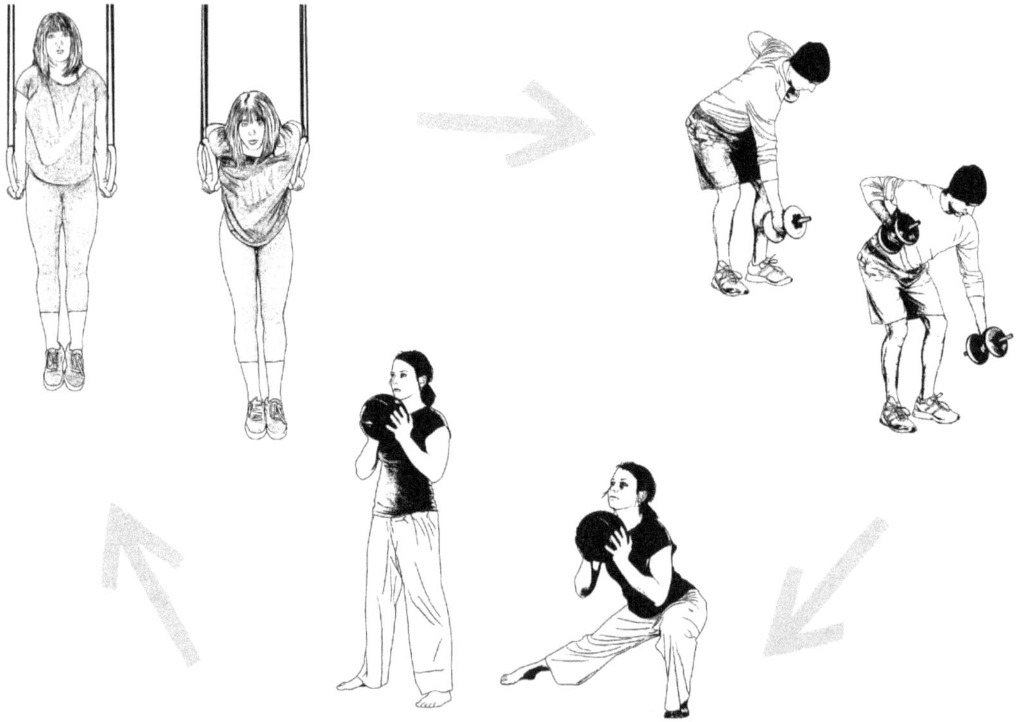

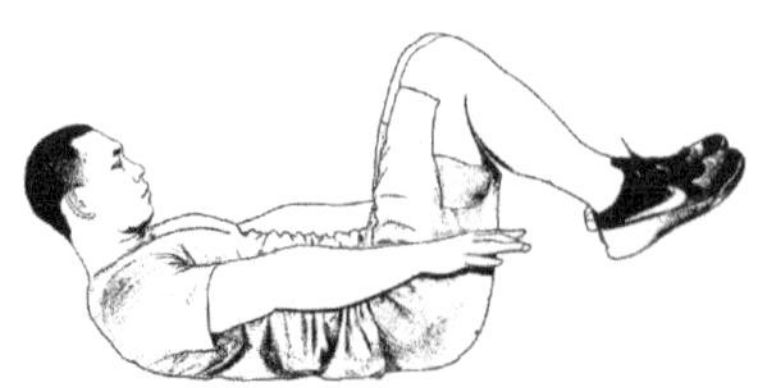

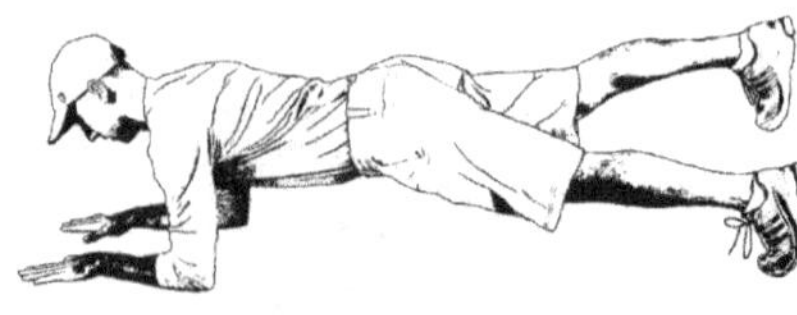

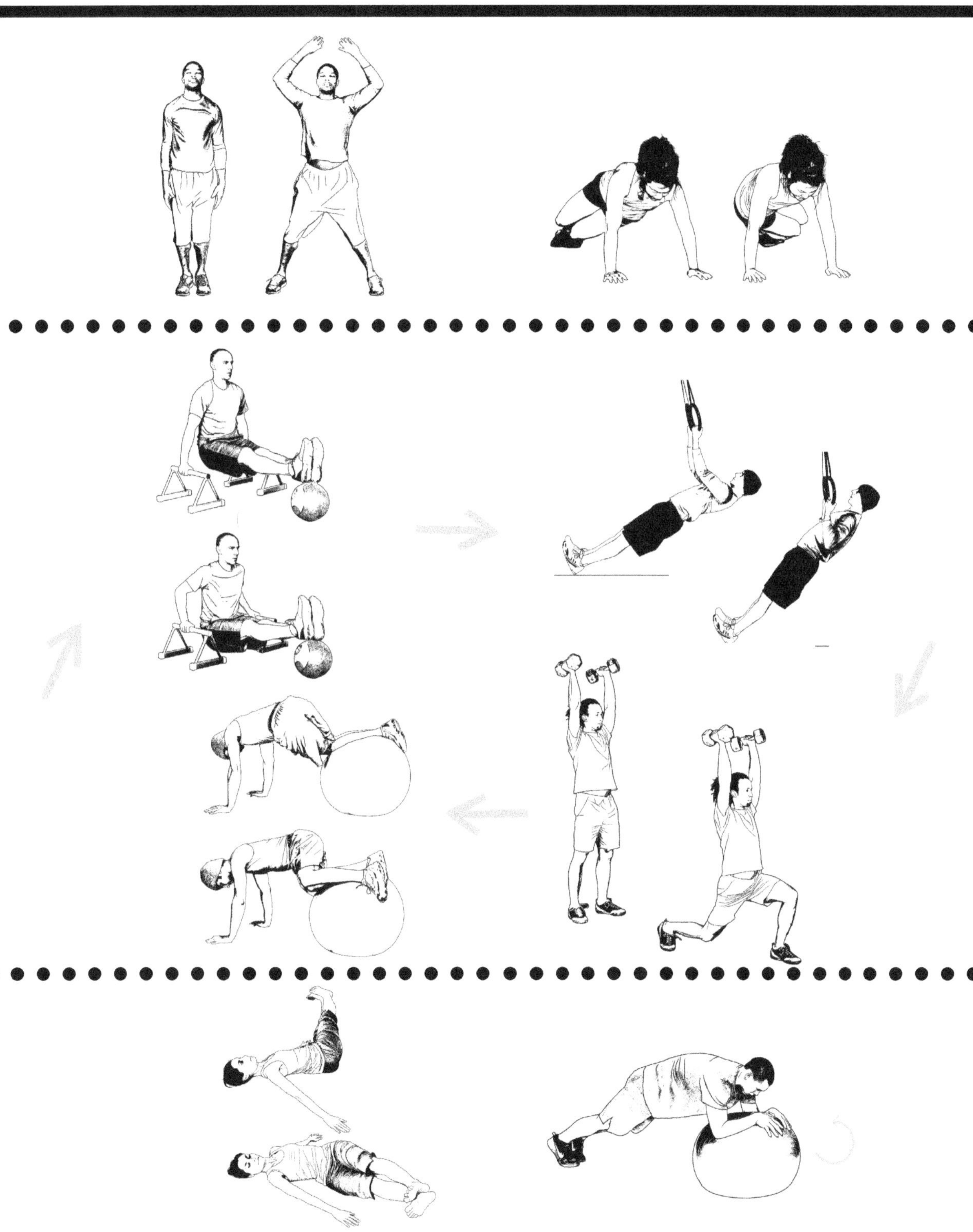

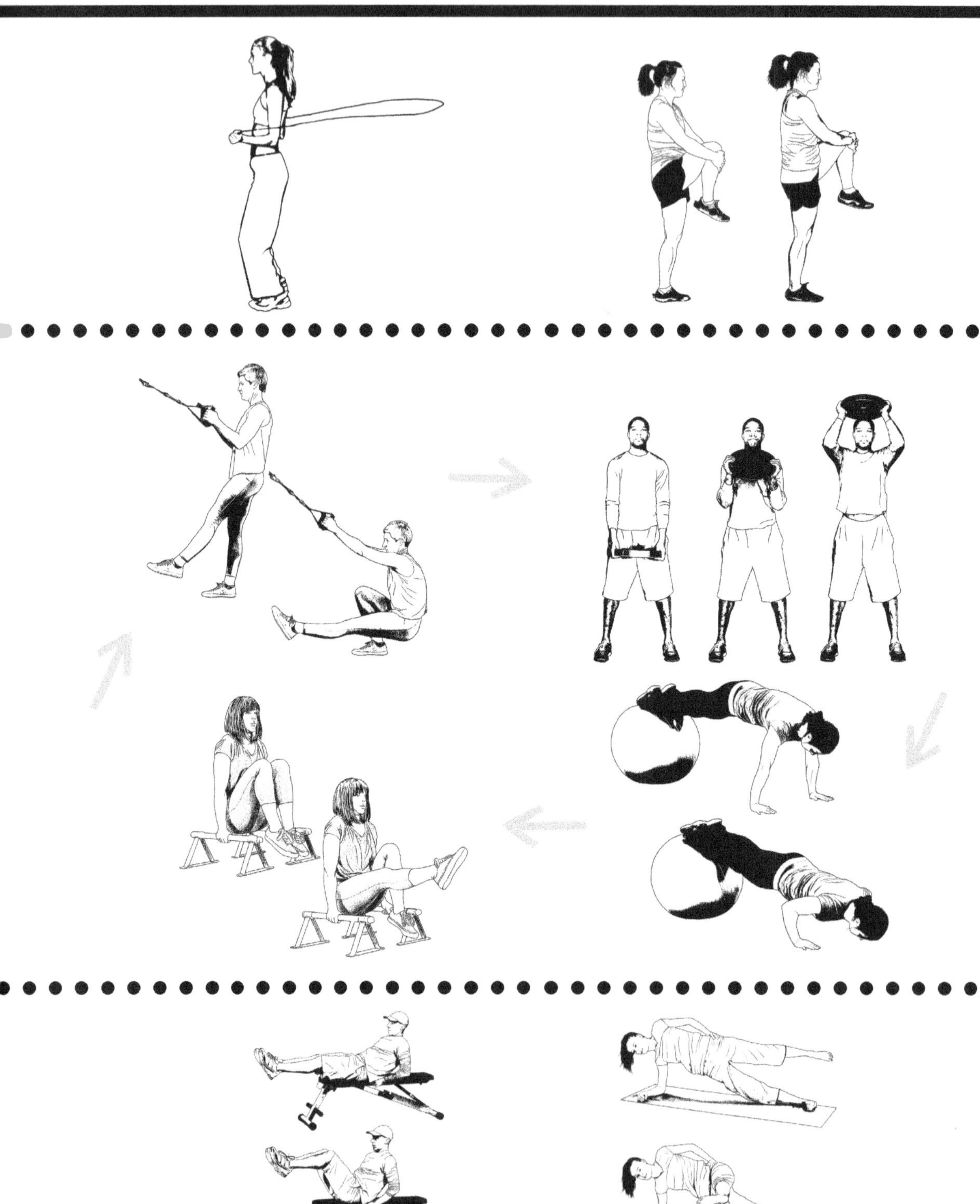

SIDE B

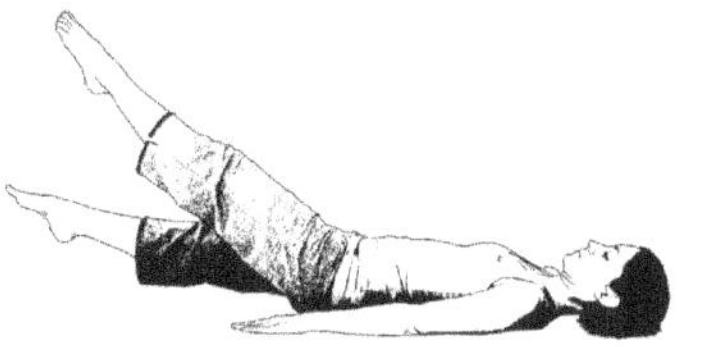

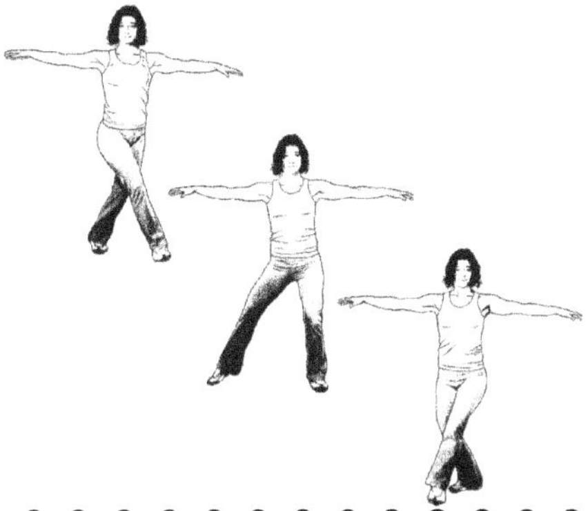

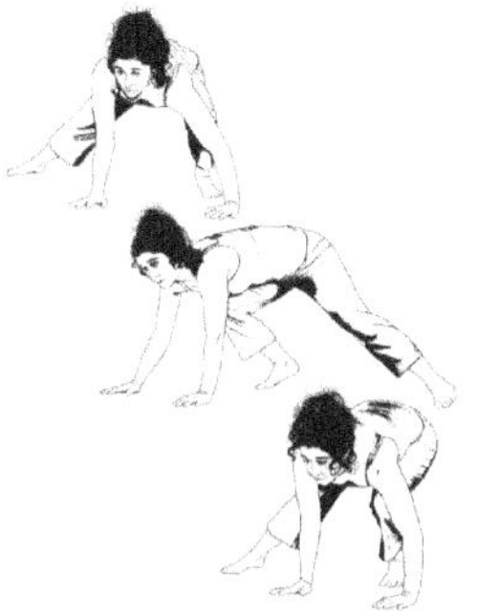

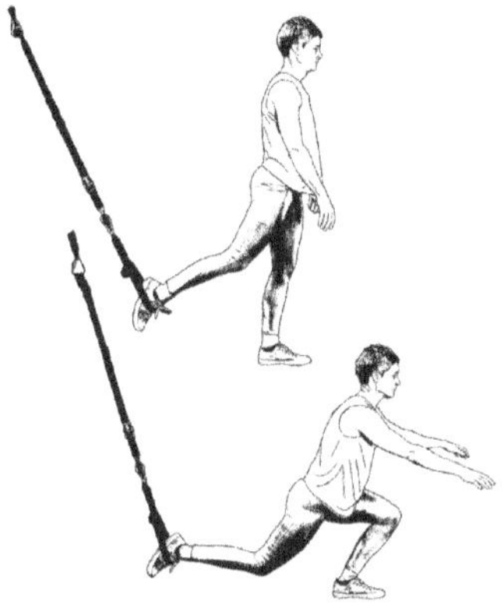

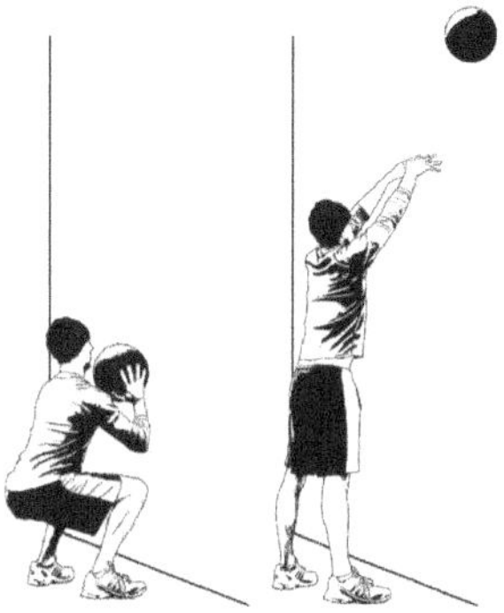

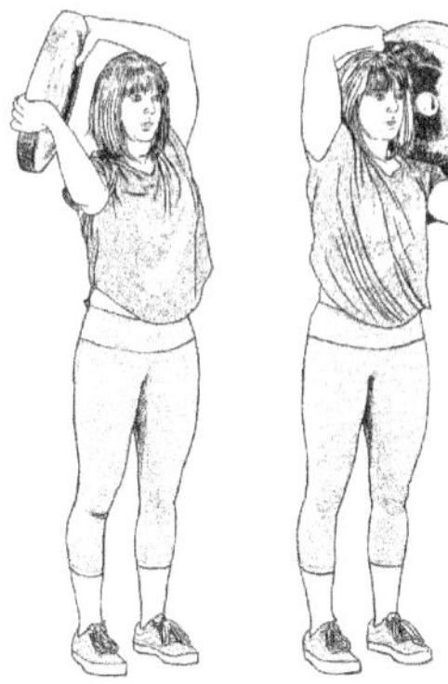

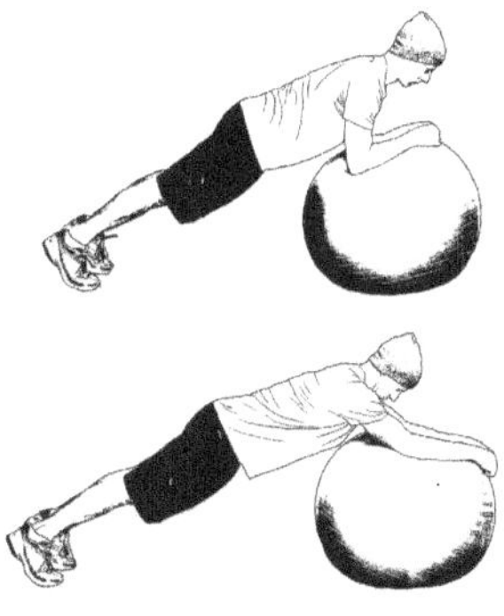

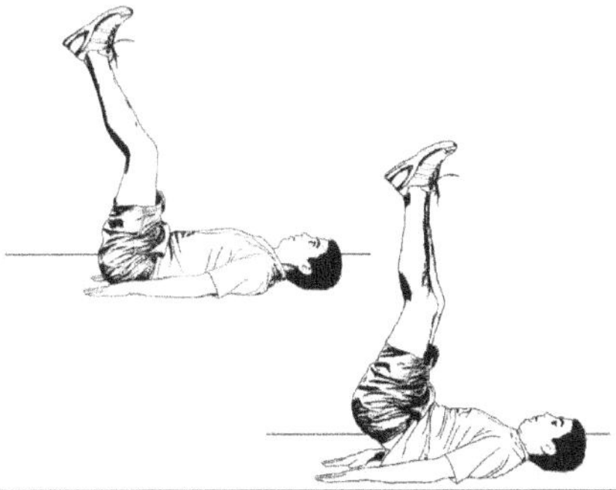

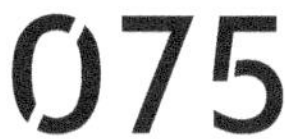

SIDE B

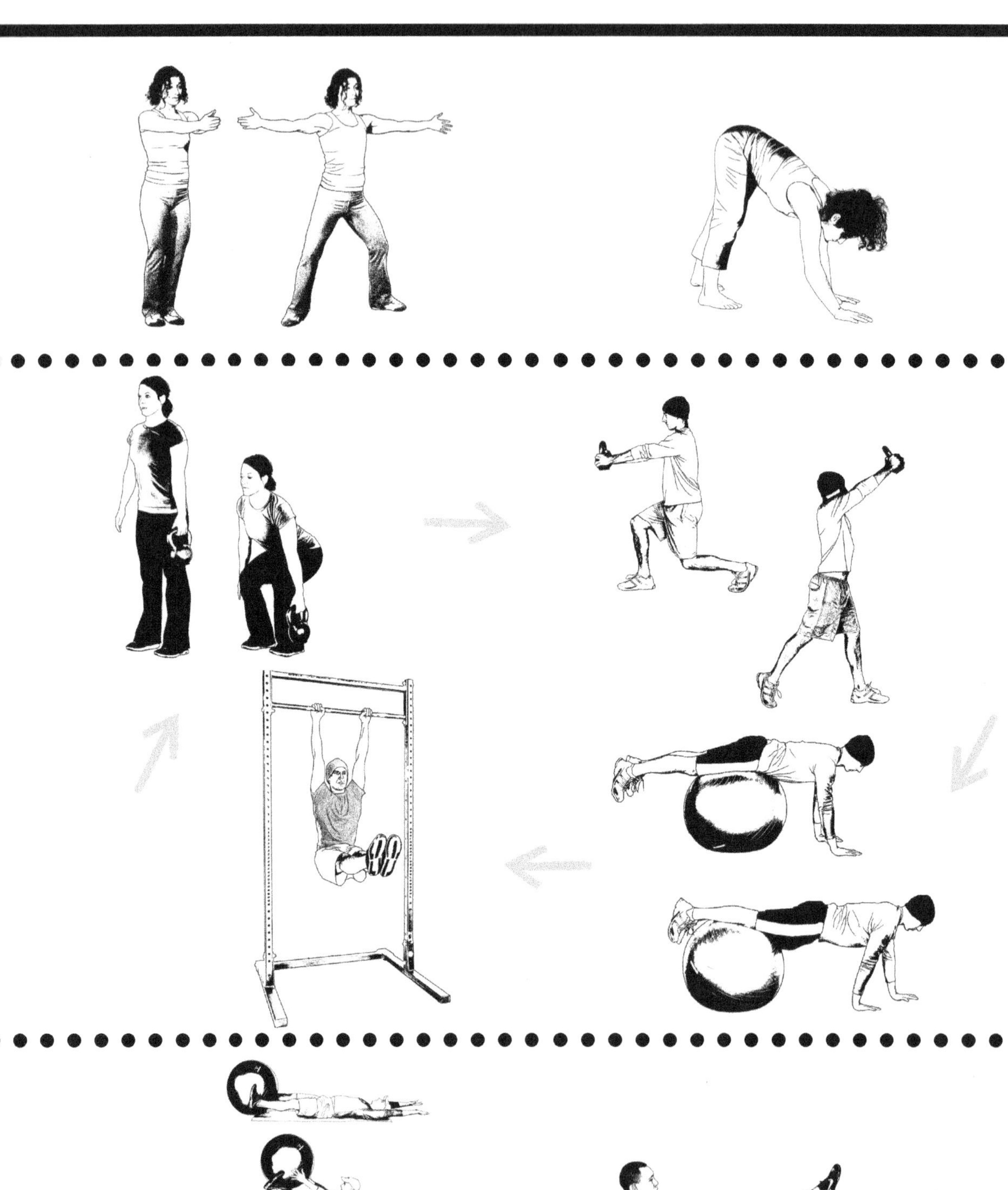

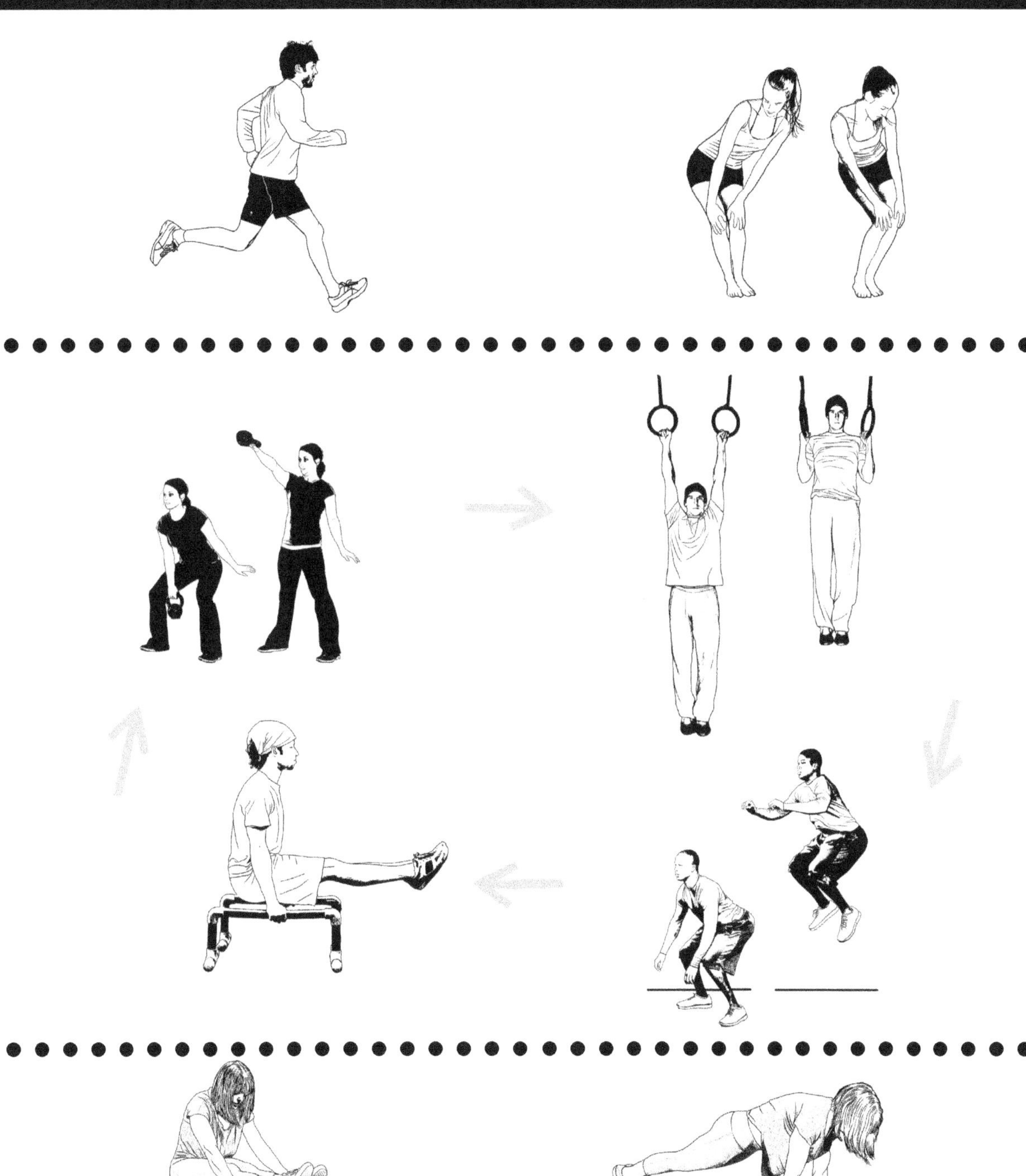

SIDE B

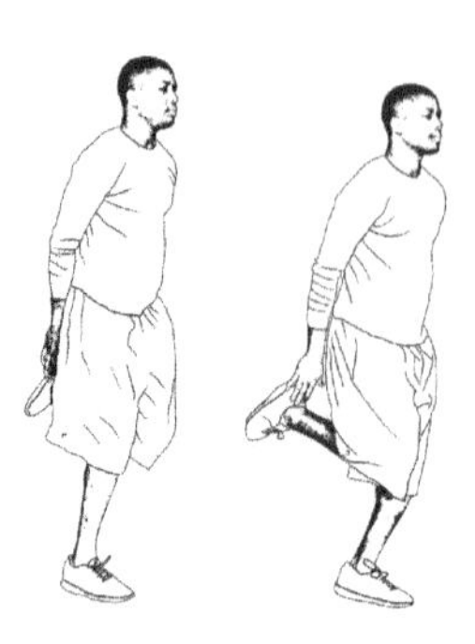

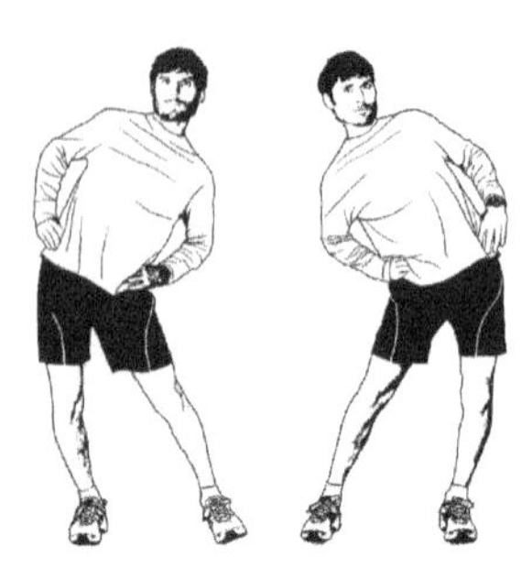

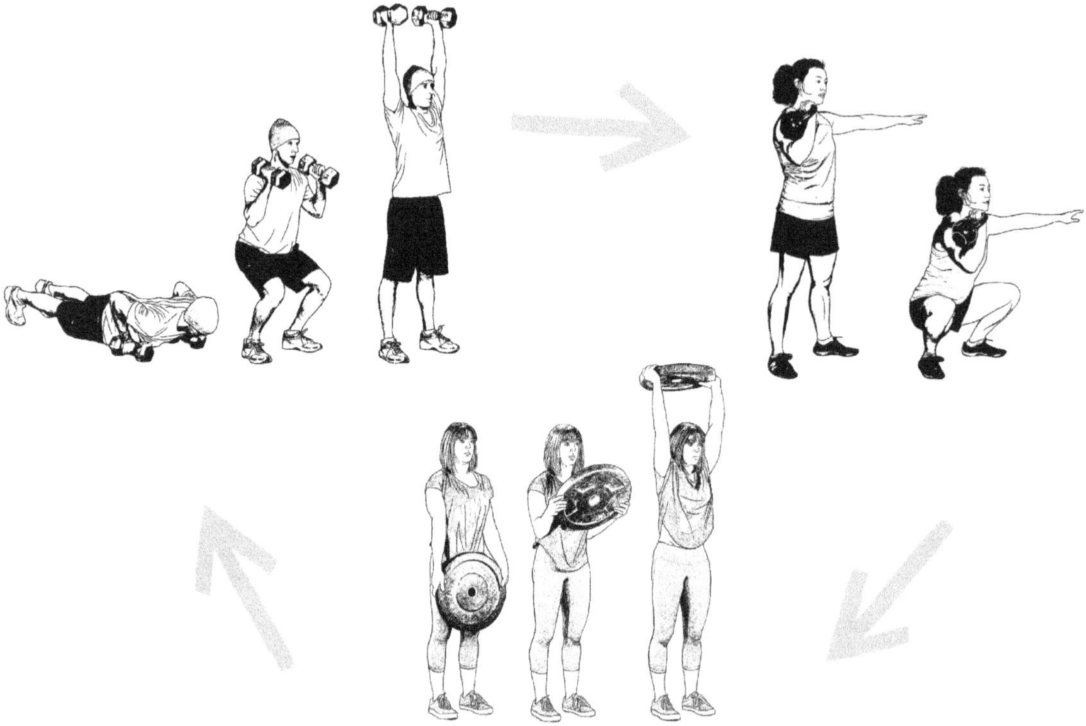

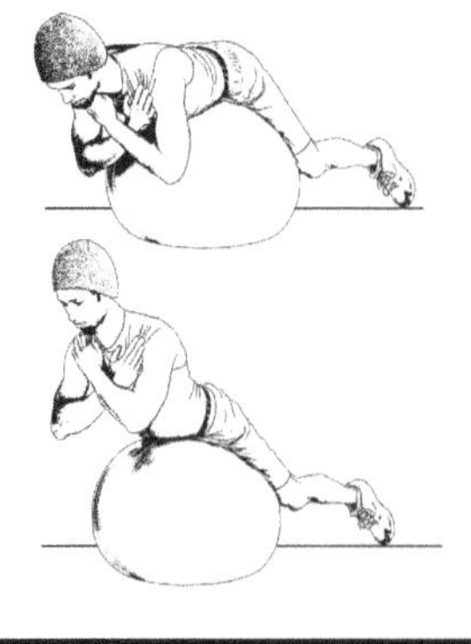

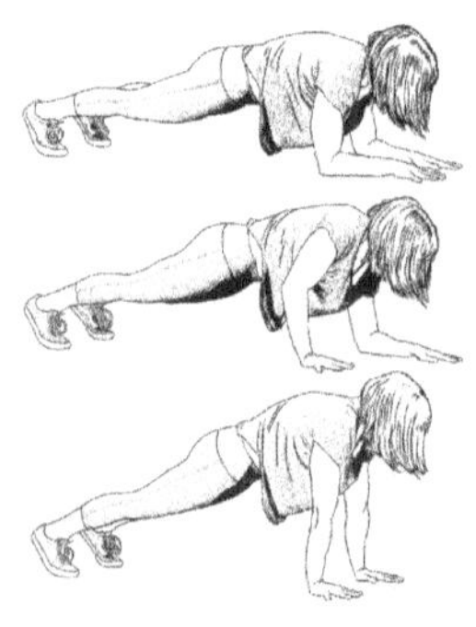

SIDE B

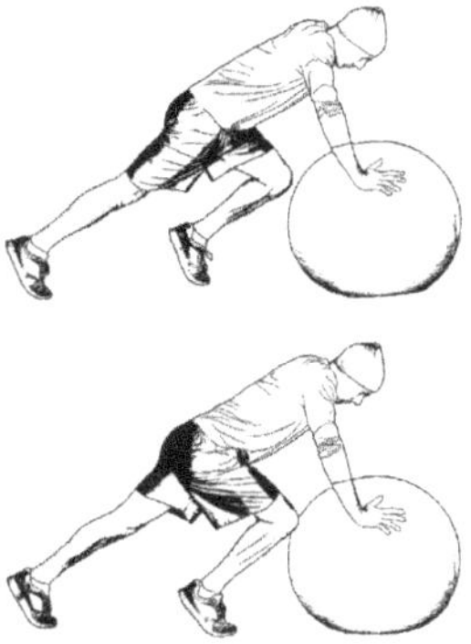

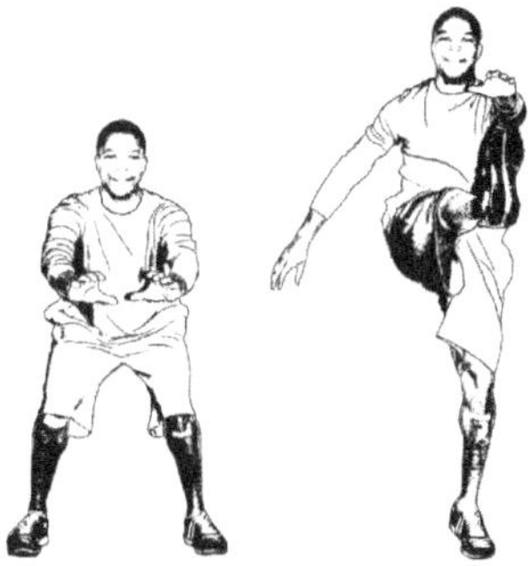

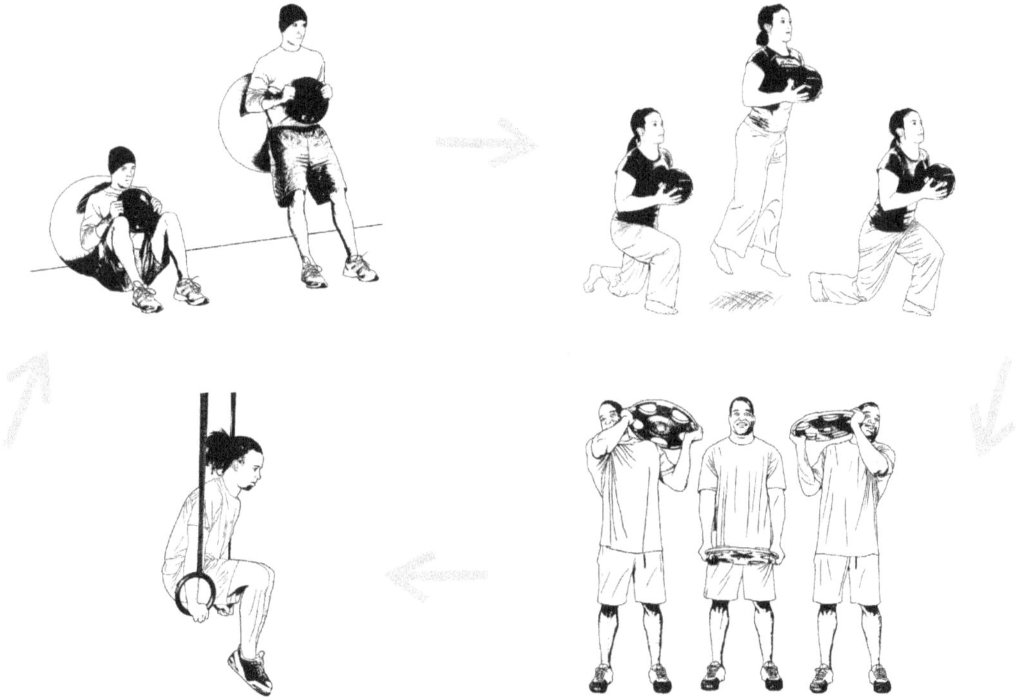

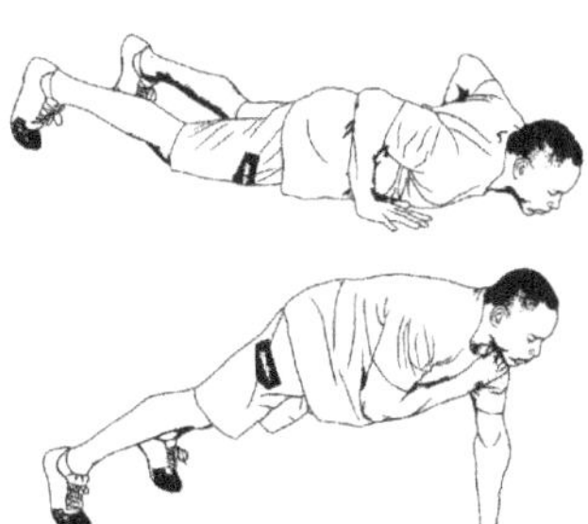

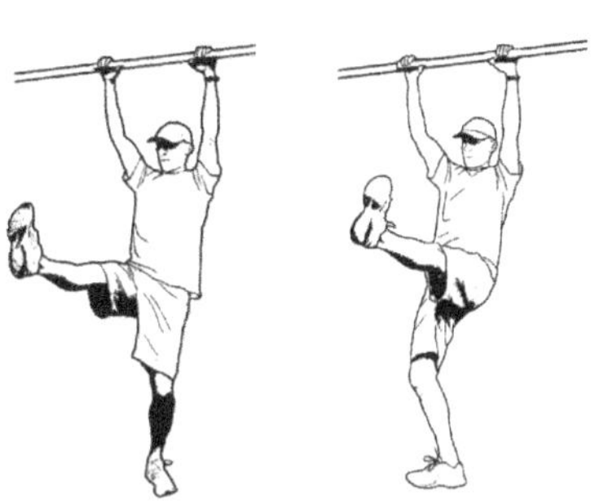

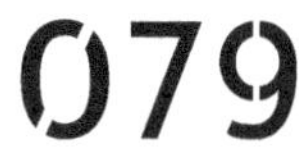

Side B

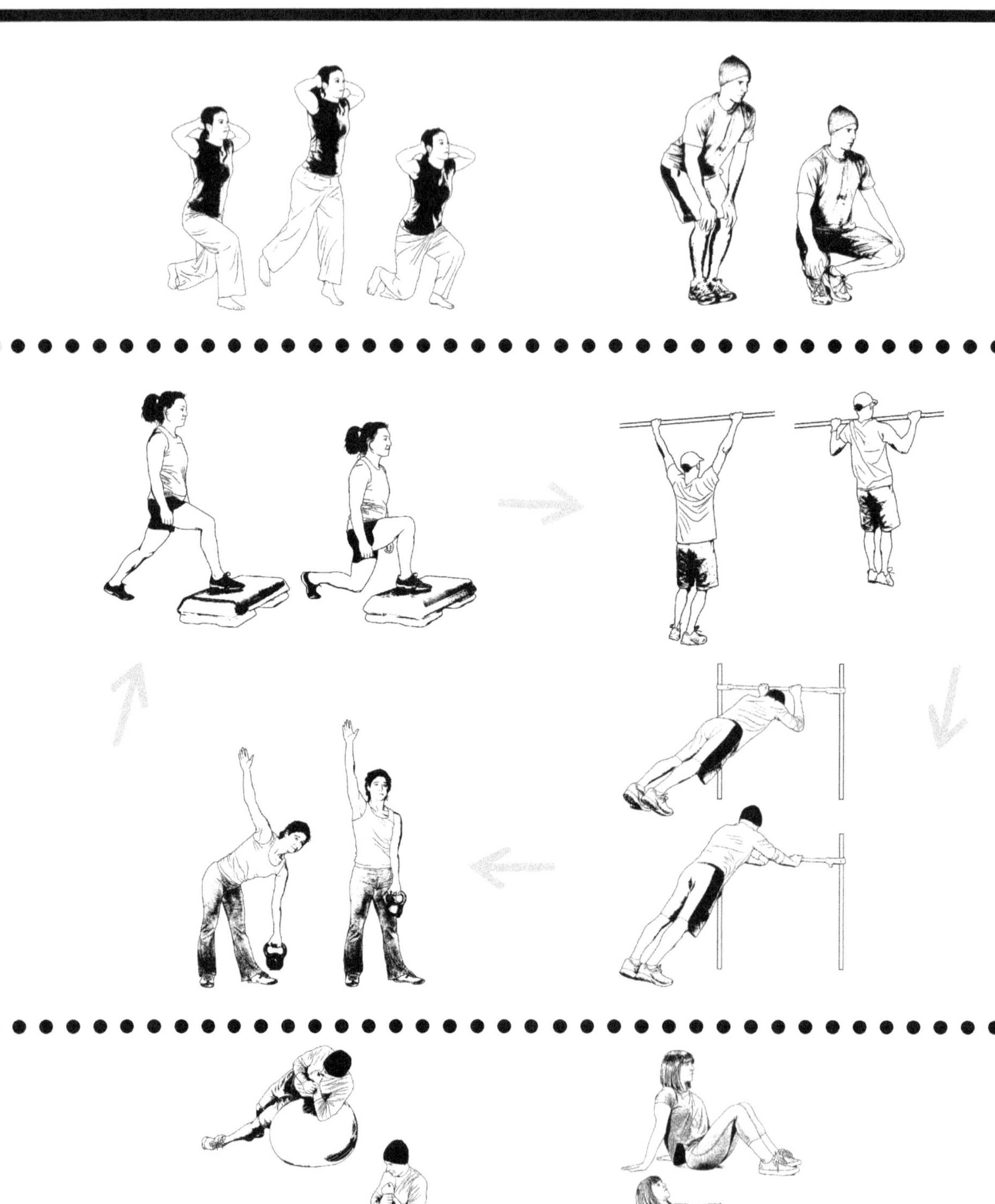

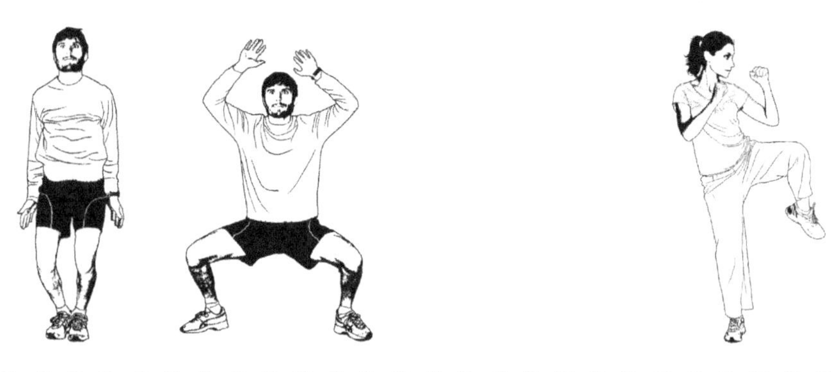

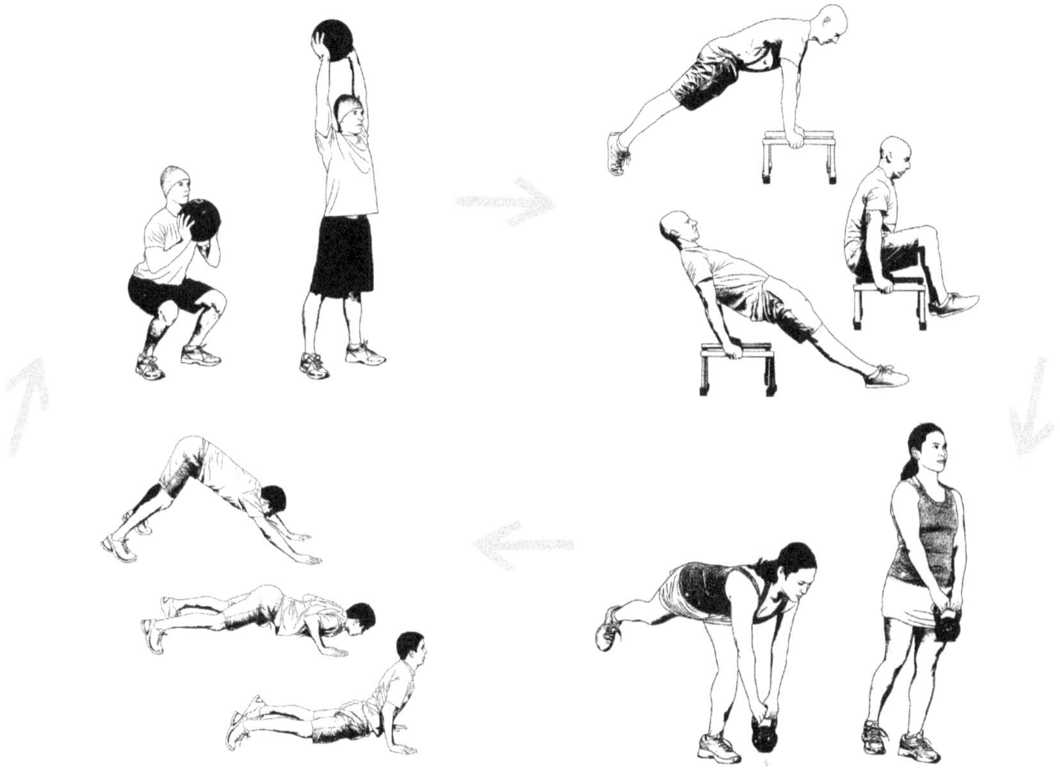

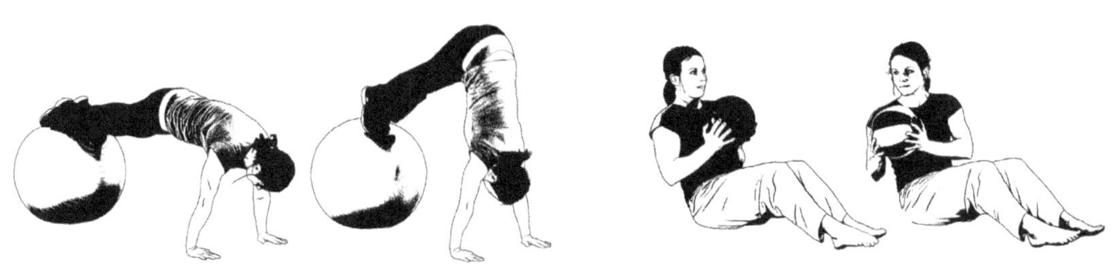

SIDE B

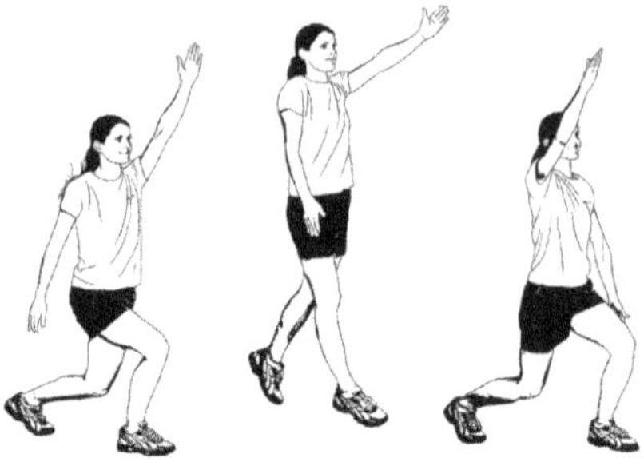

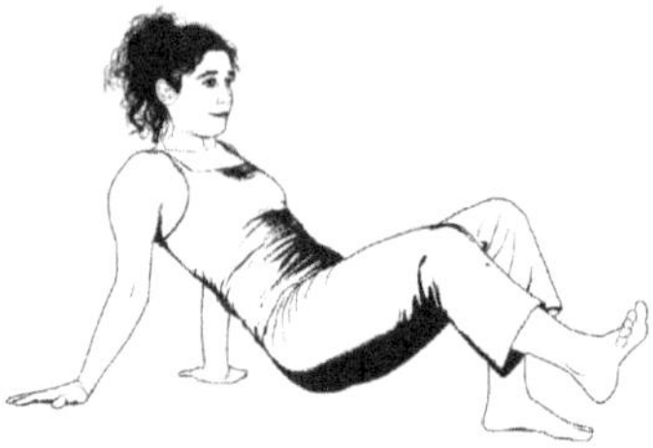

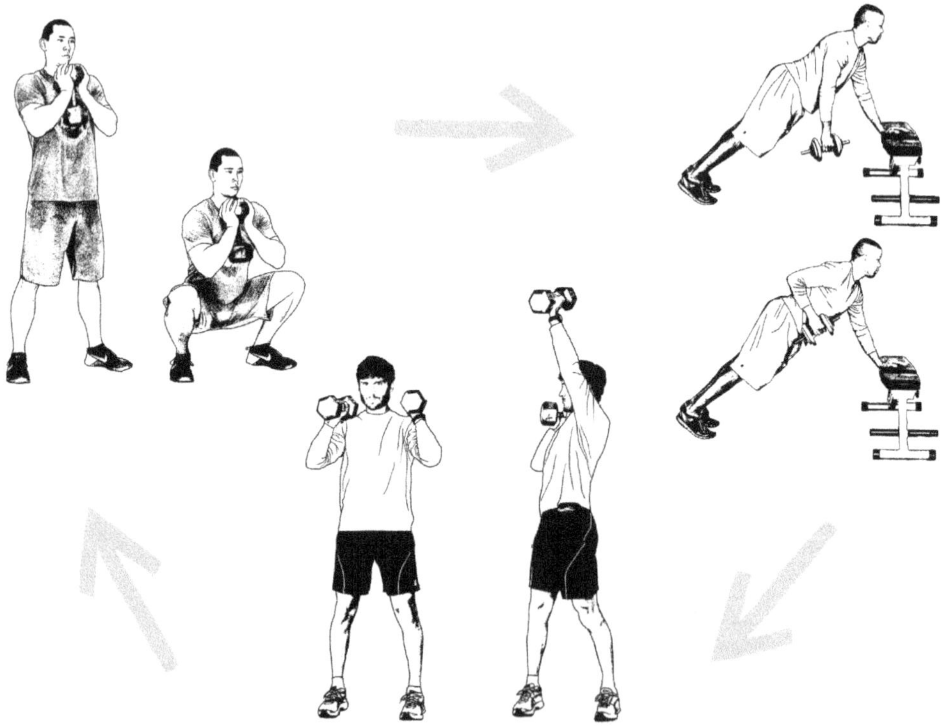

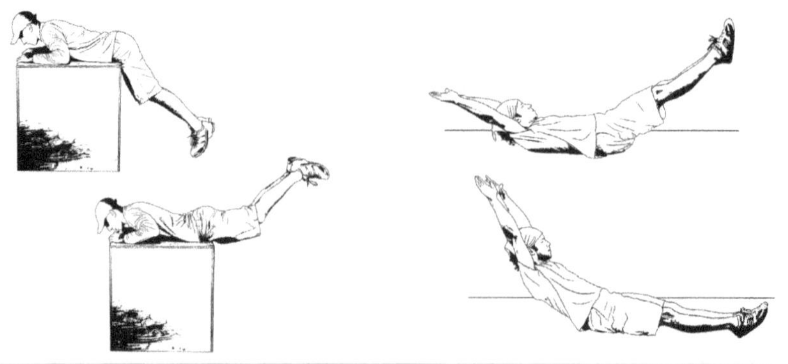

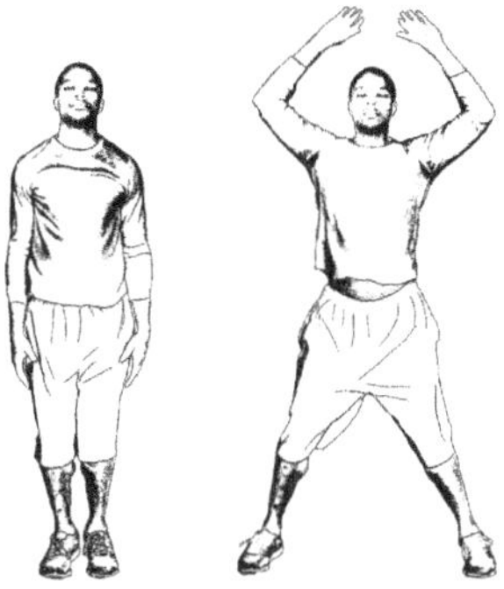

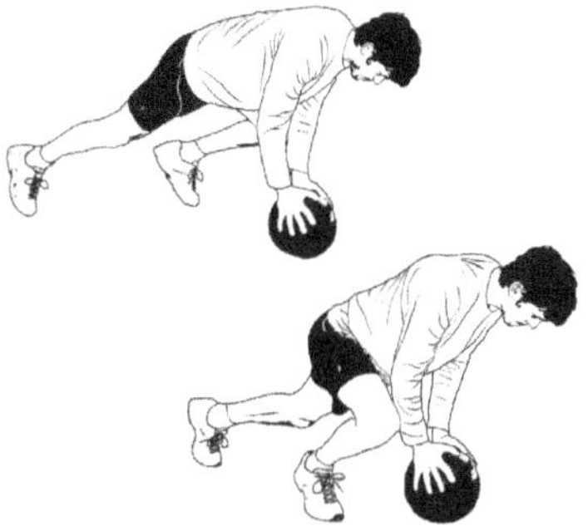

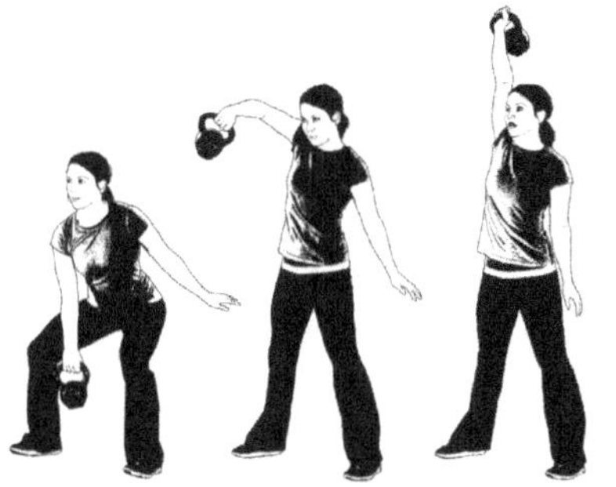

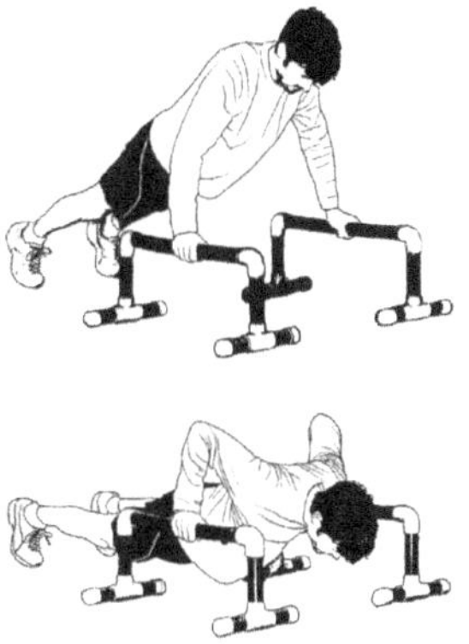

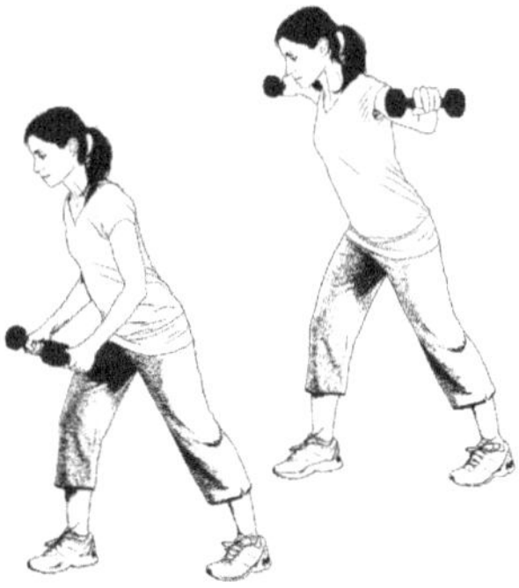

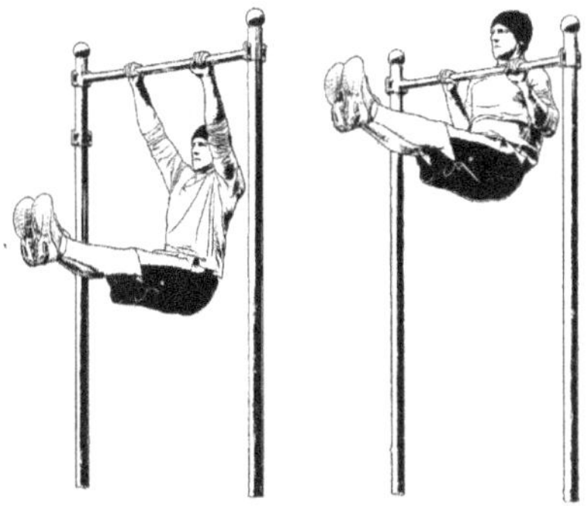

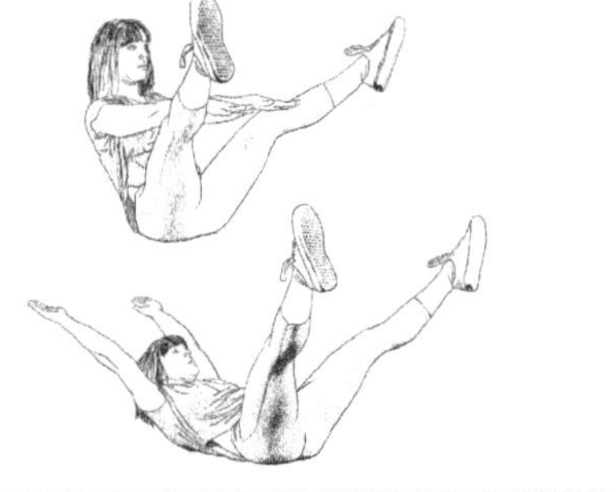

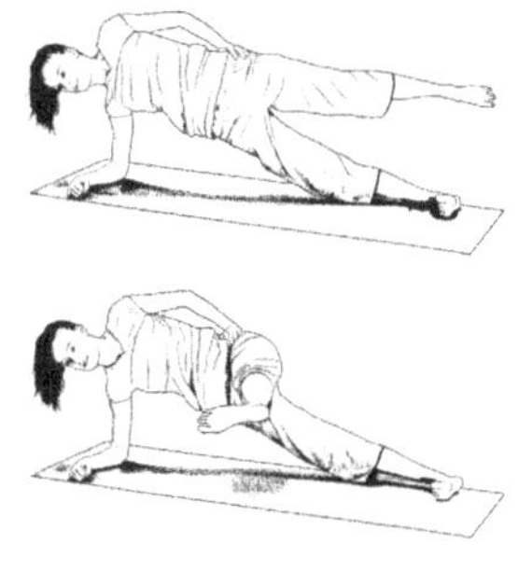

SIDE B

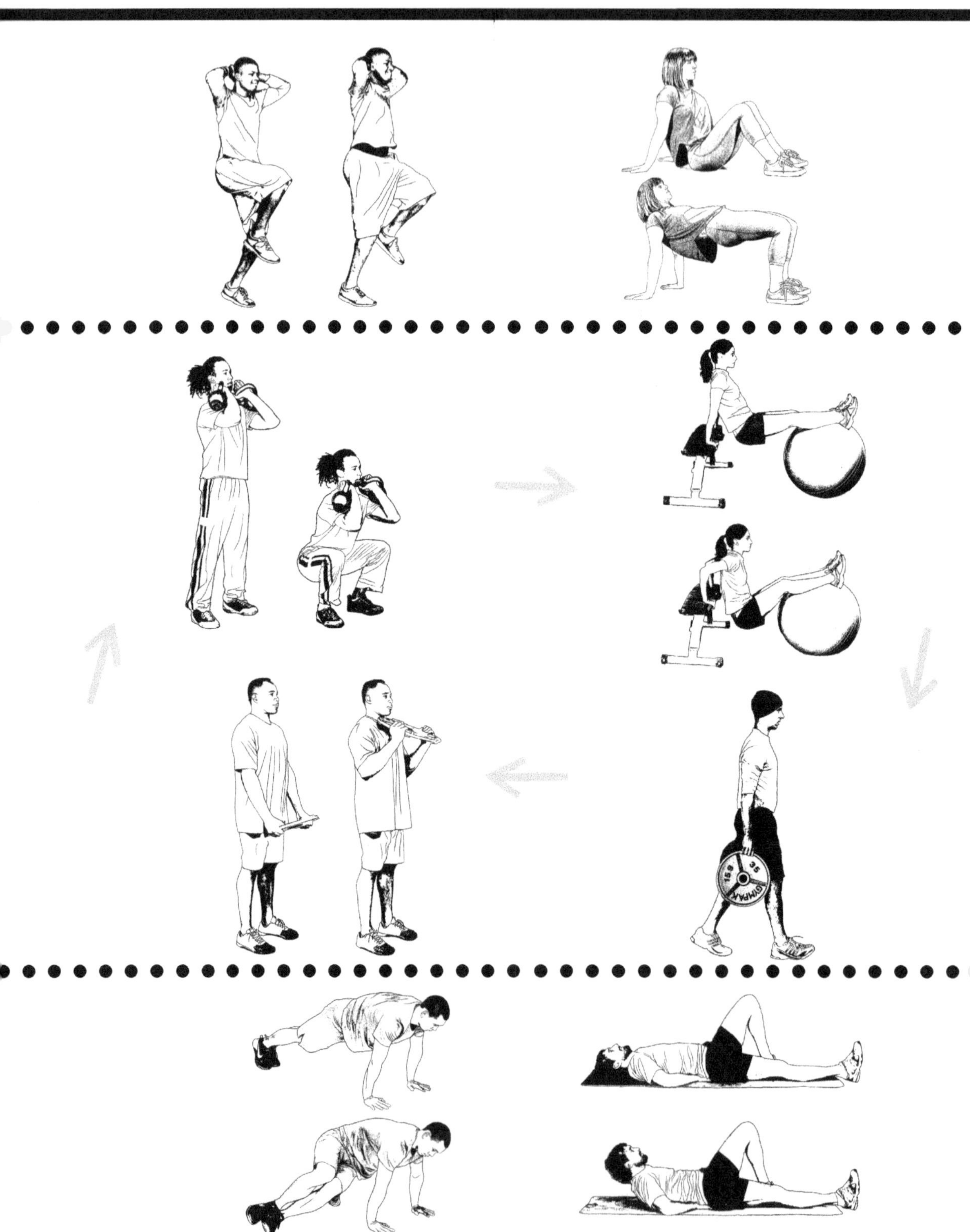

SIDE B

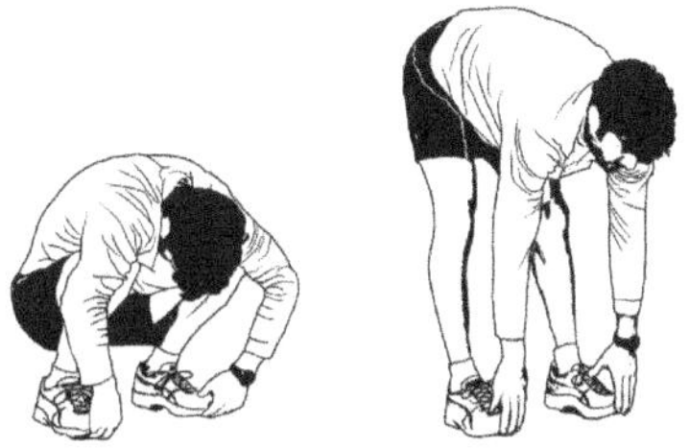

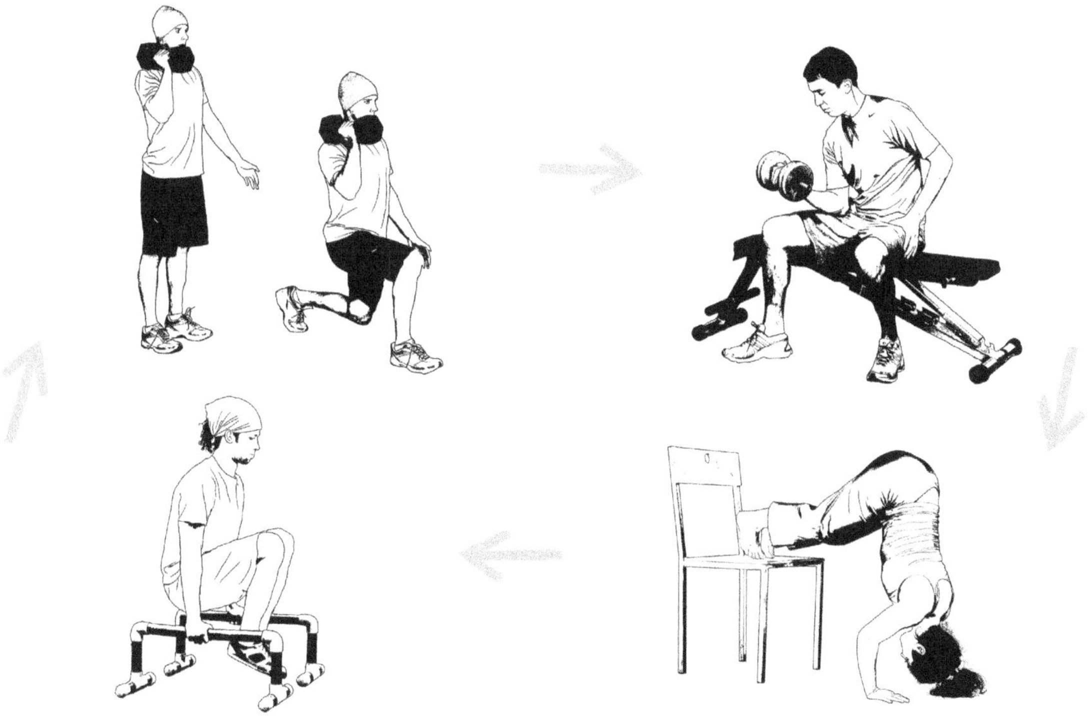

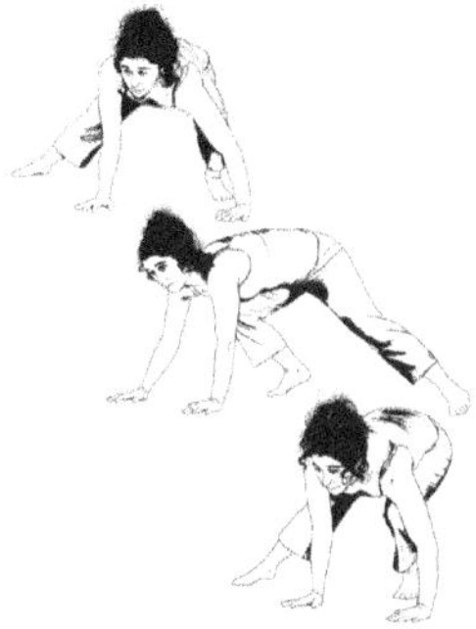

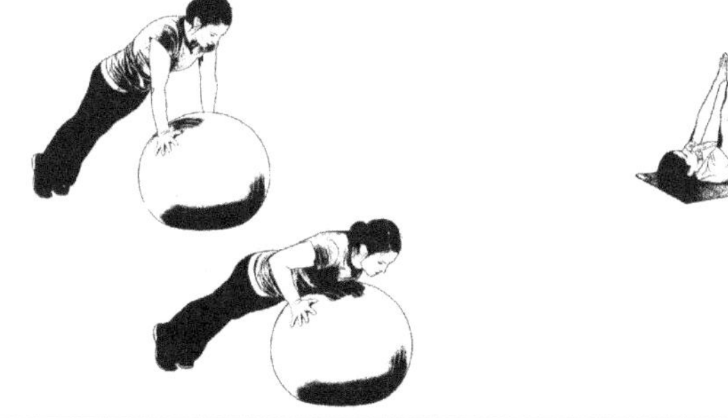

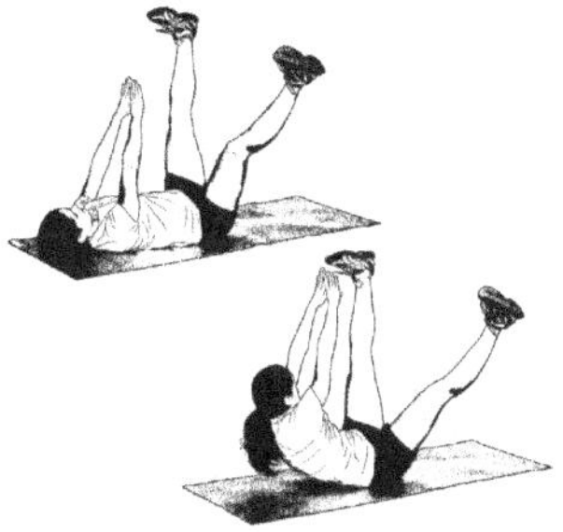

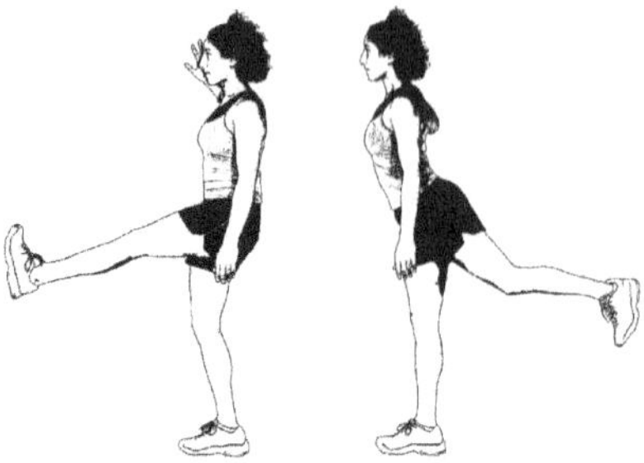

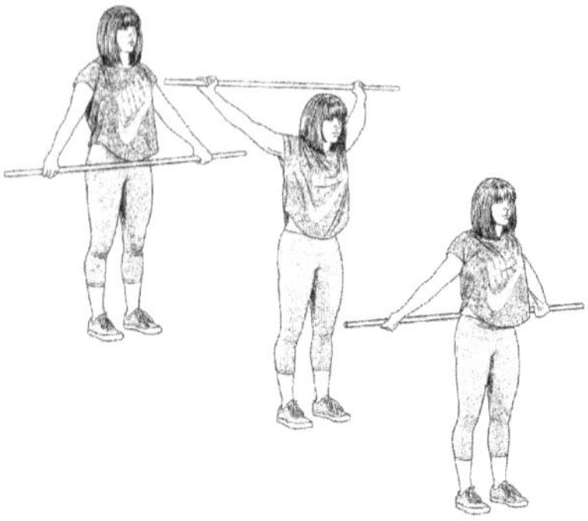

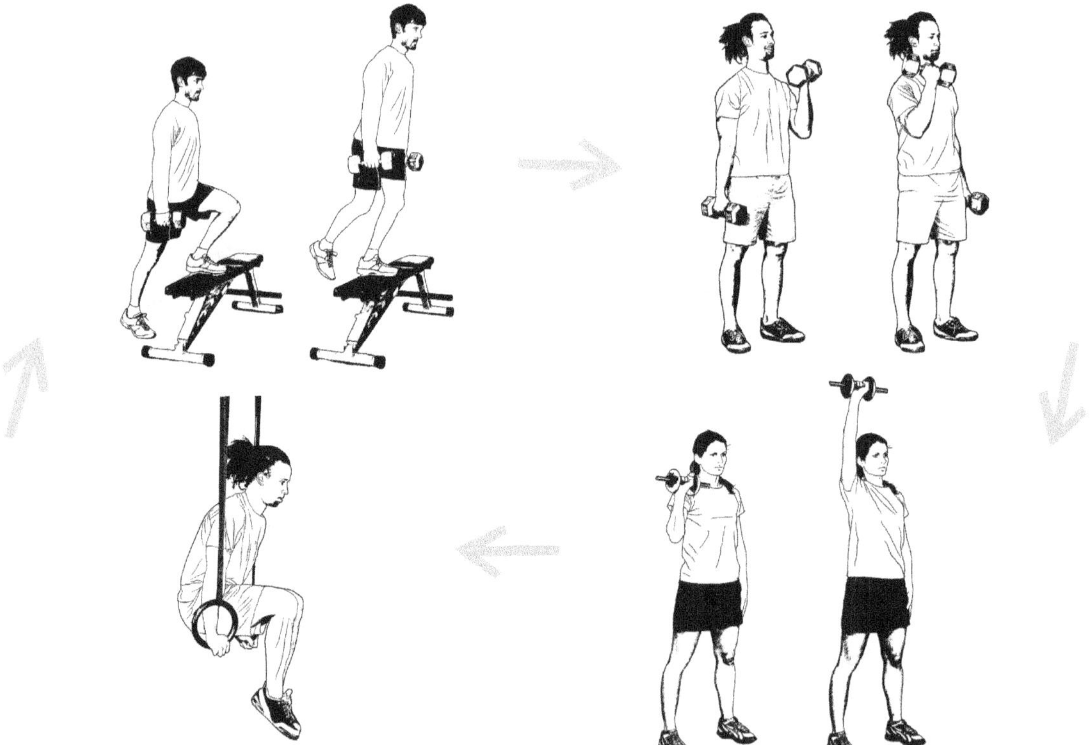

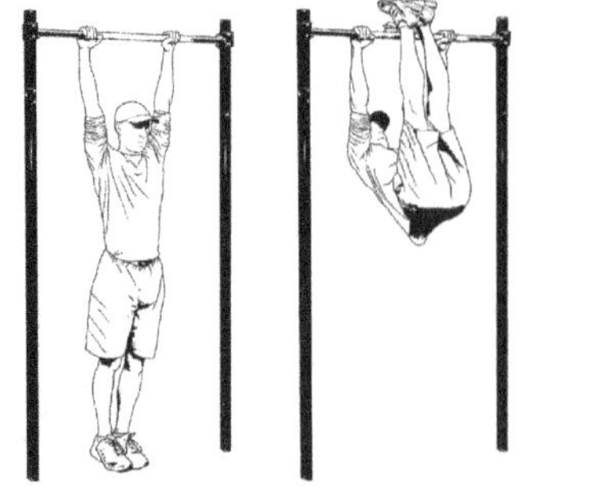

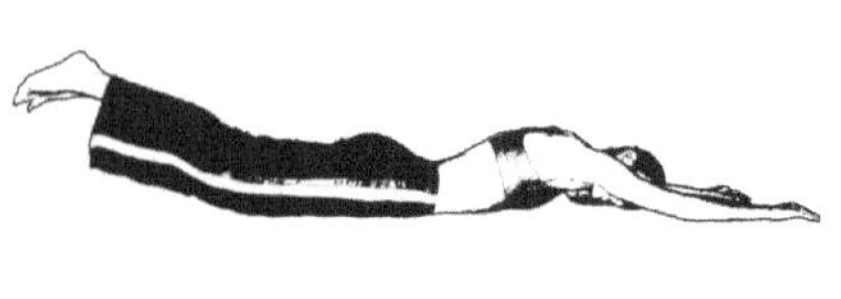

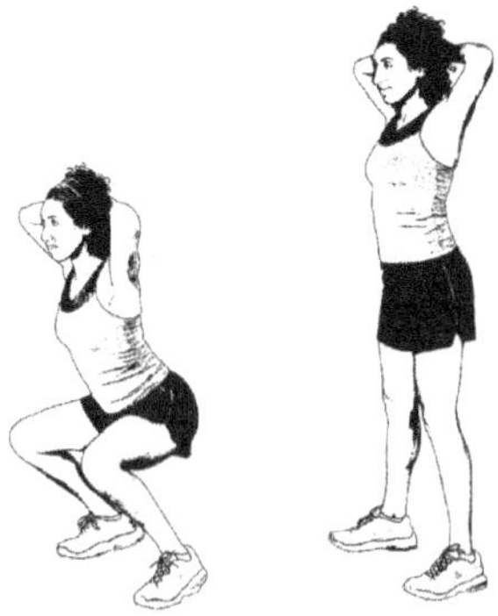

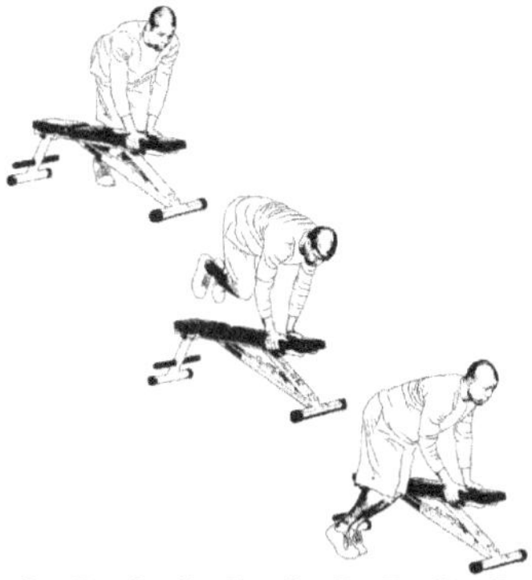

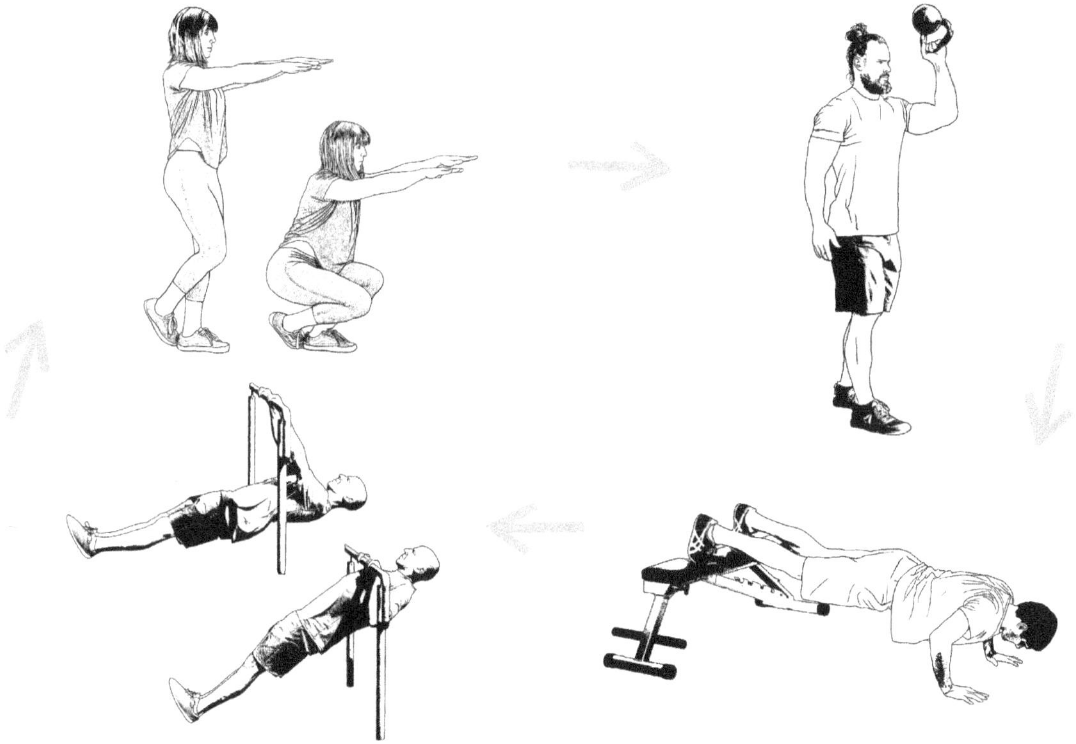

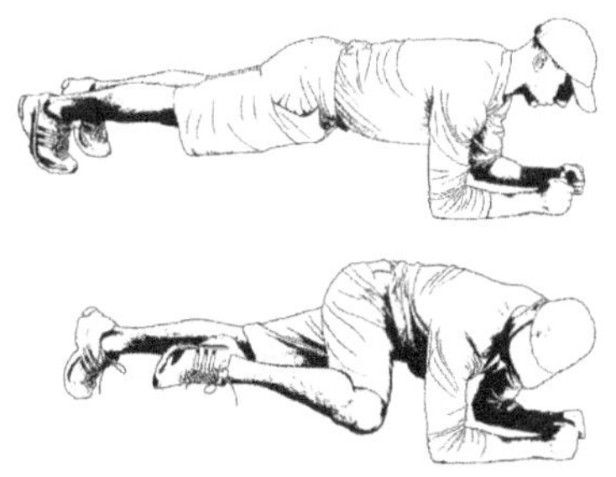
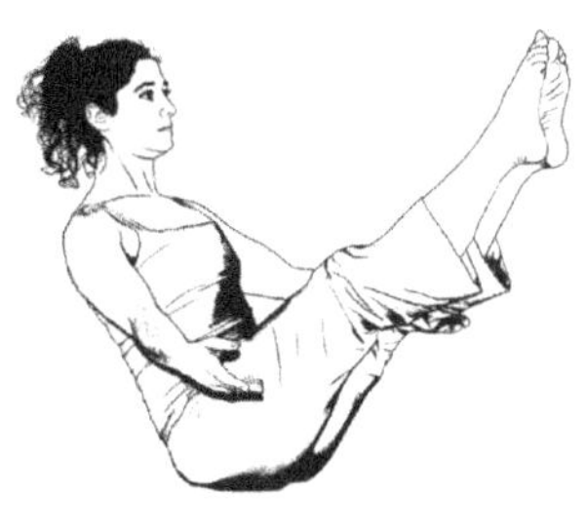

Side B

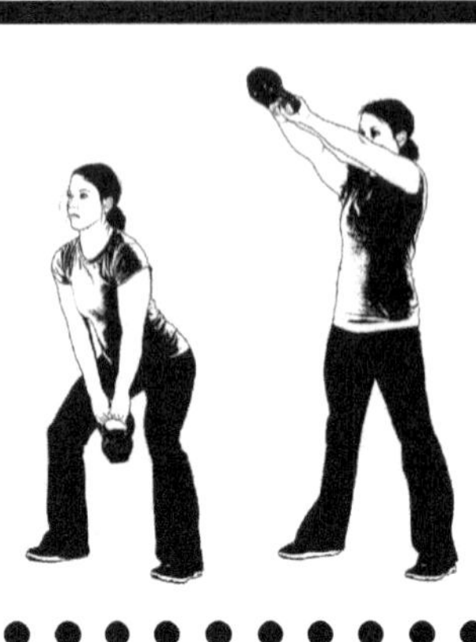

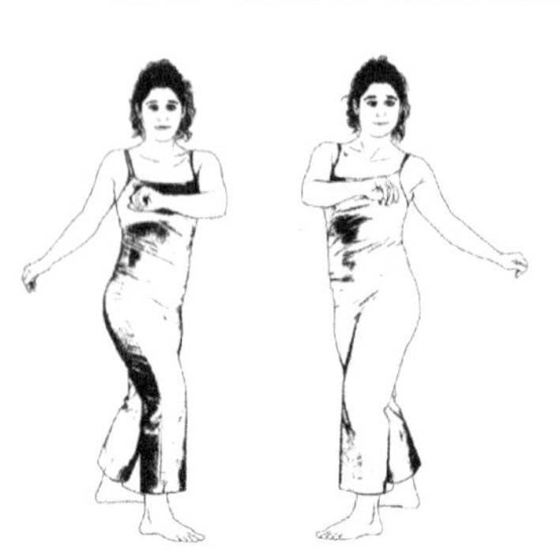

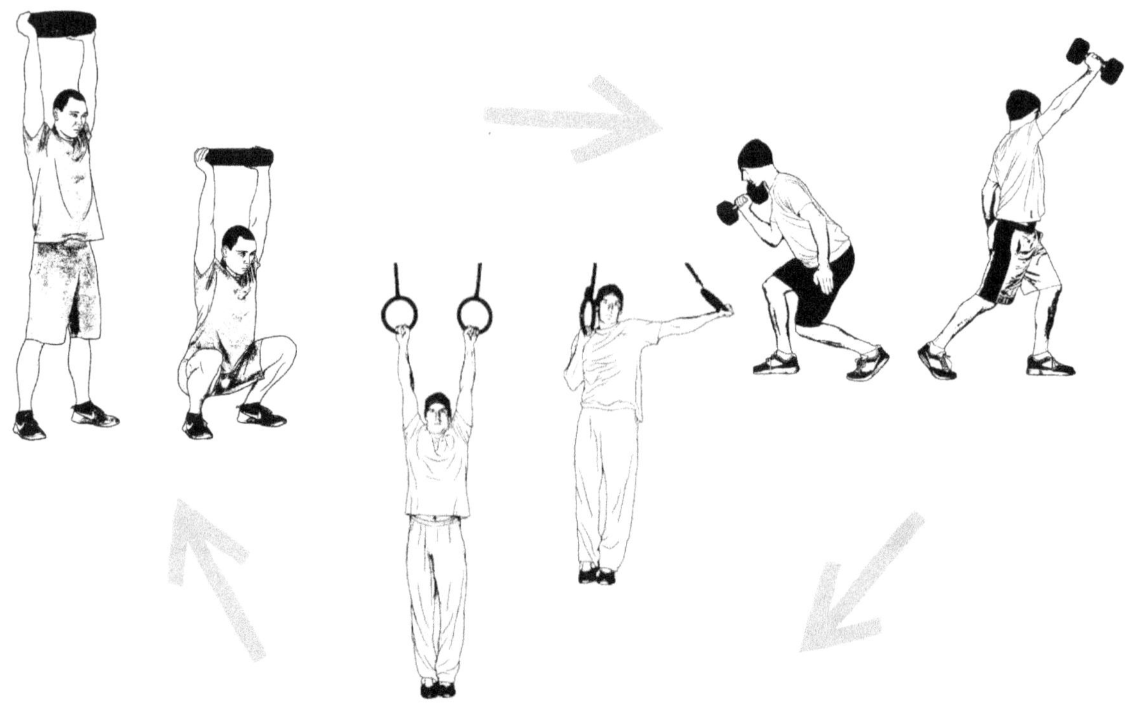

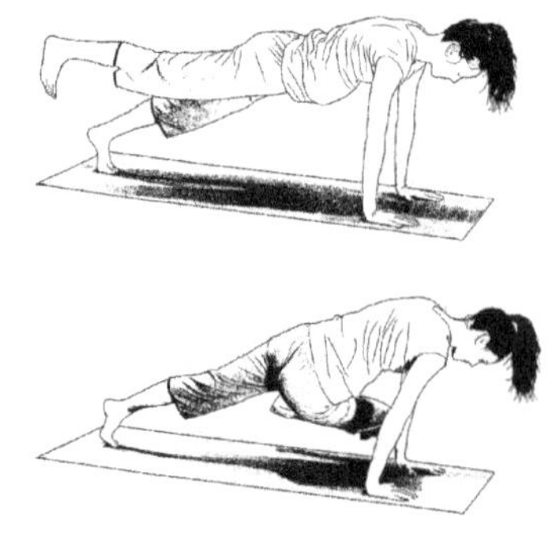

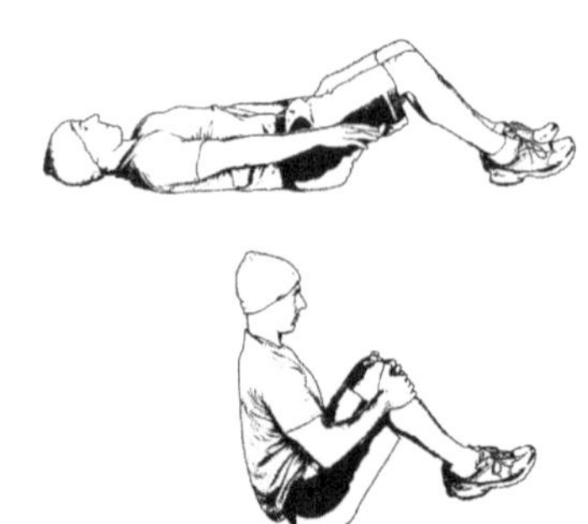

SIDE B

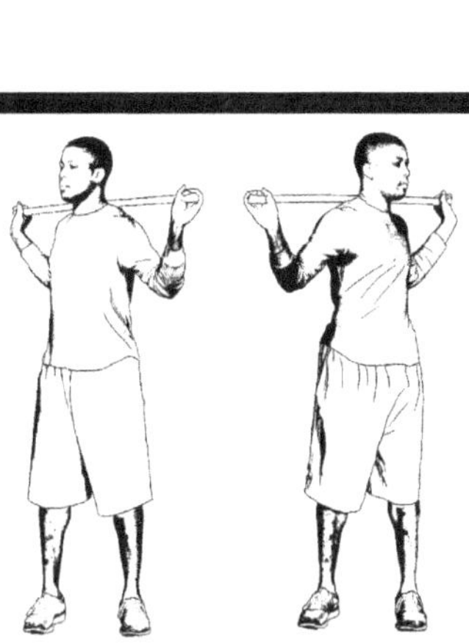

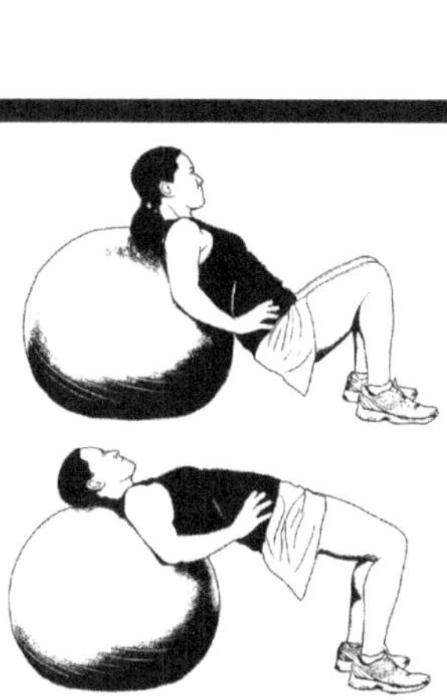

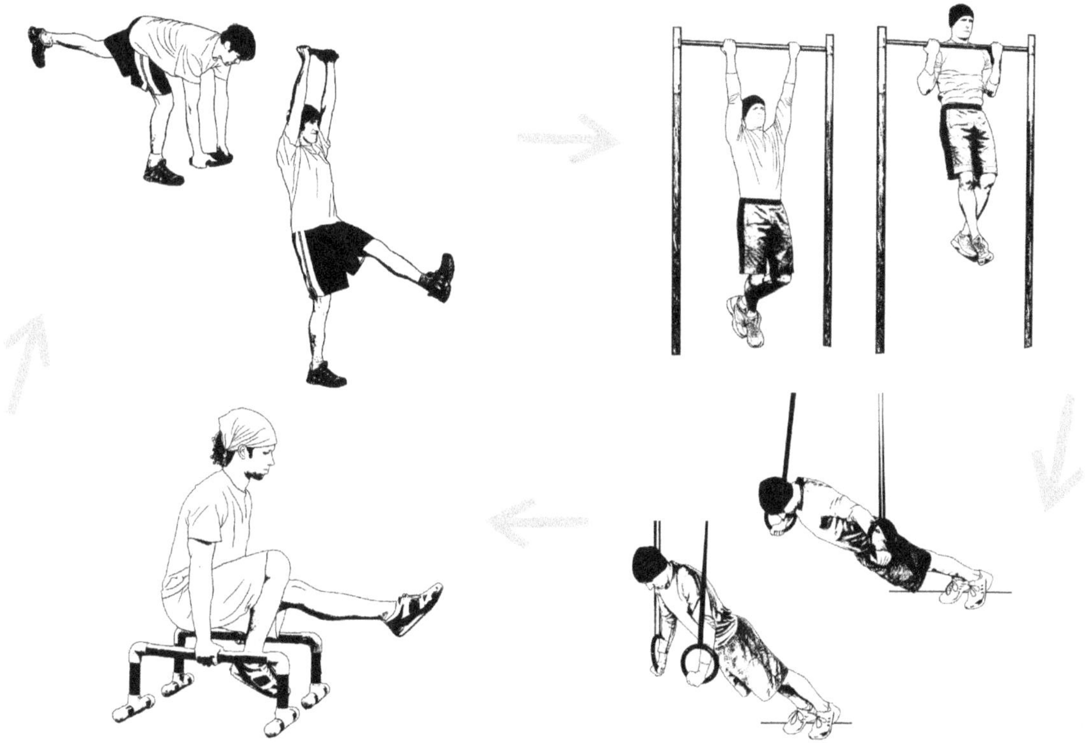

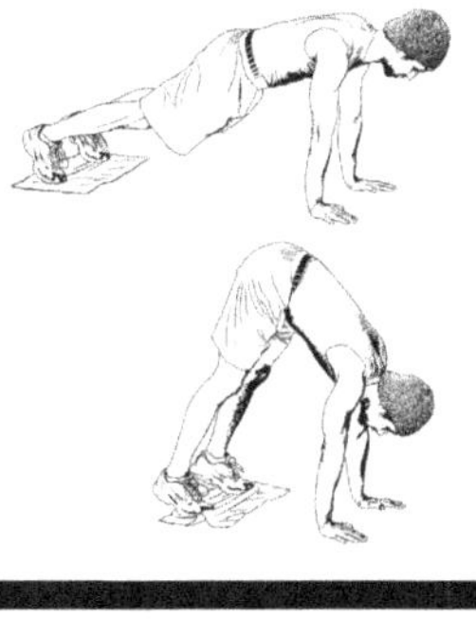

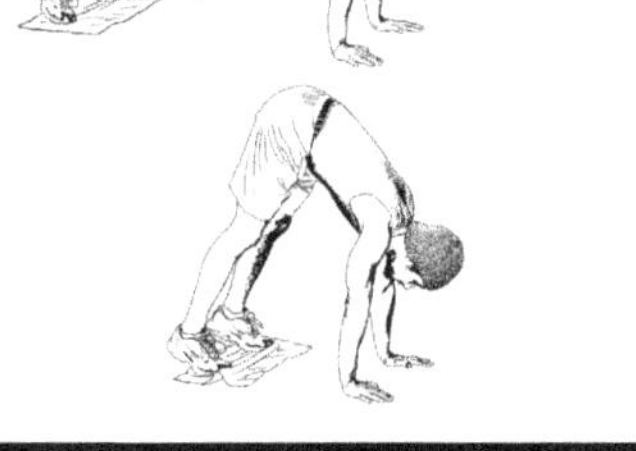
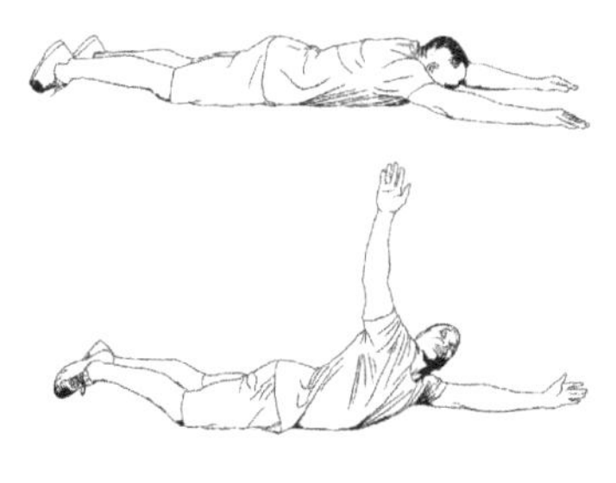

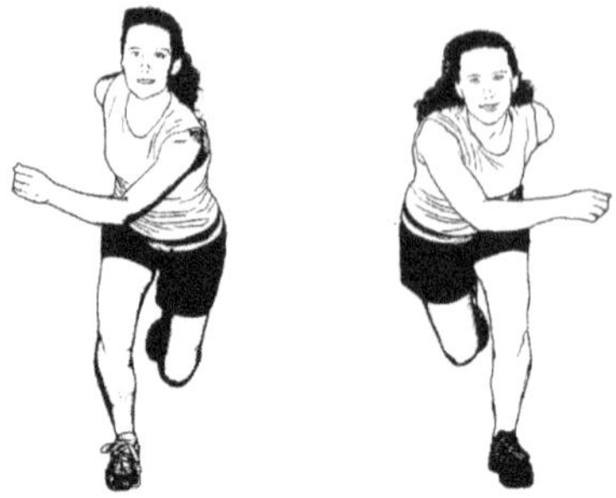

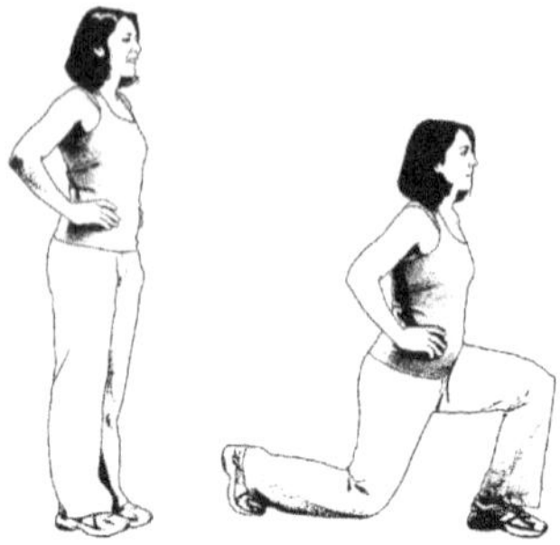

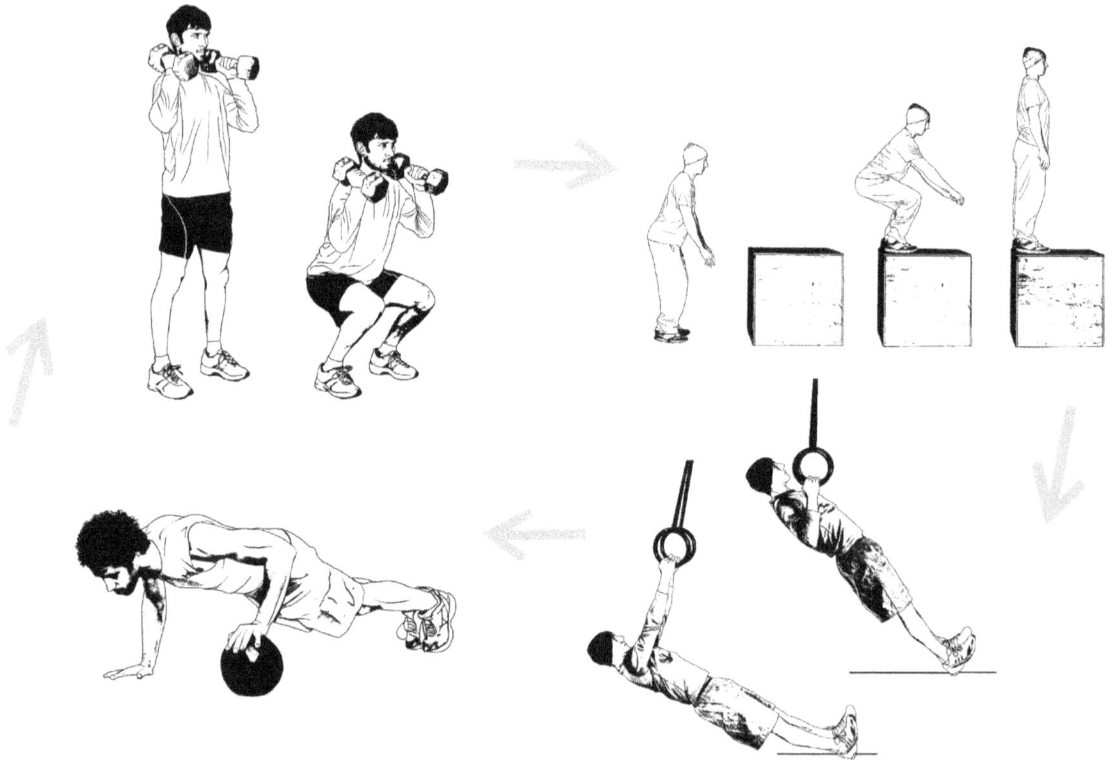

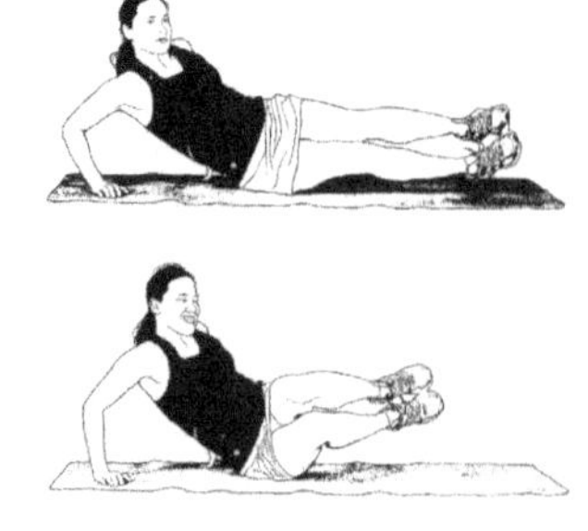

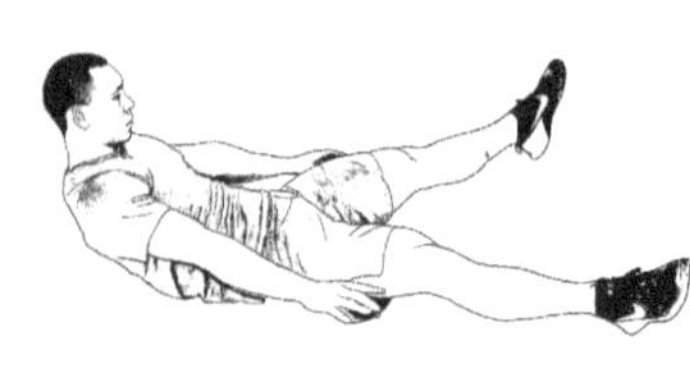

Side B

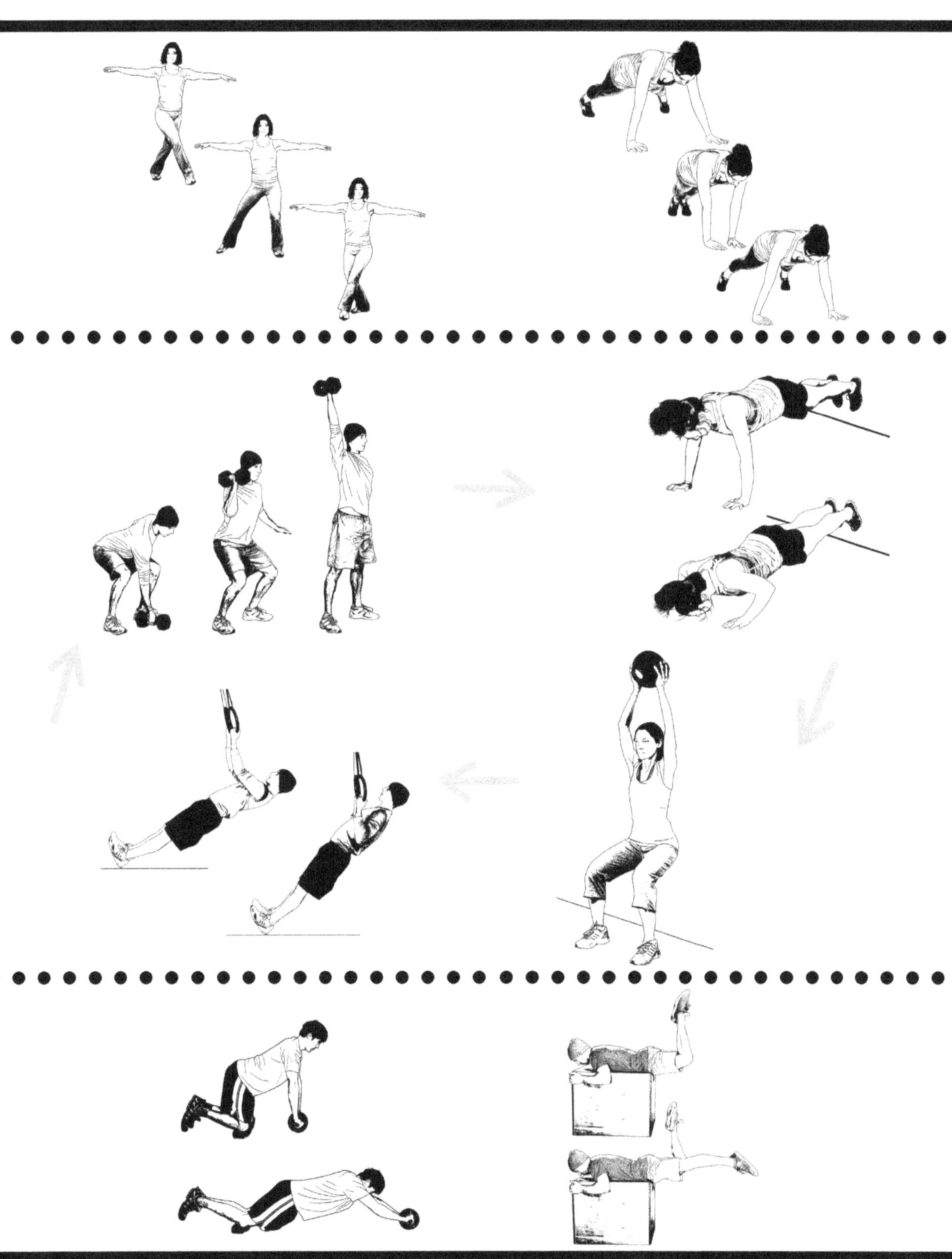

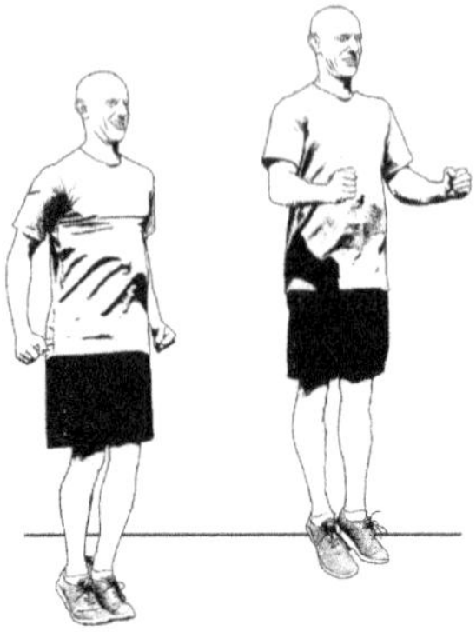

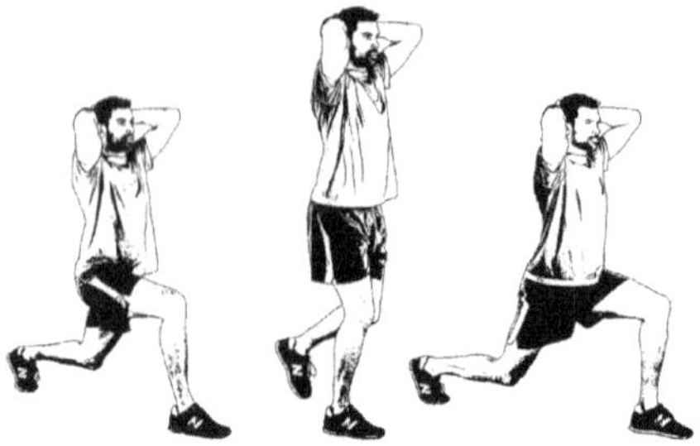

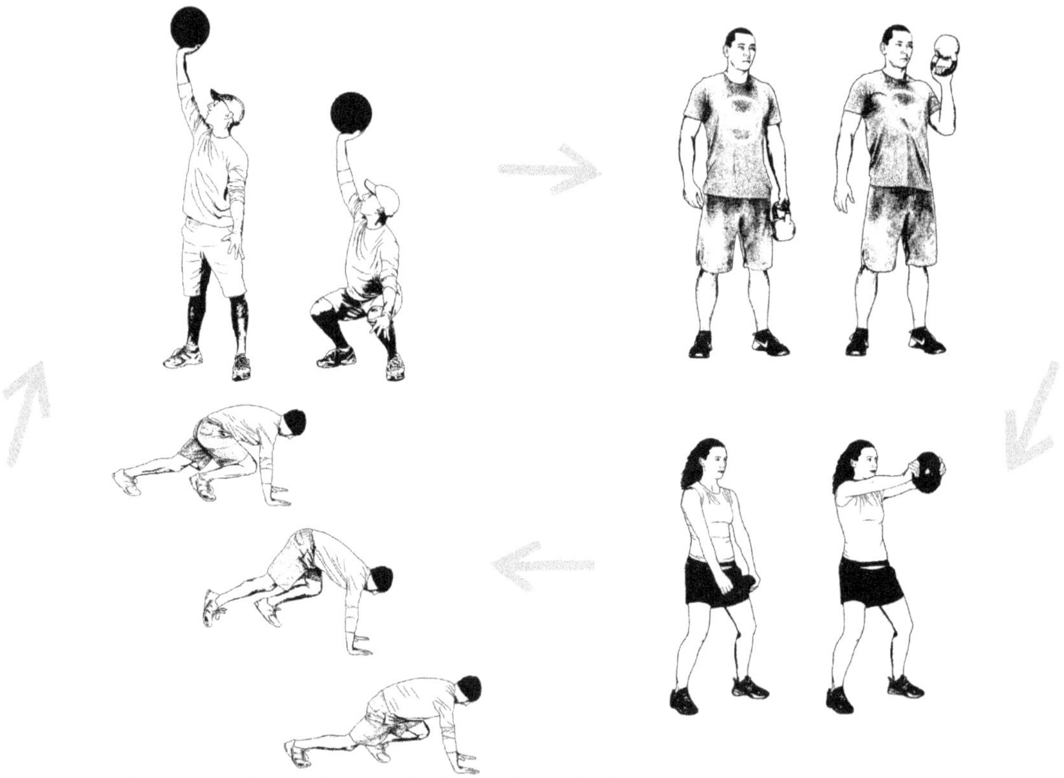

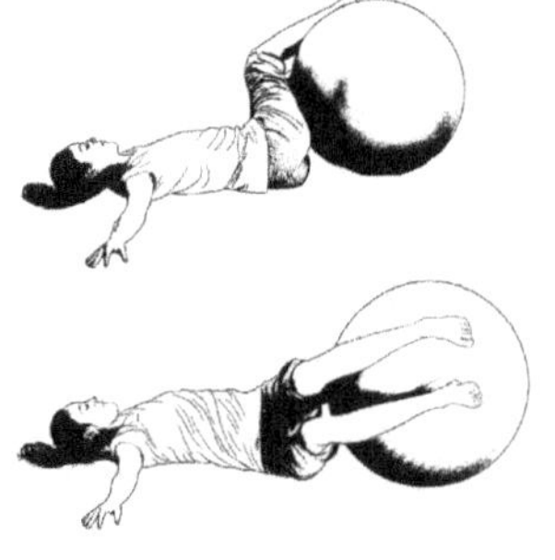
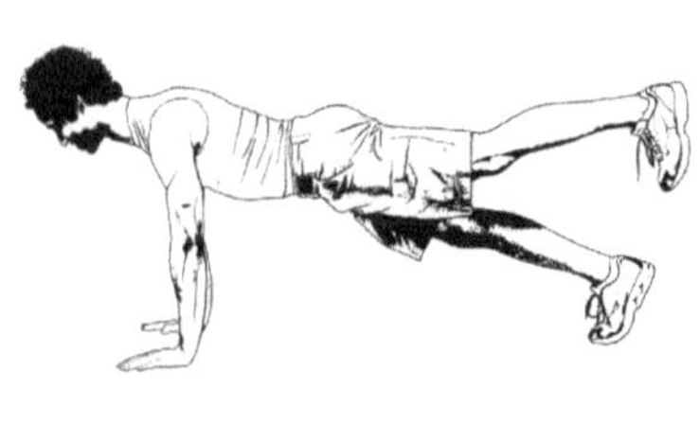

SIDE B

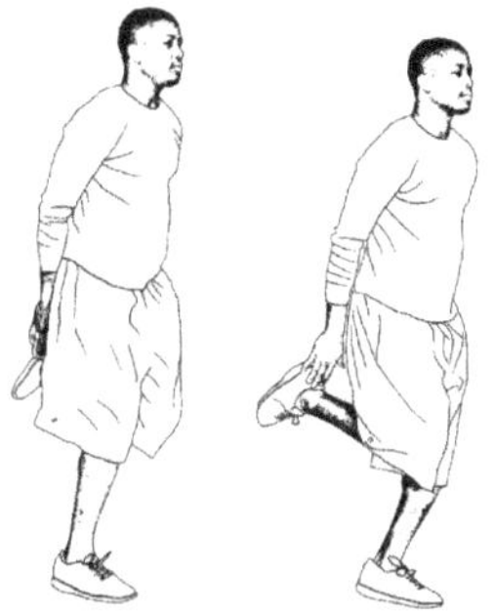

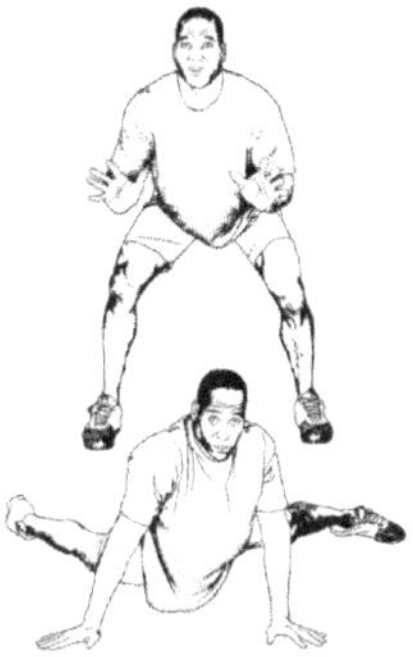

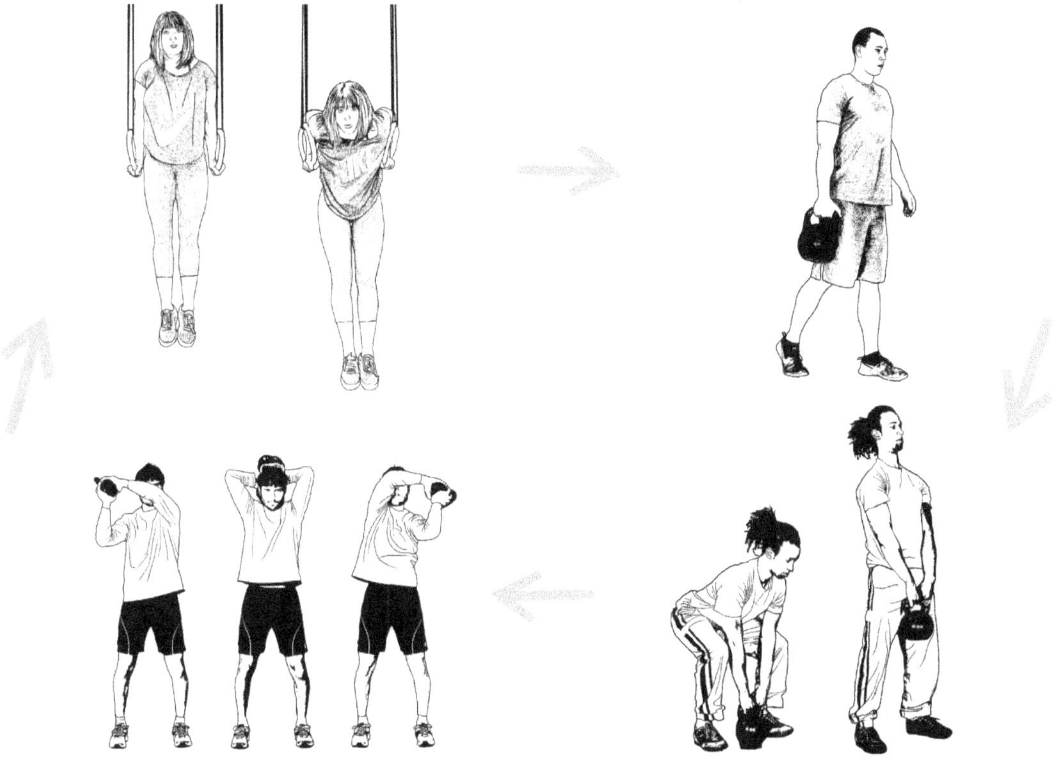

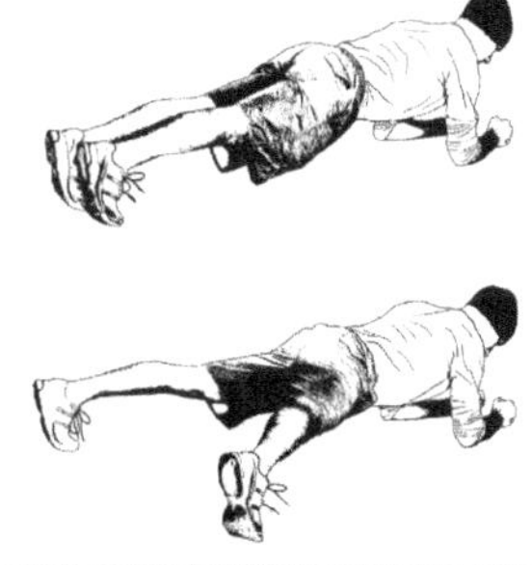

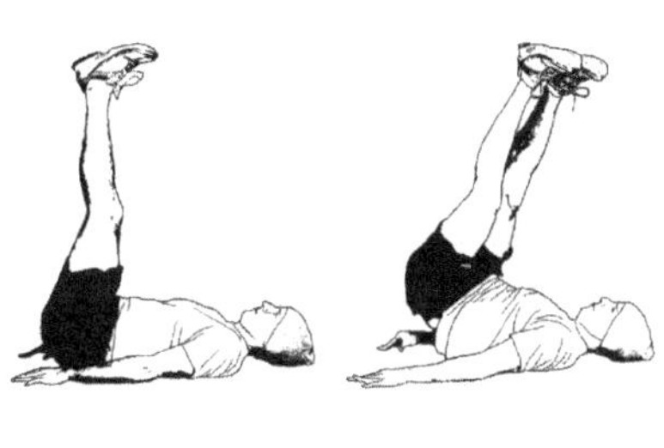

Side B

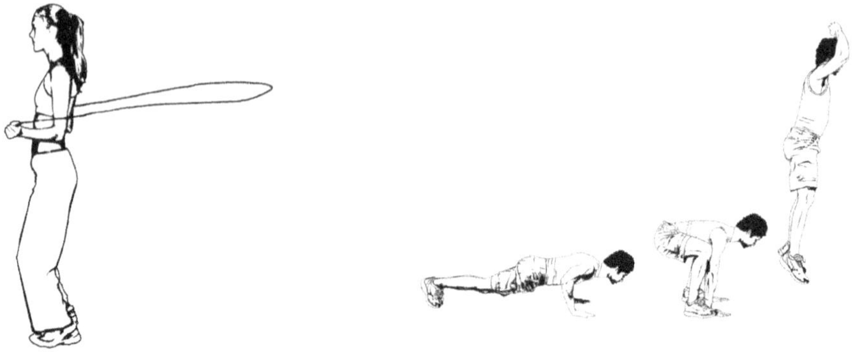

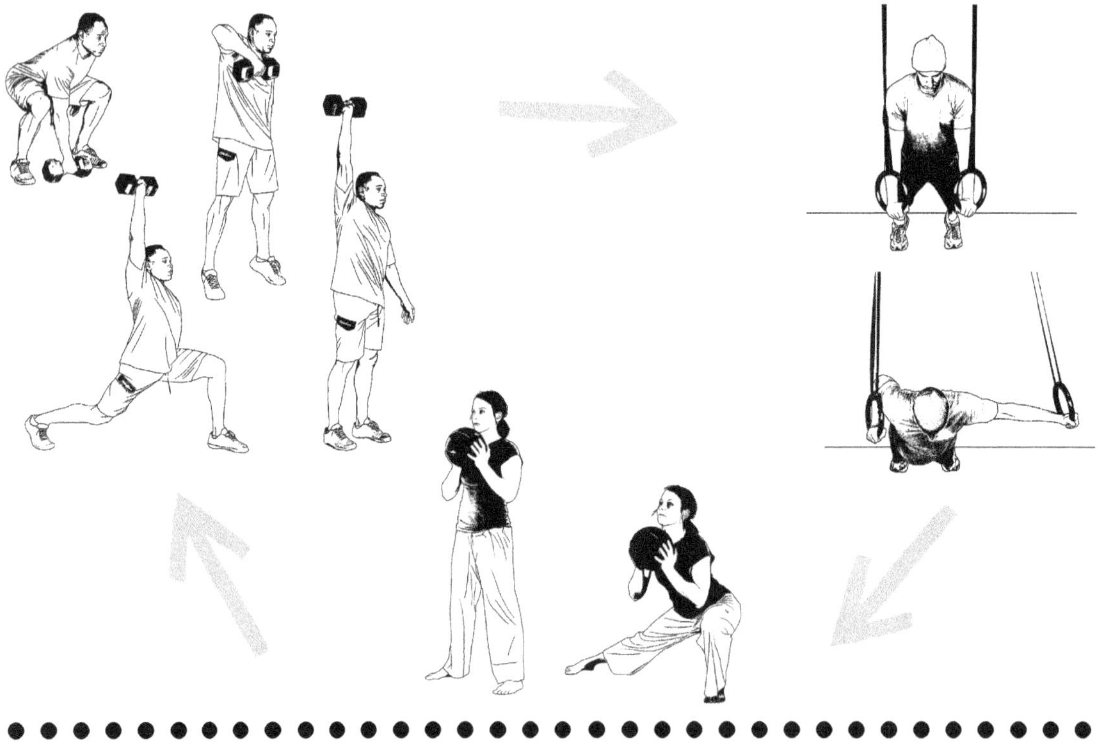

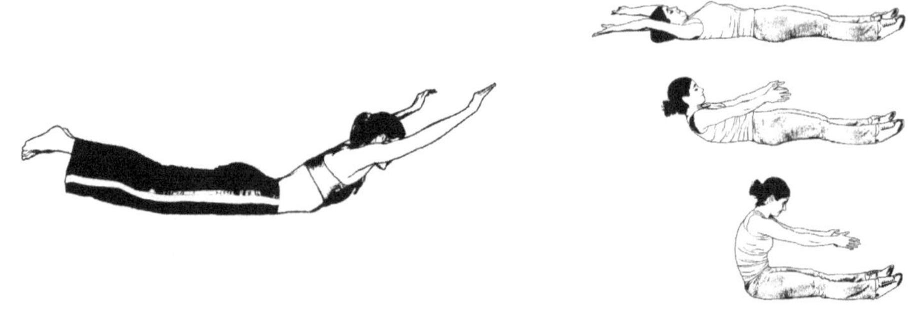

SIDE B

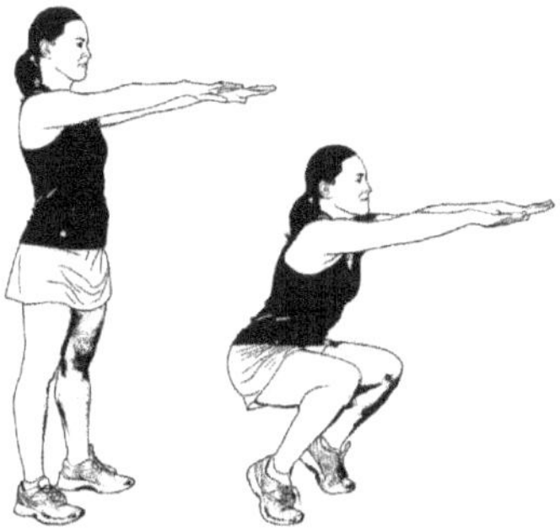

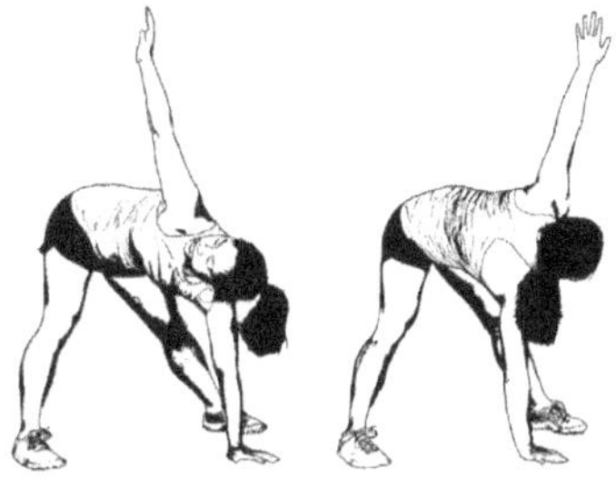

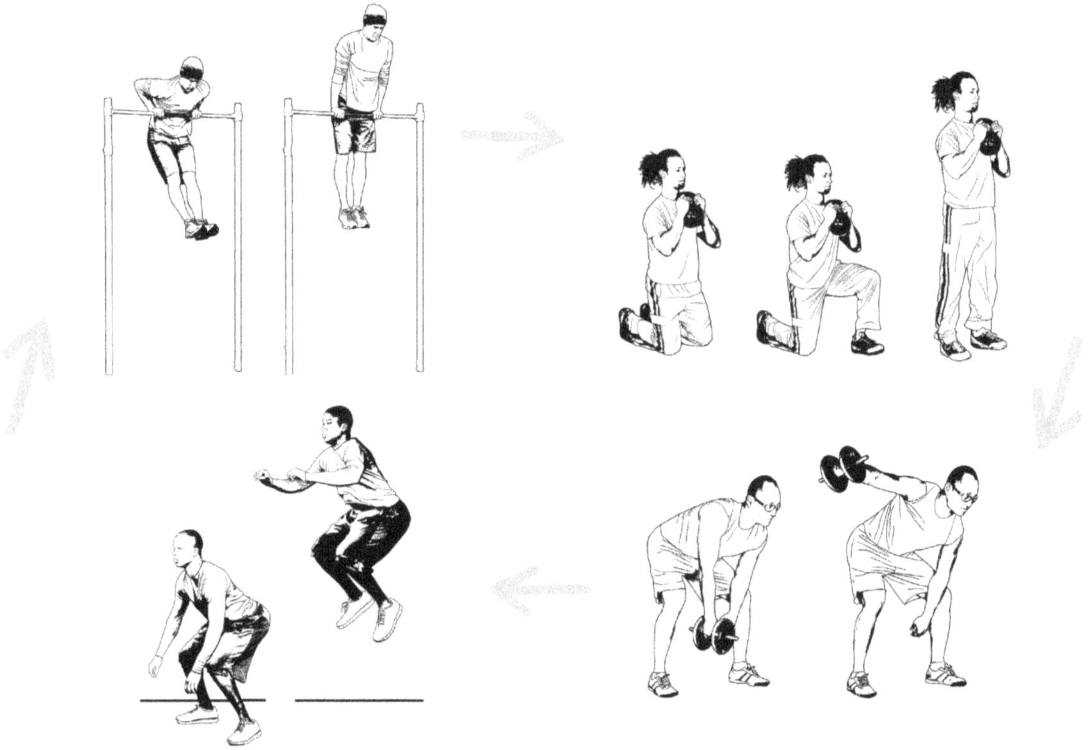

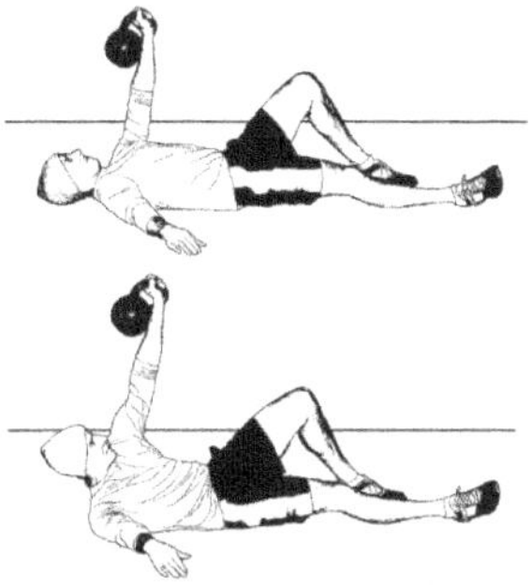

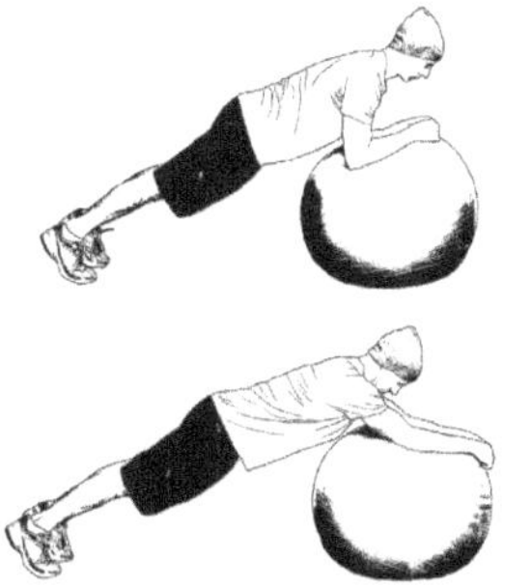

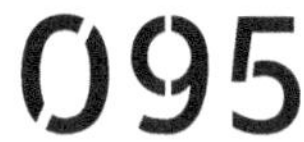

SIDE B

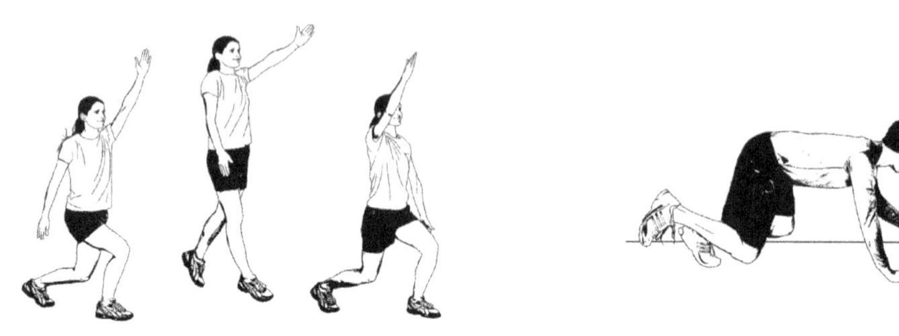

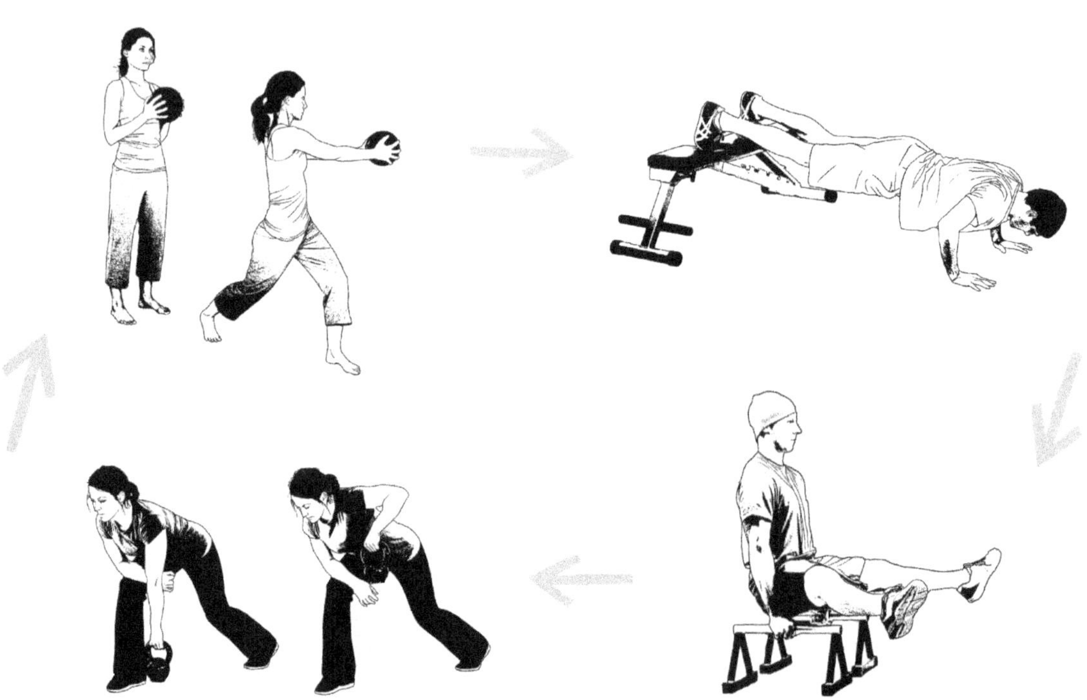

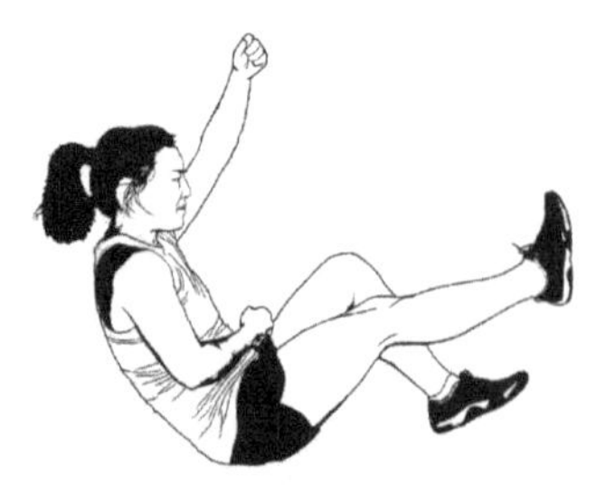

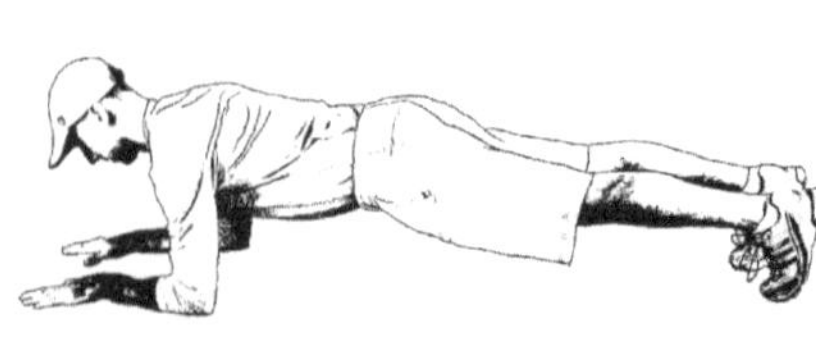

SIDE B

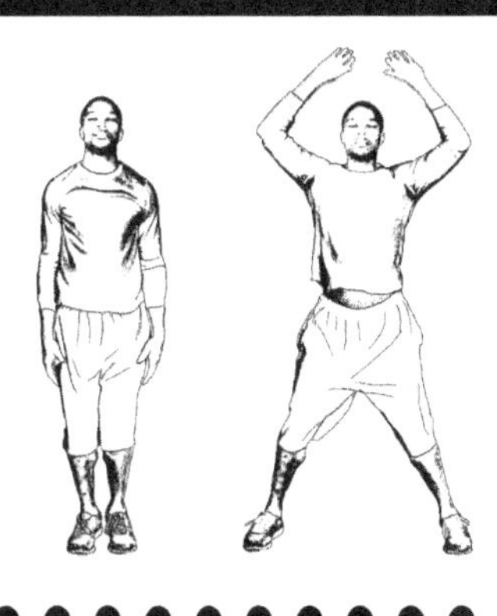

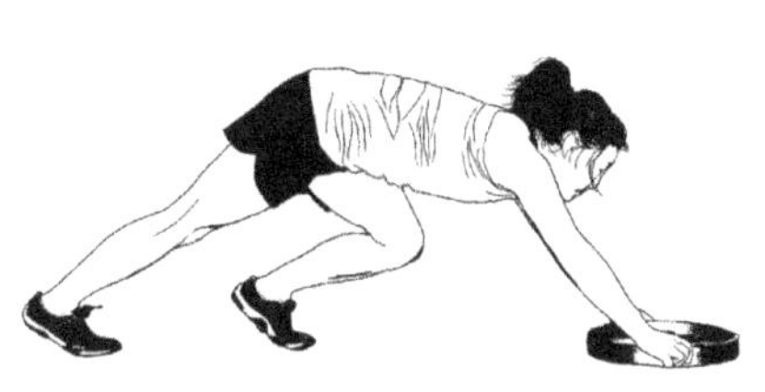

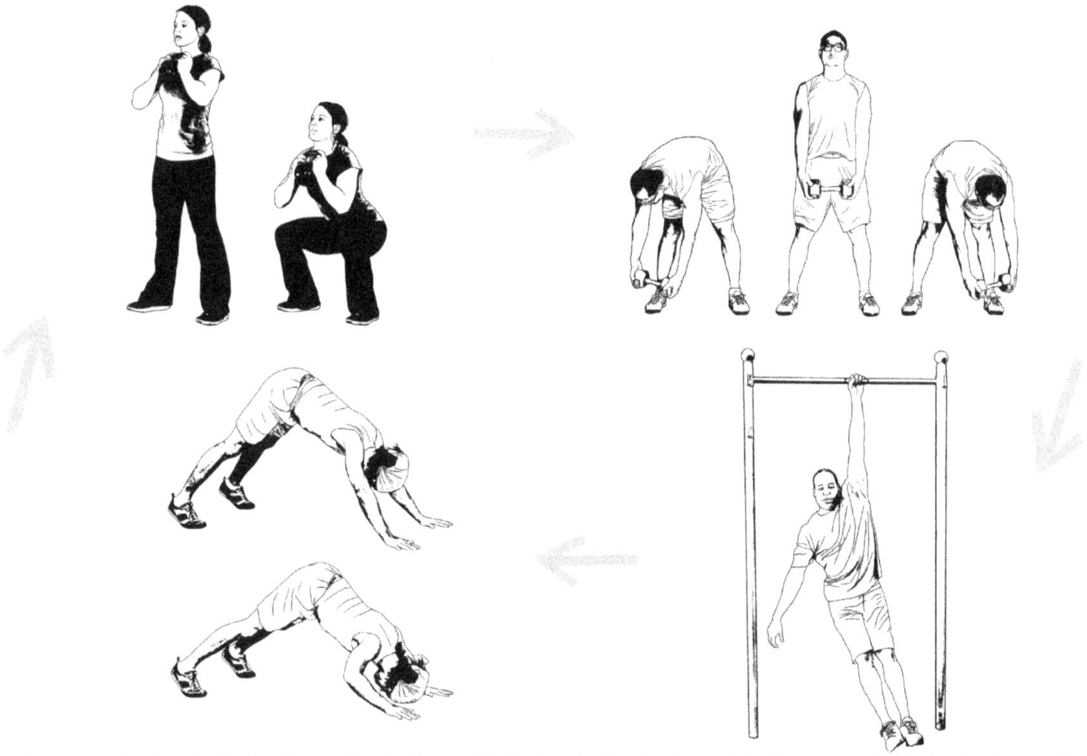

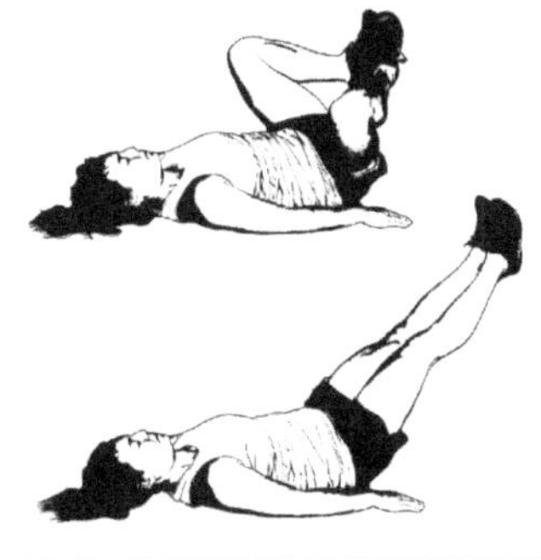

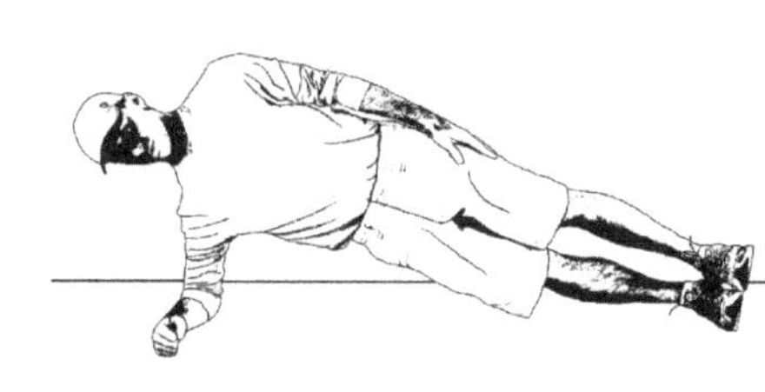

SIDE B

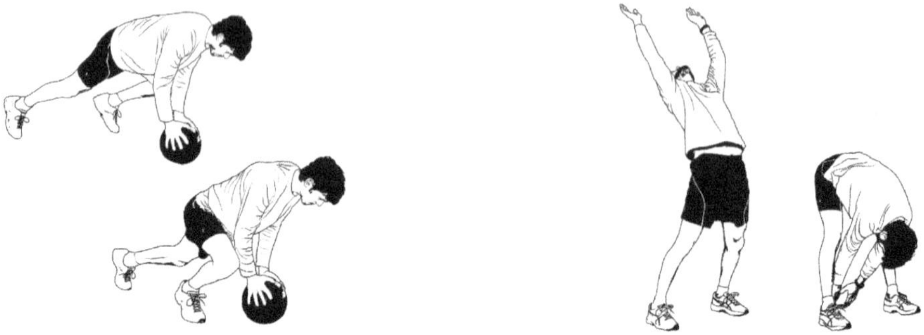

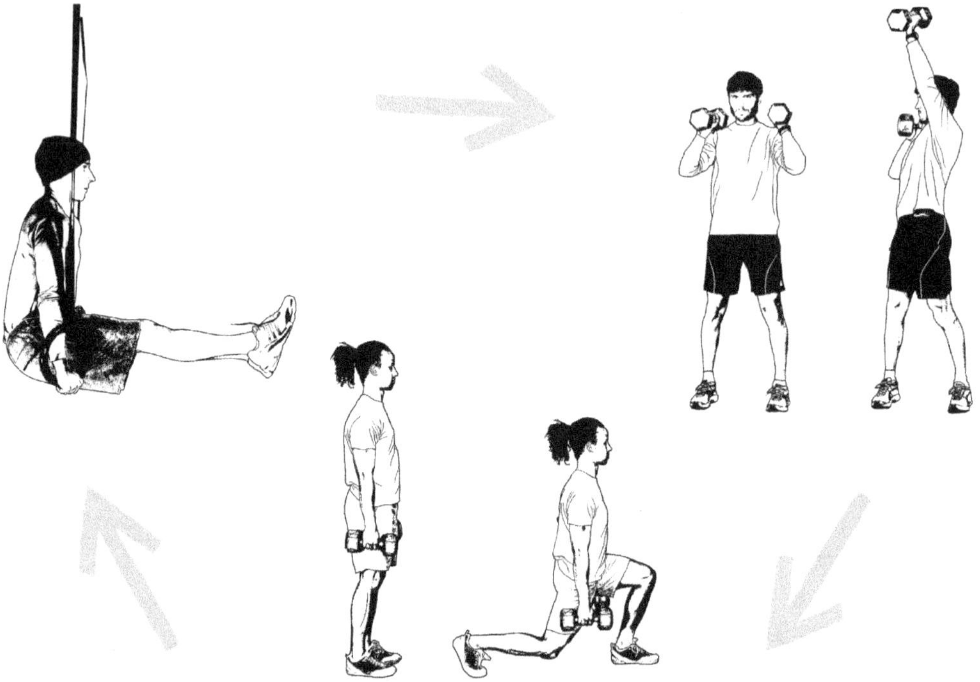

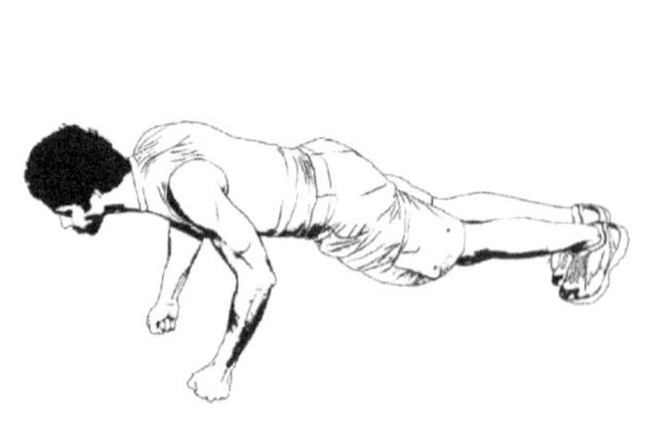

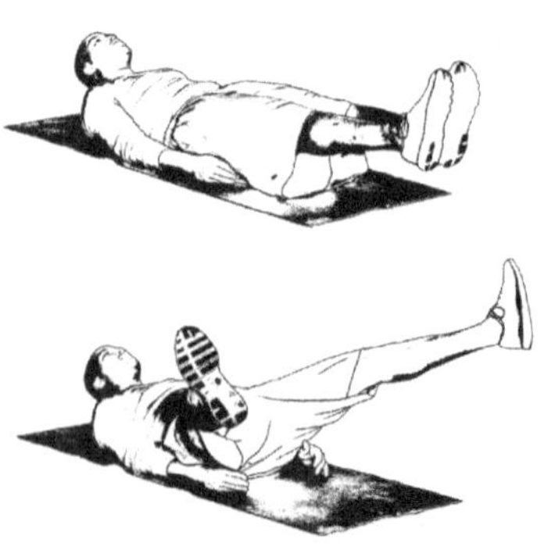

SIDE B

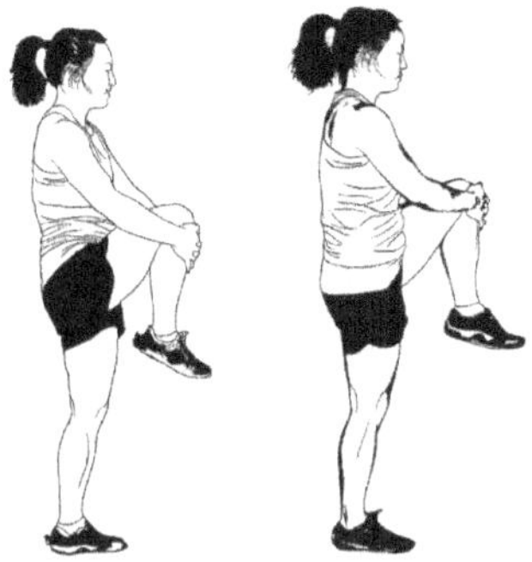

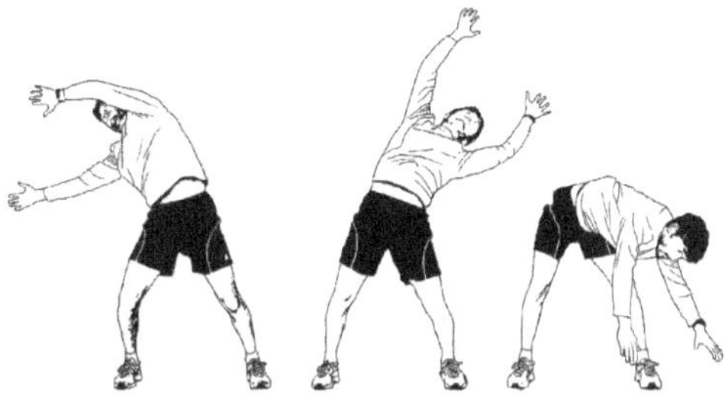

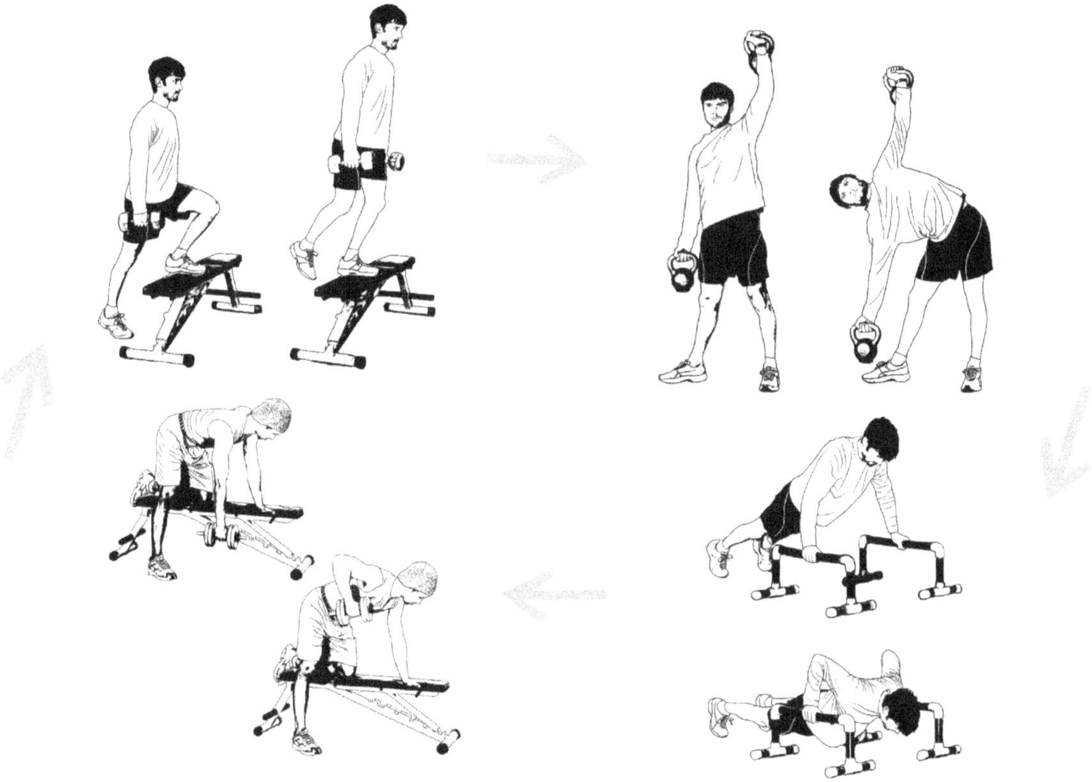

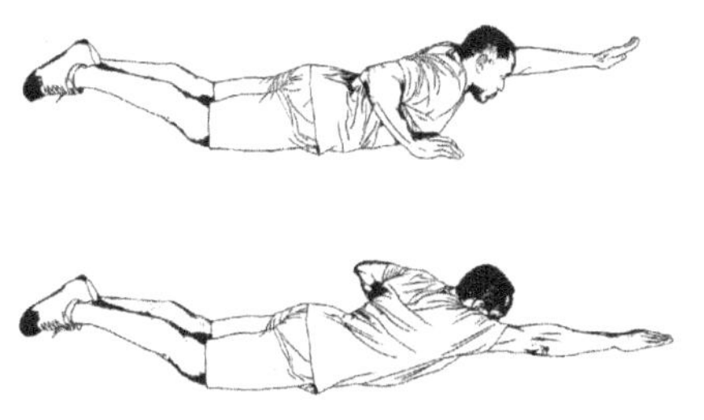

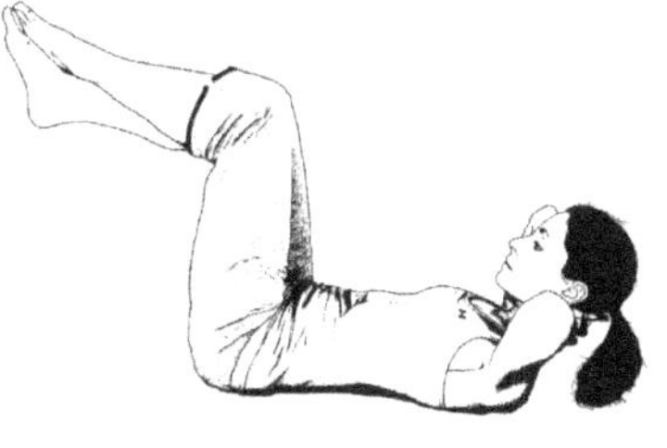

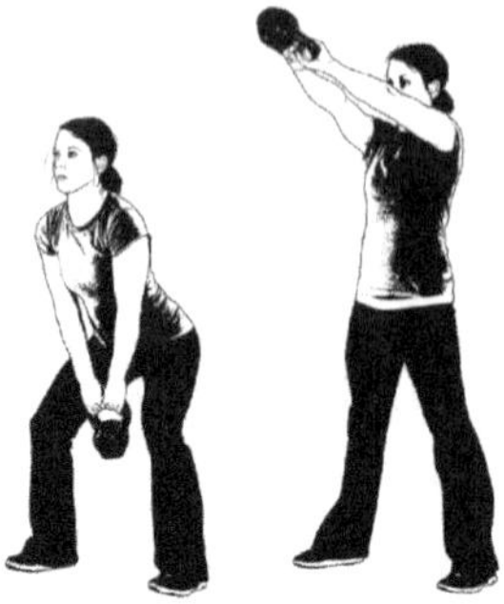

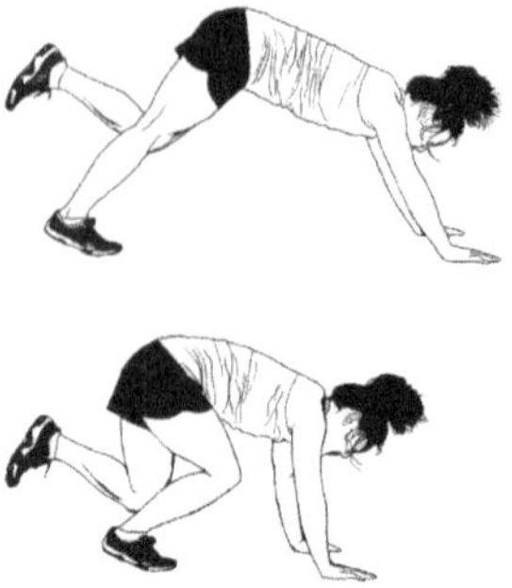

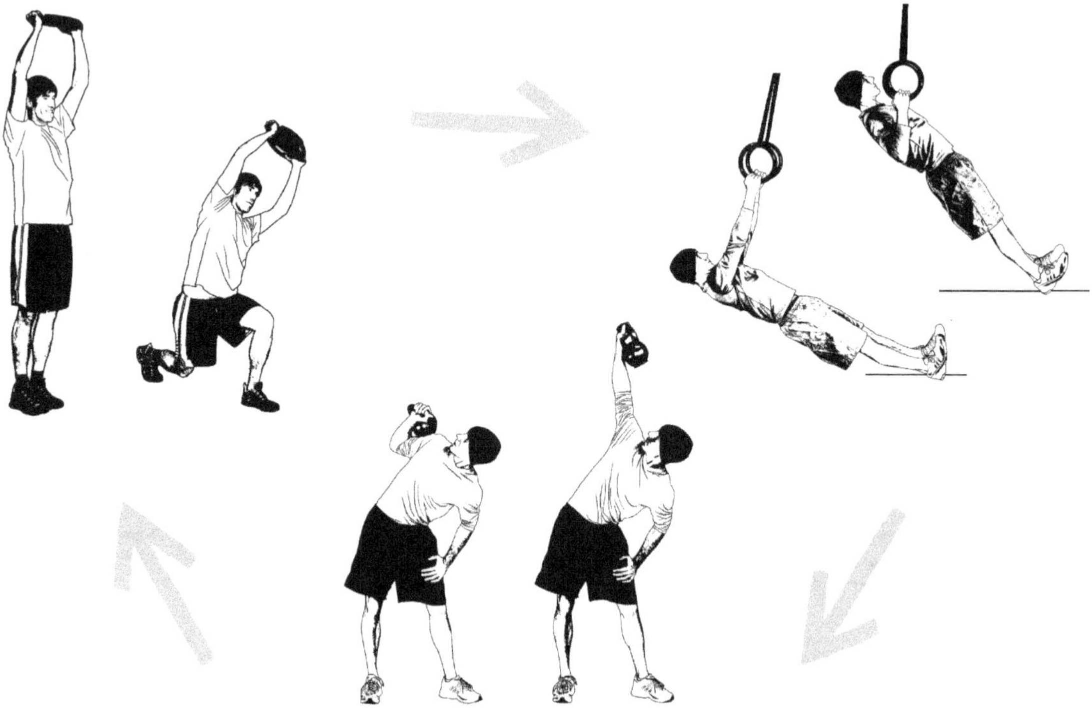

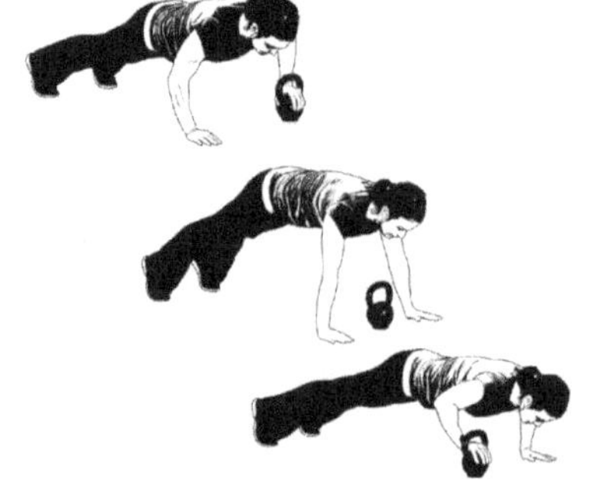

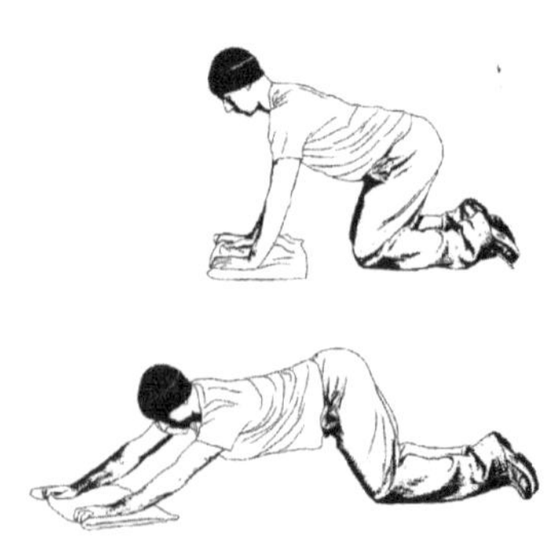

SIDE B

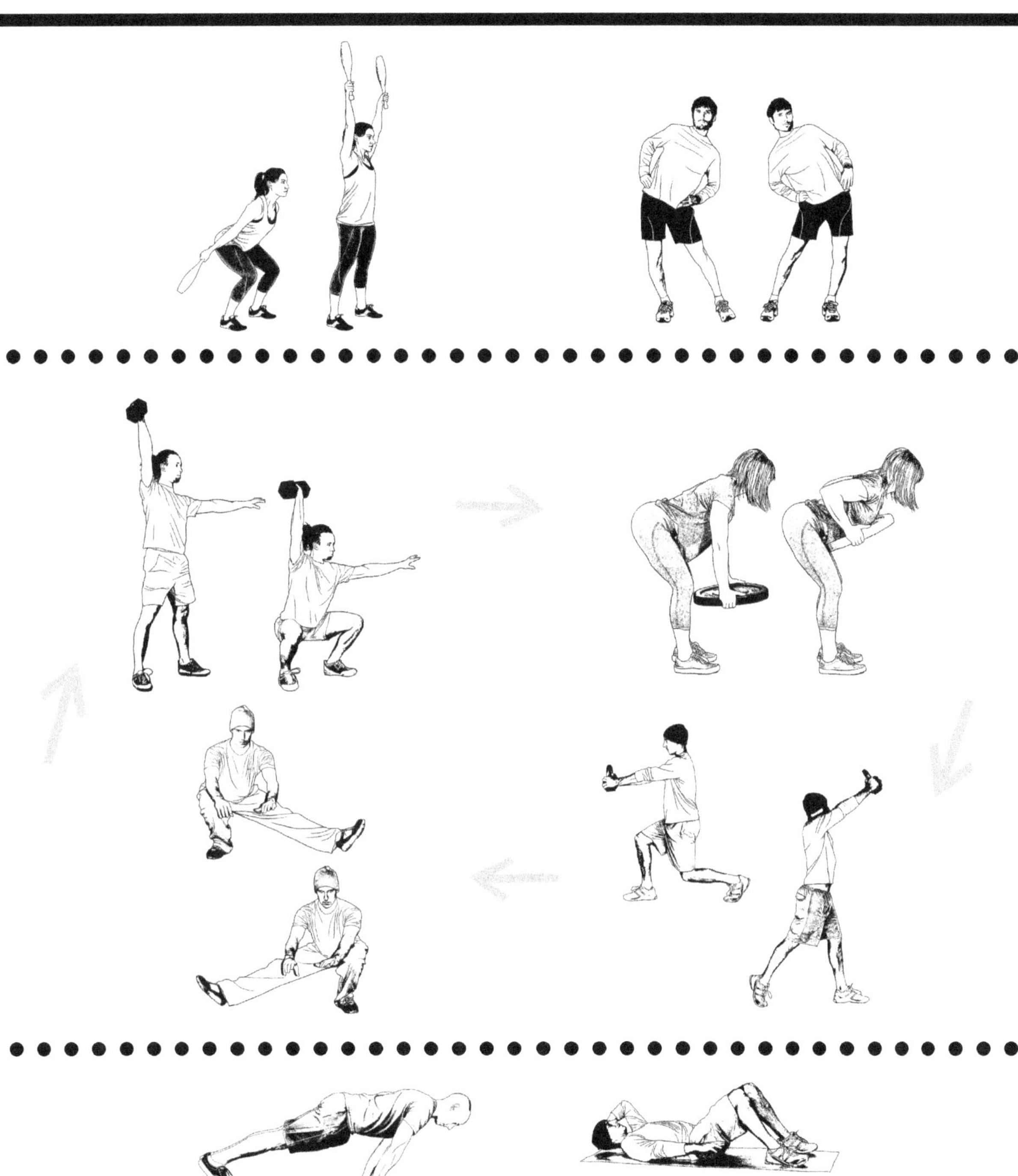

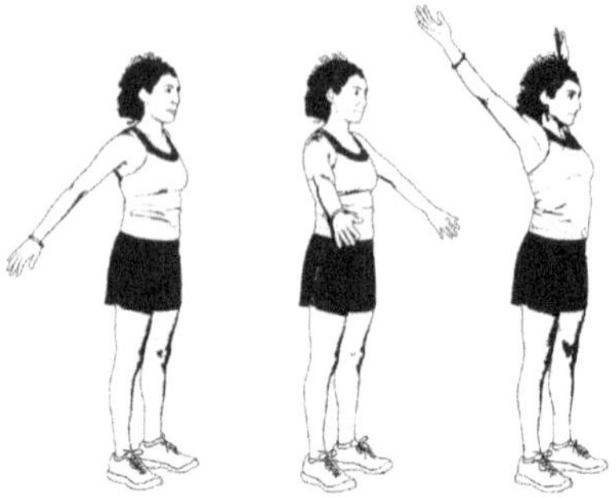

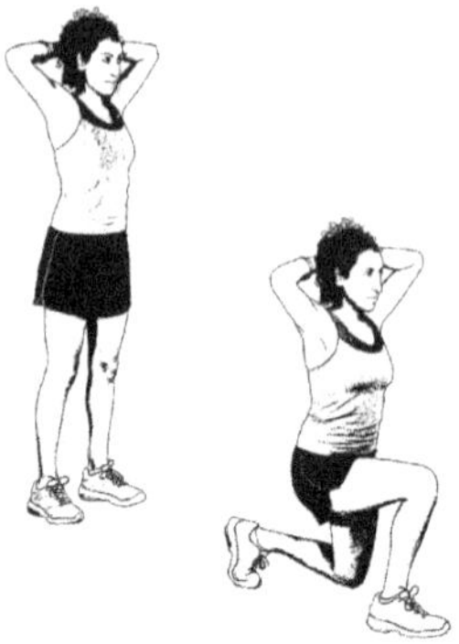

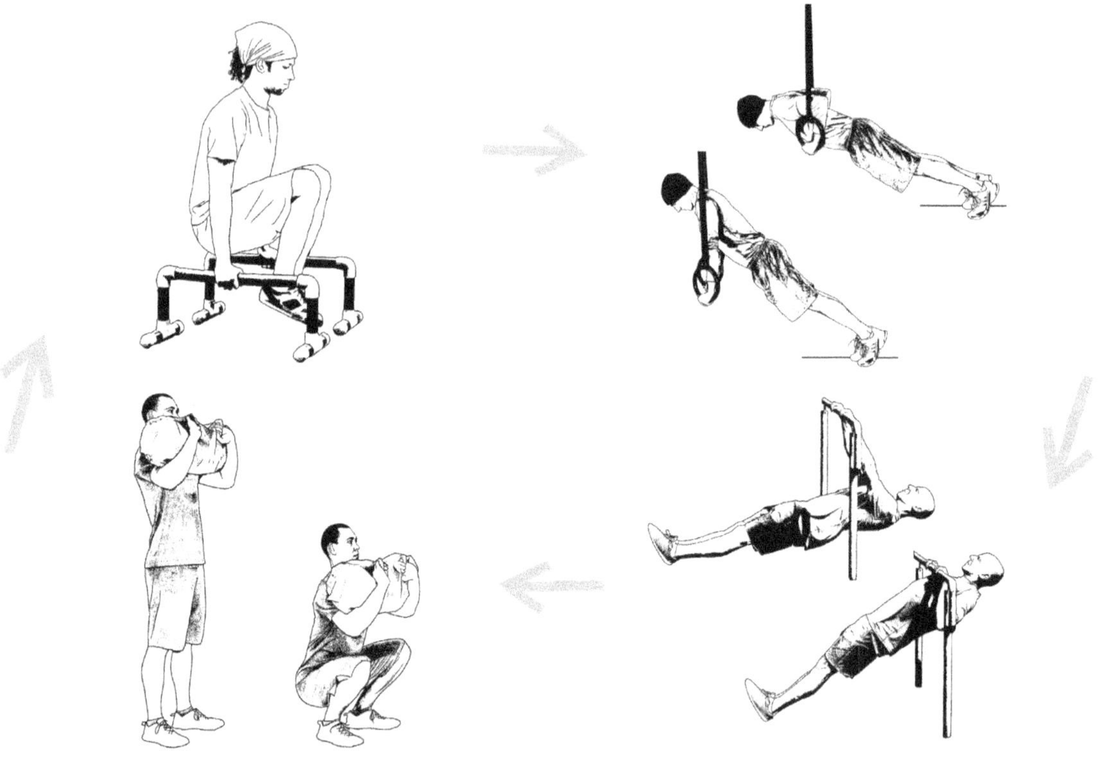

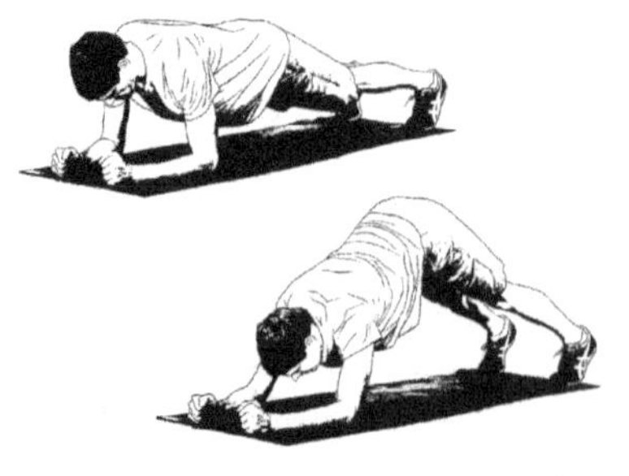
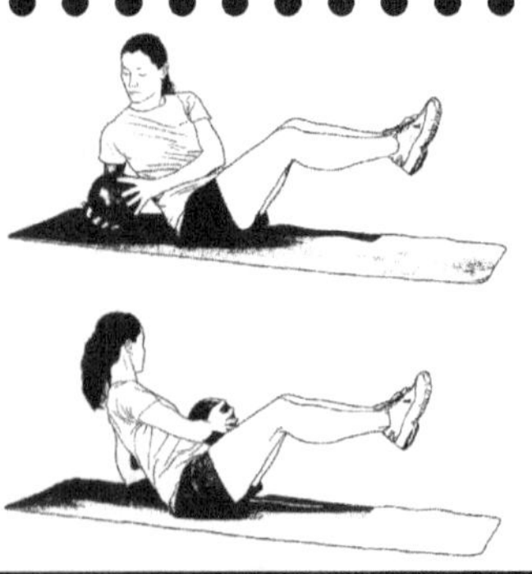

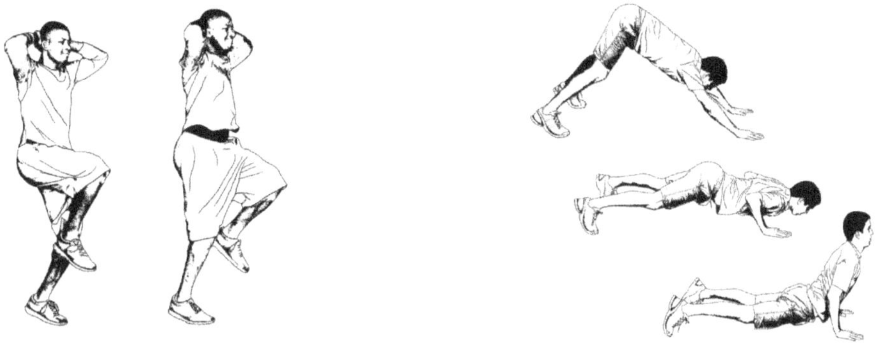

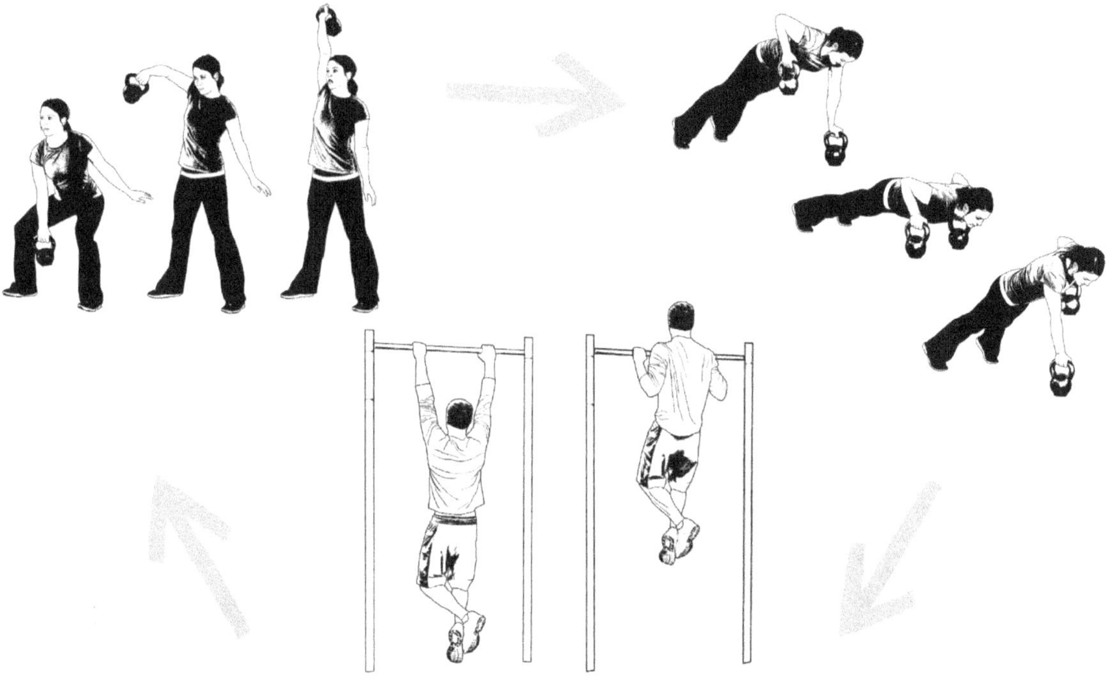

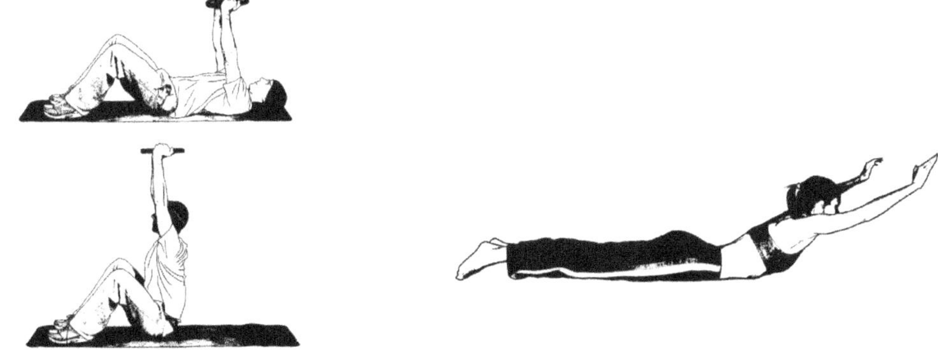

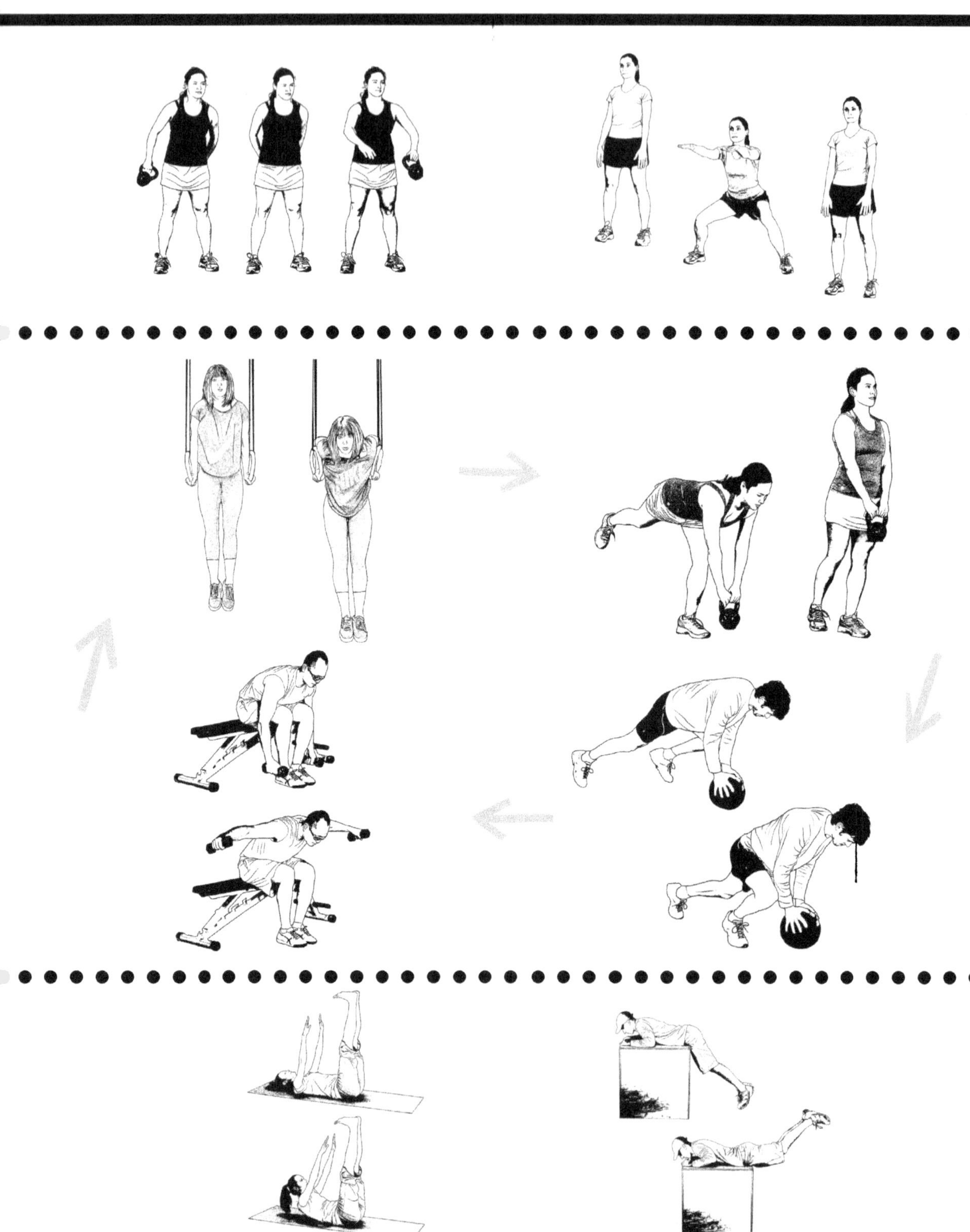

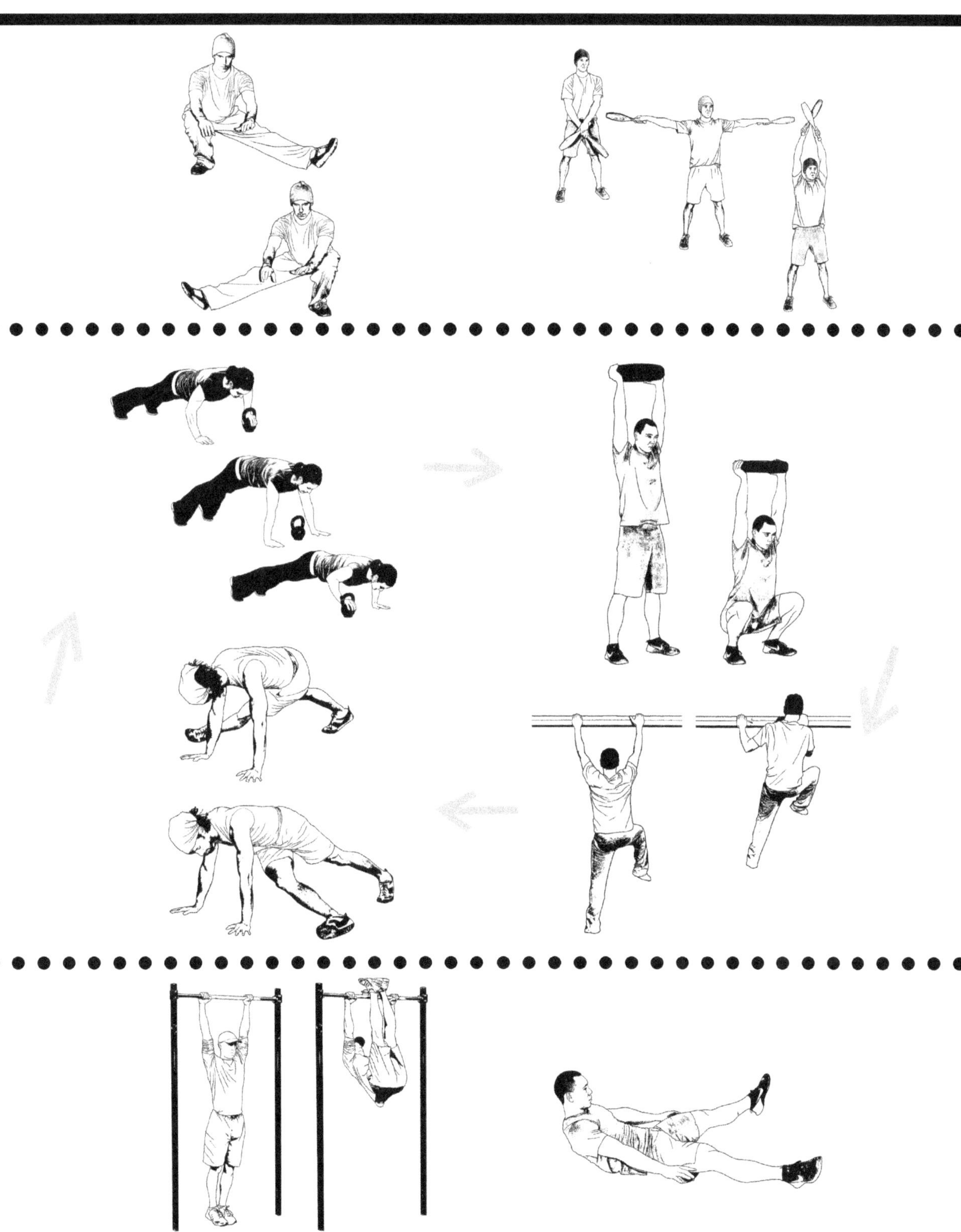

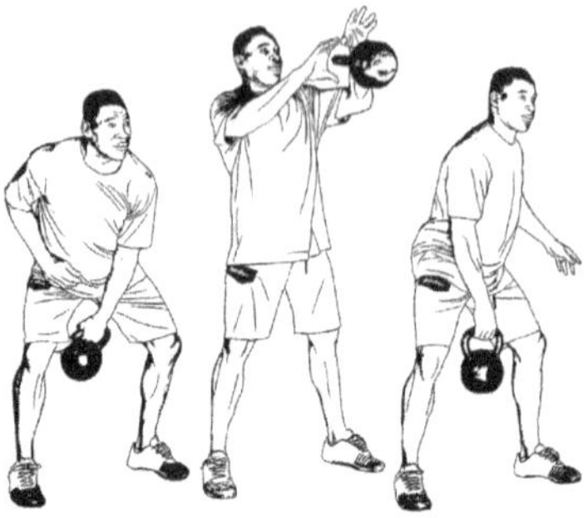

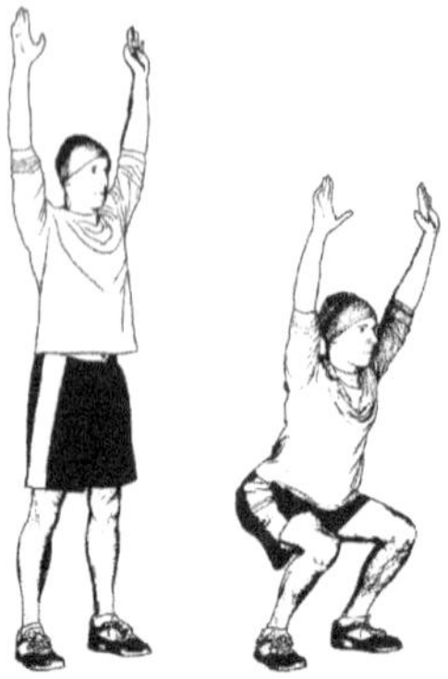

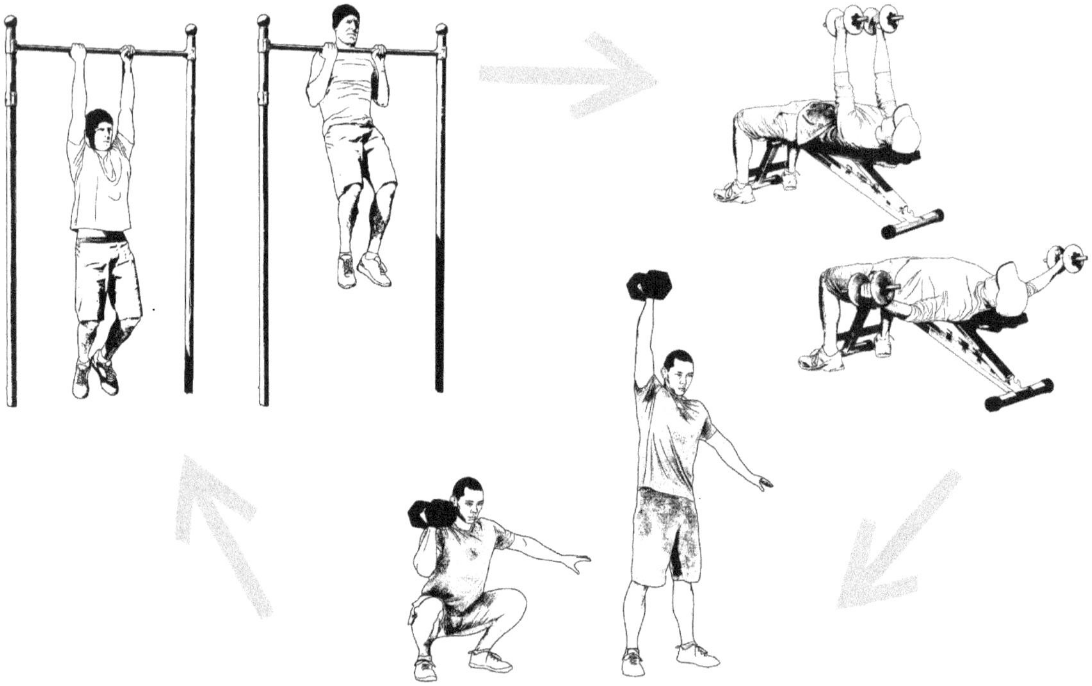

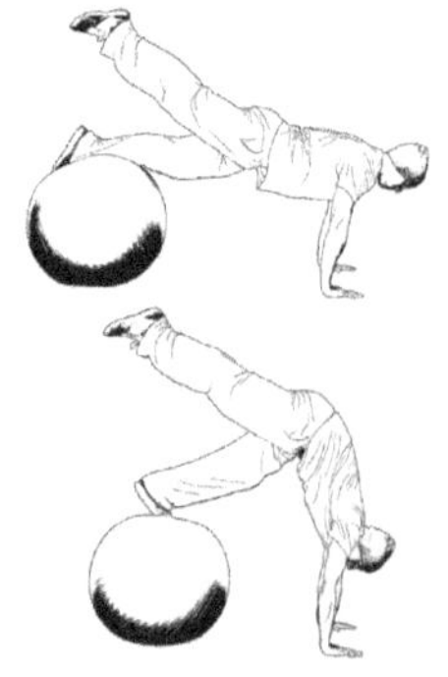
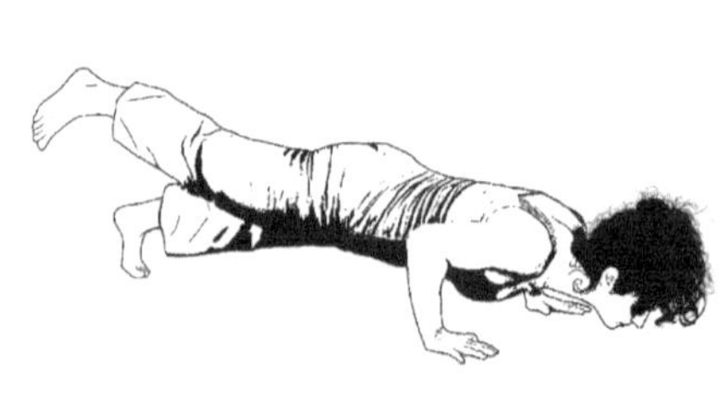

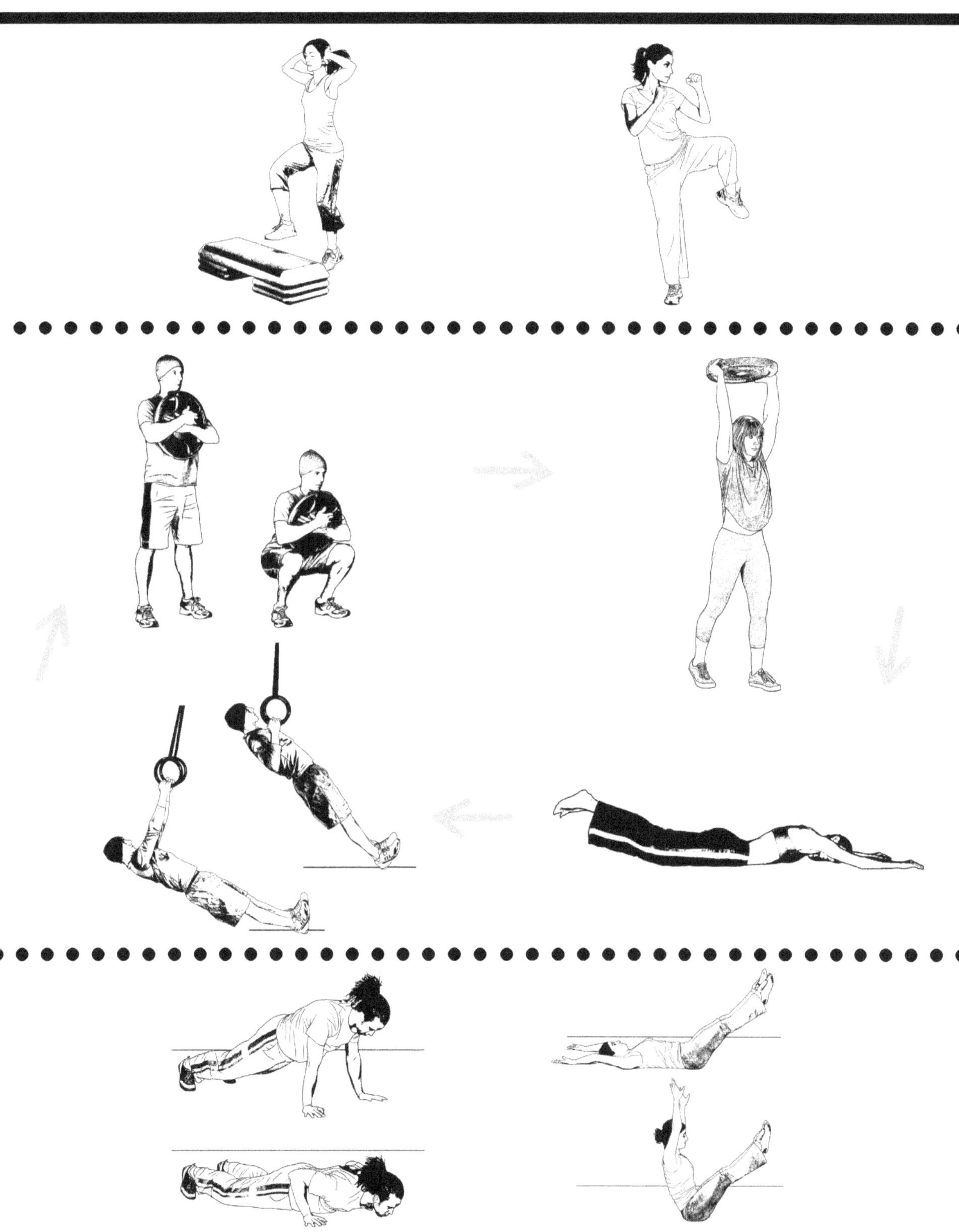

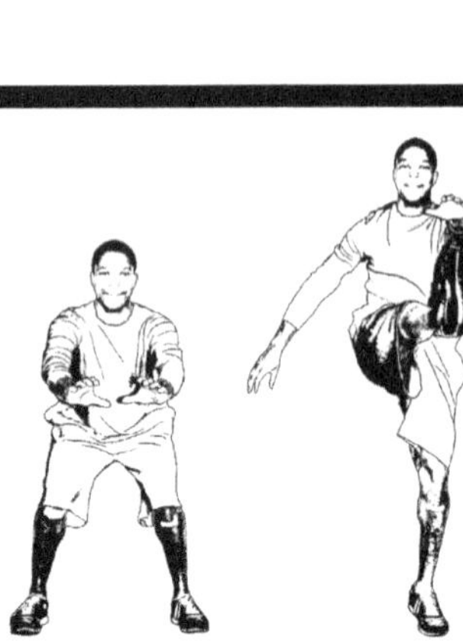

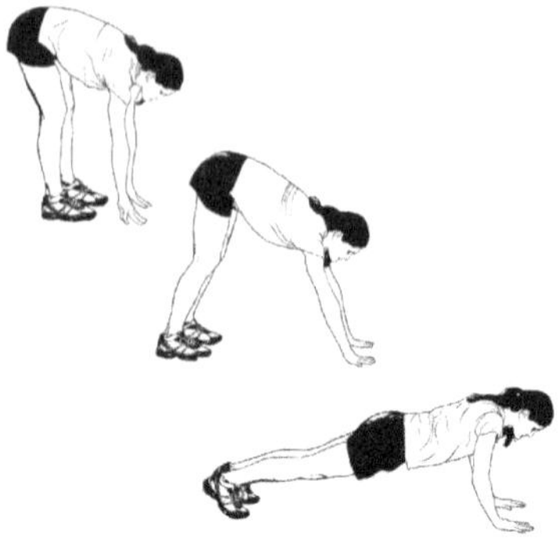

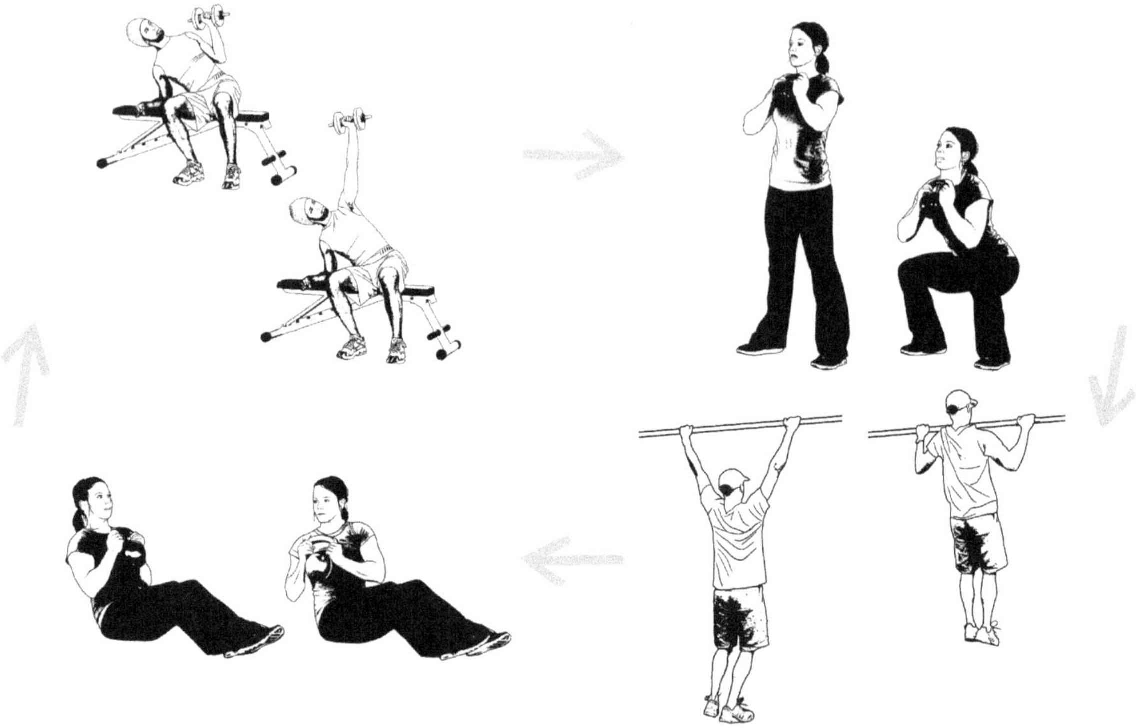

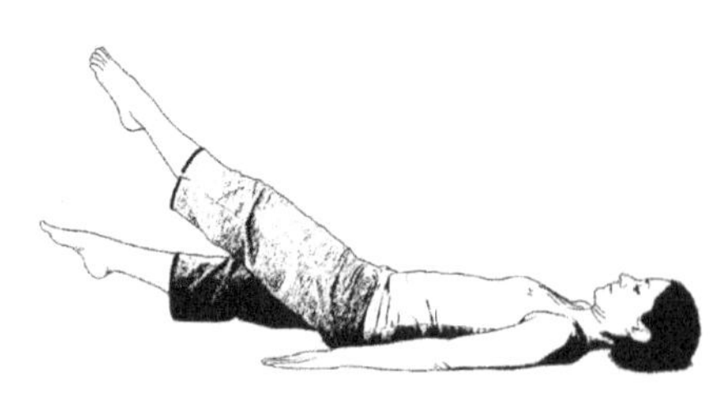
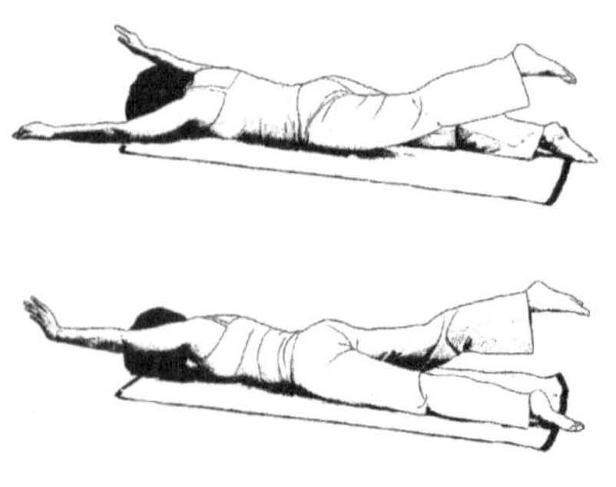

SIDE B

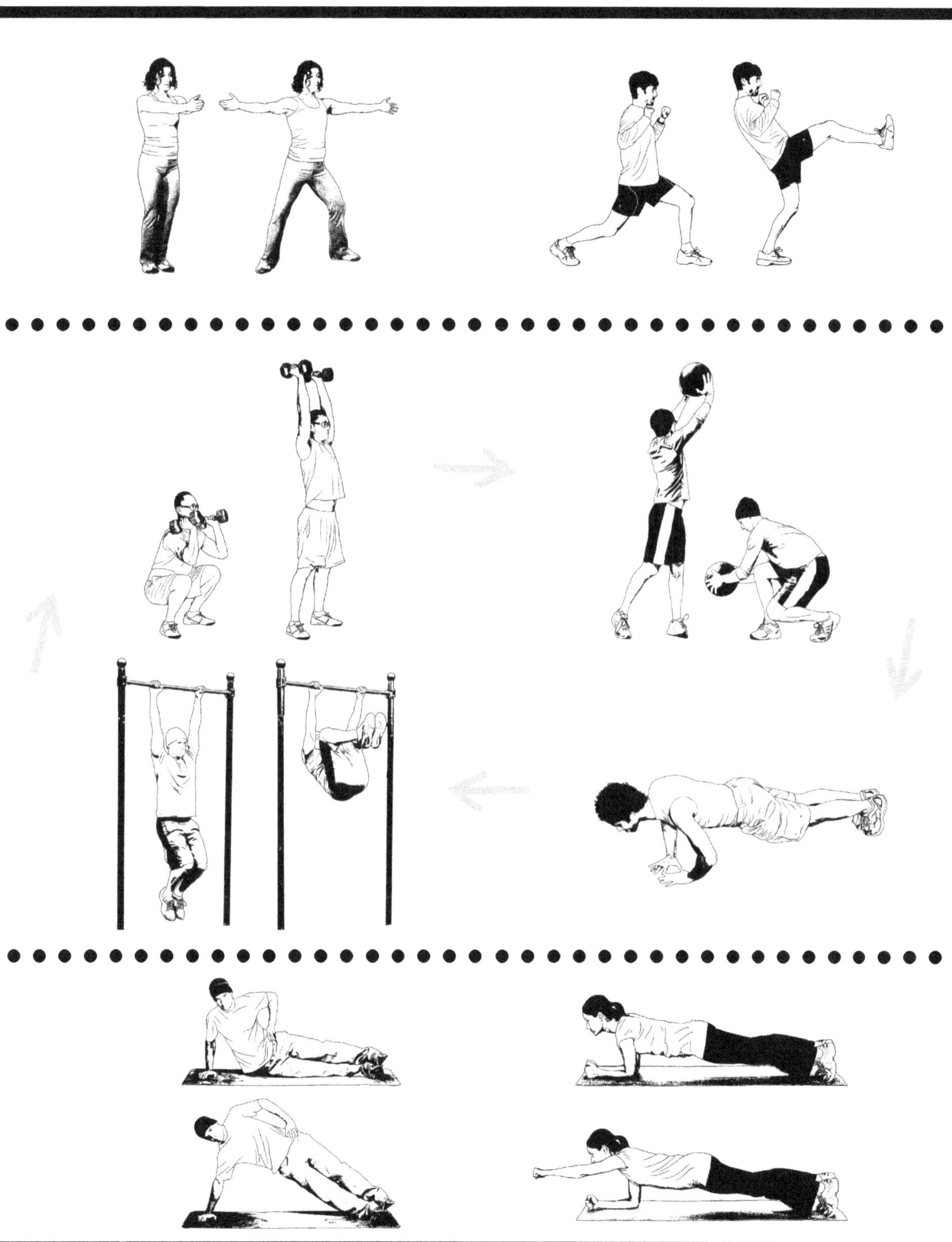

SIDE B

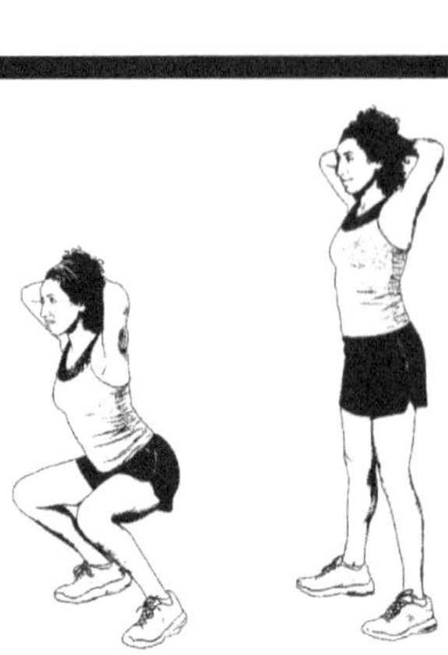

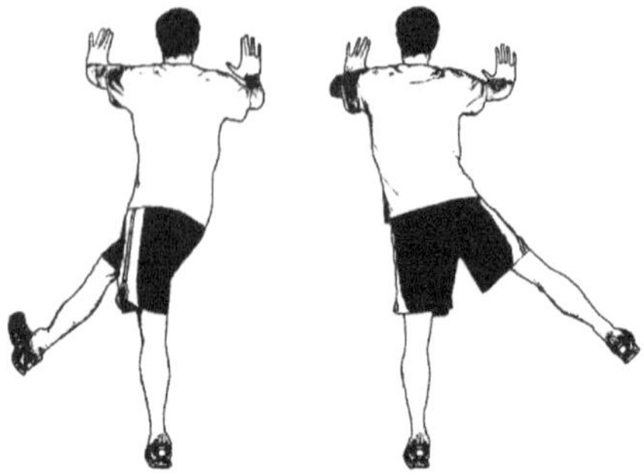

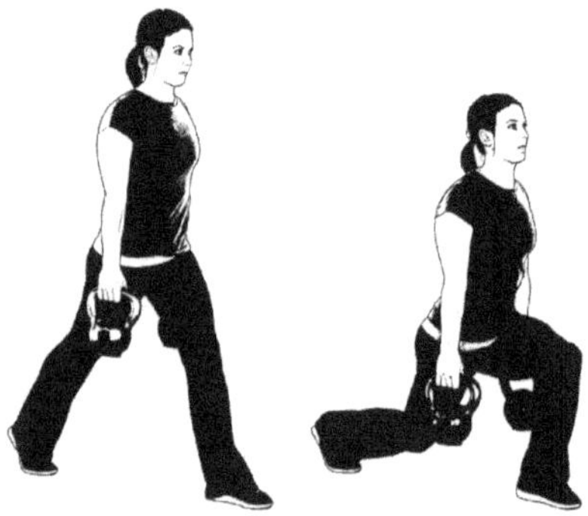

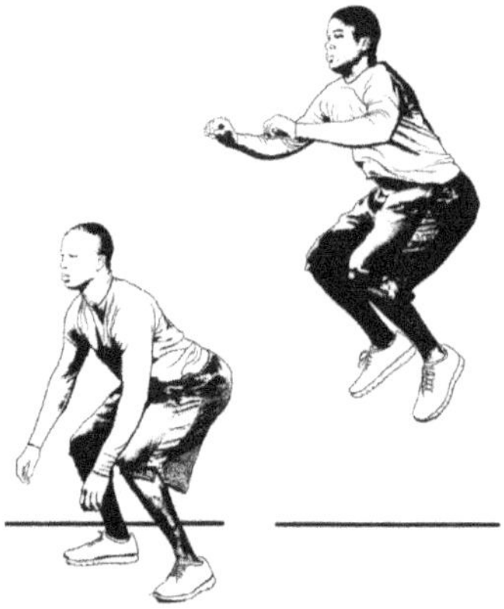

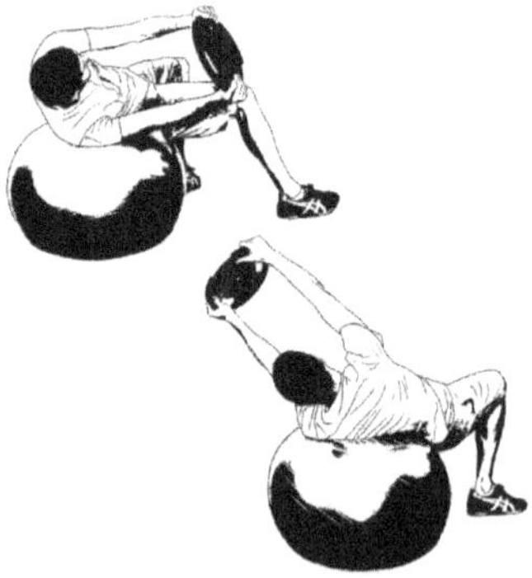

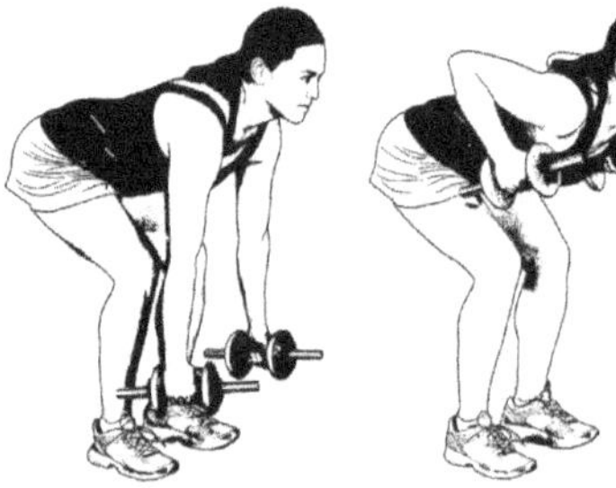

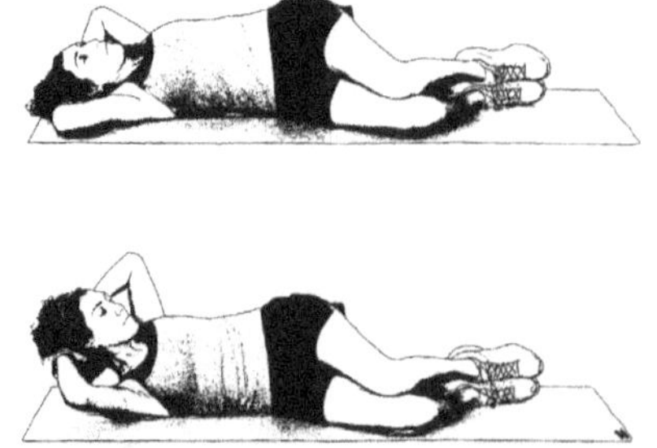

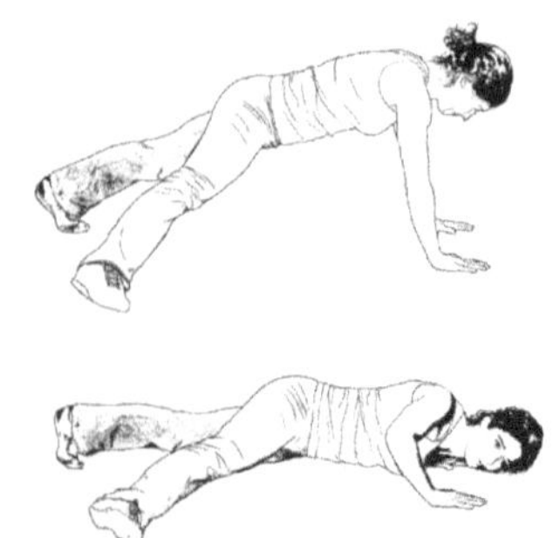

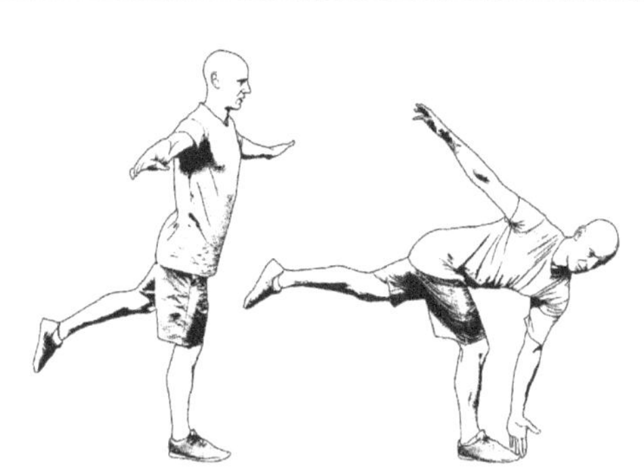
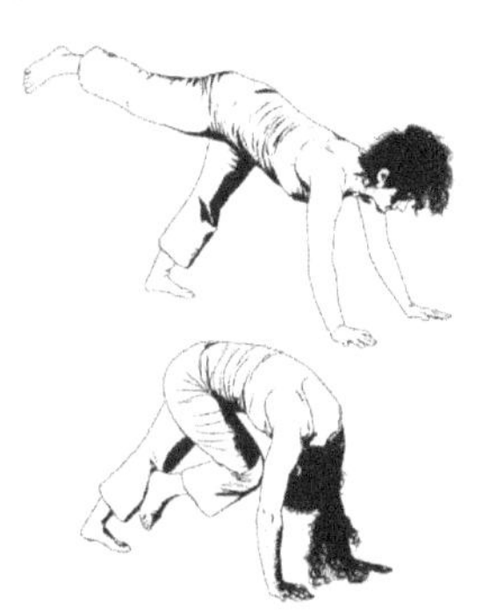
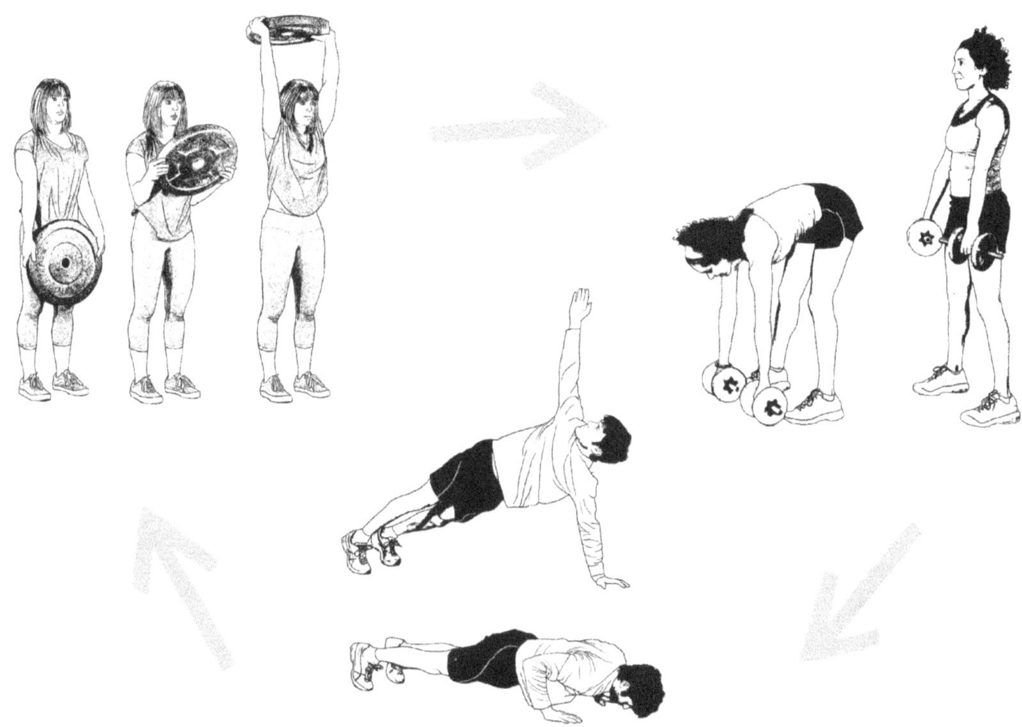
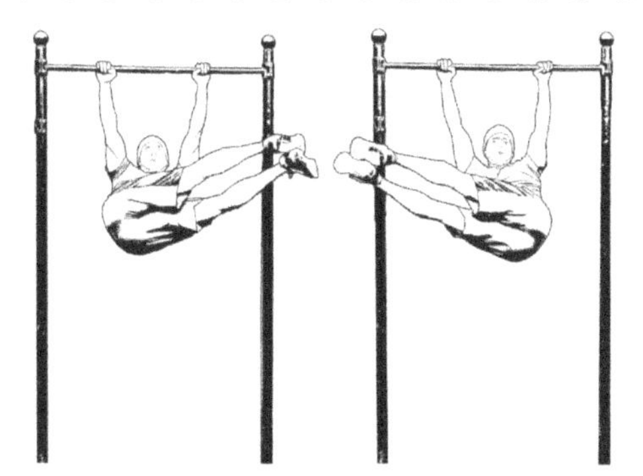
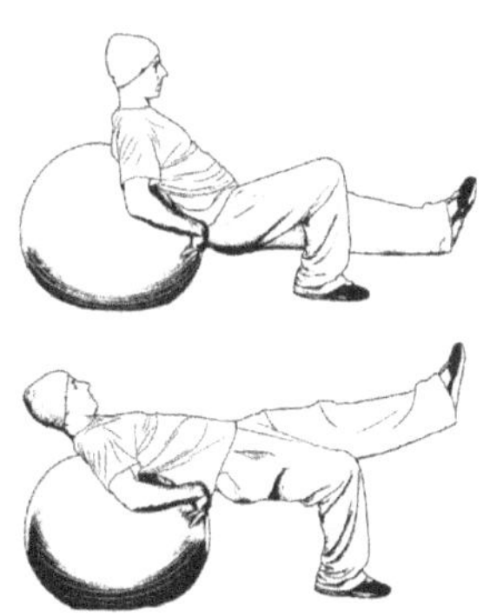

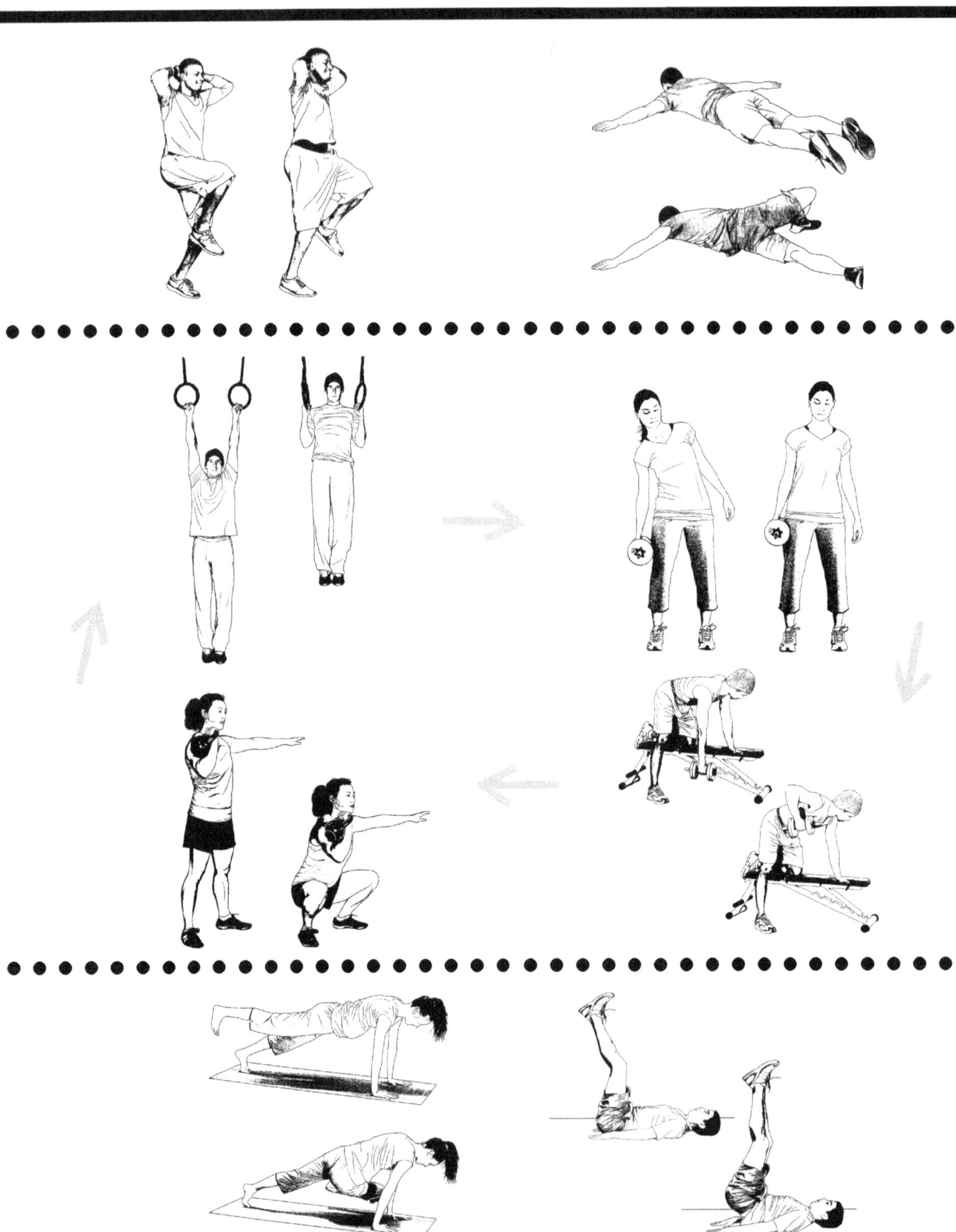

SIDE B

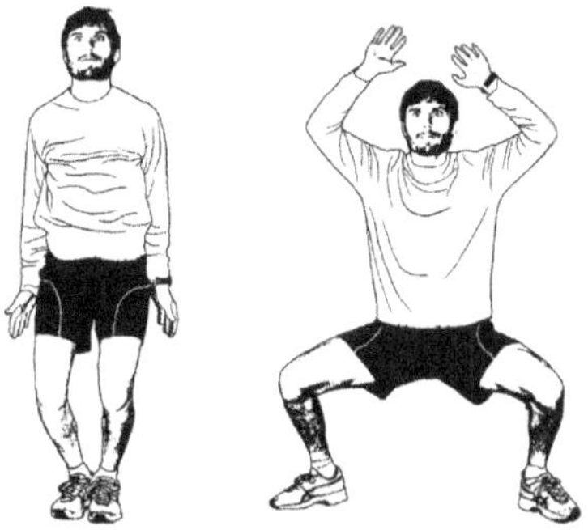

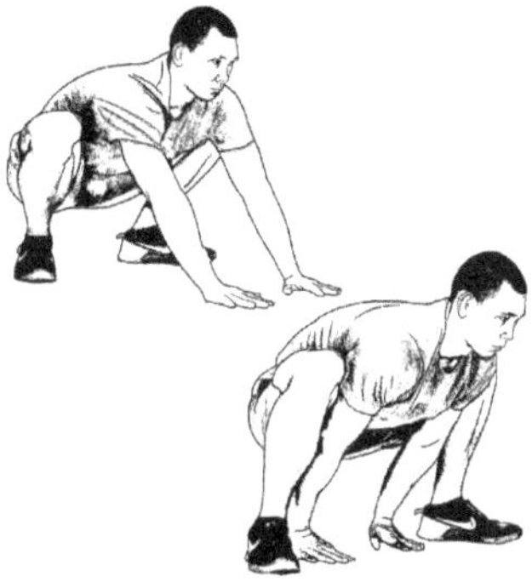

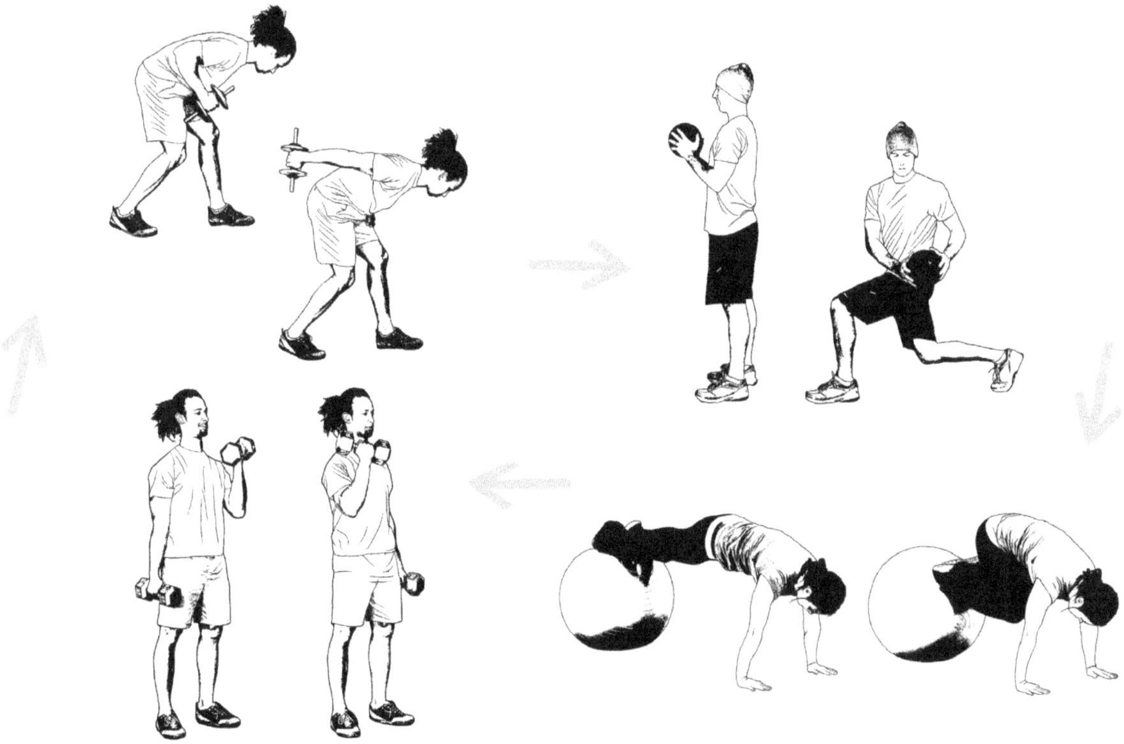

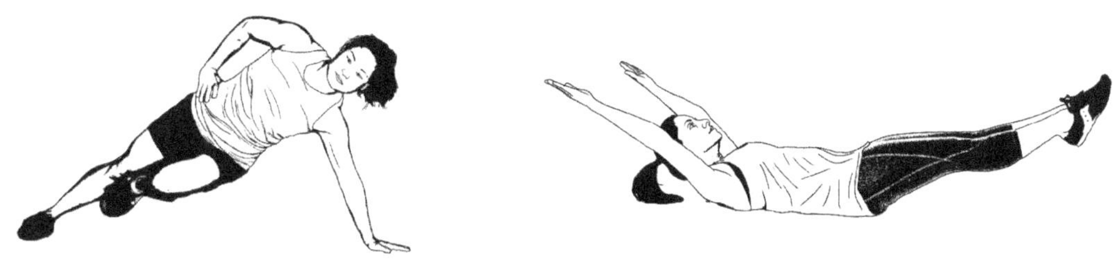

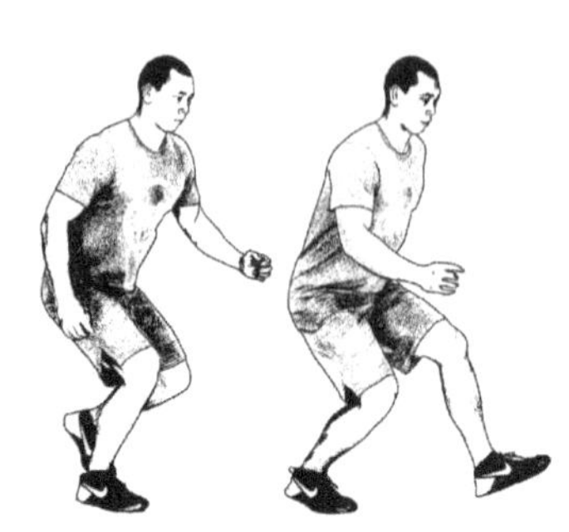

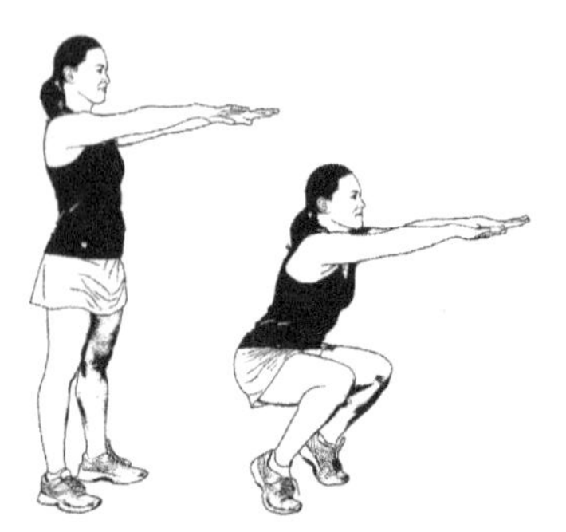

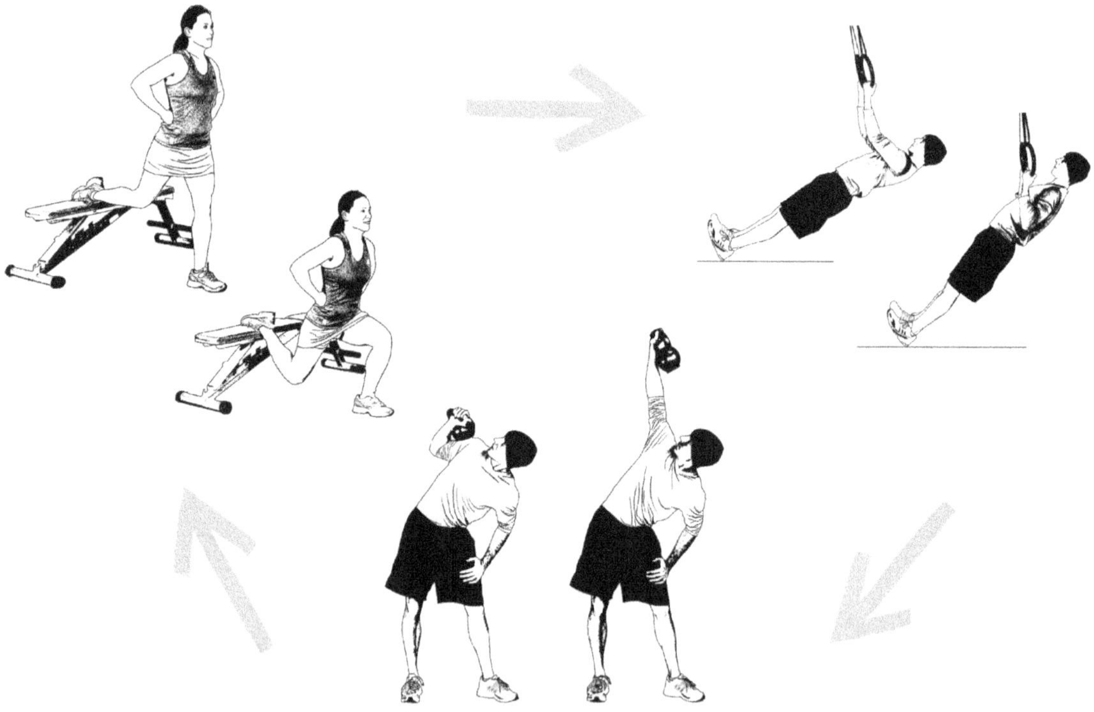

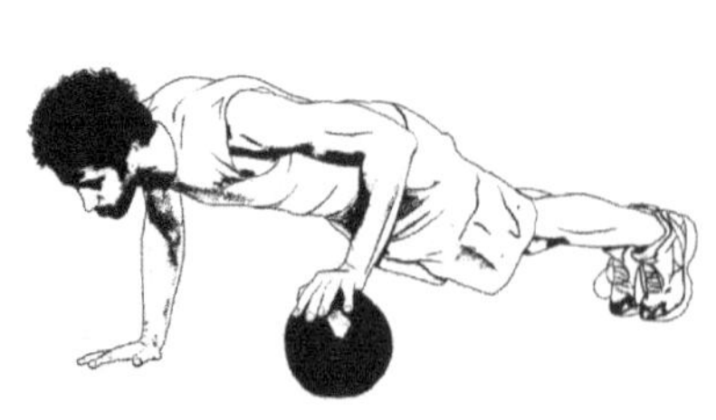

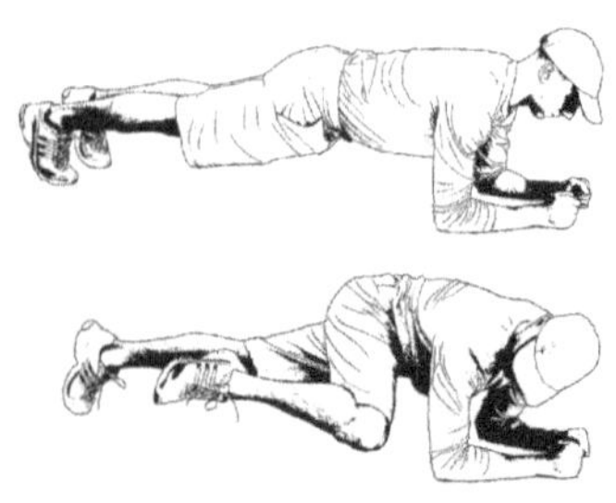

SIDE B

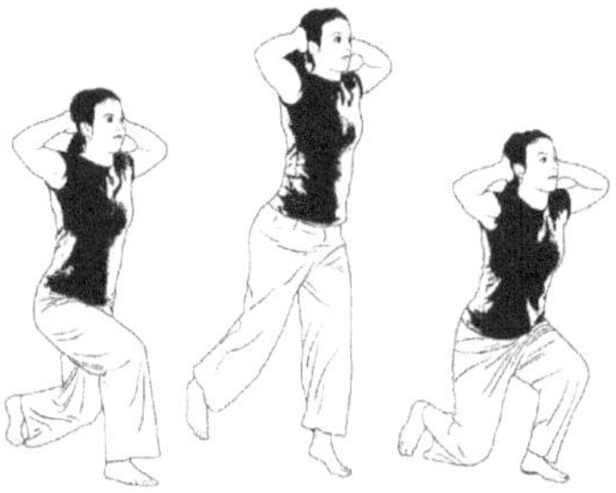

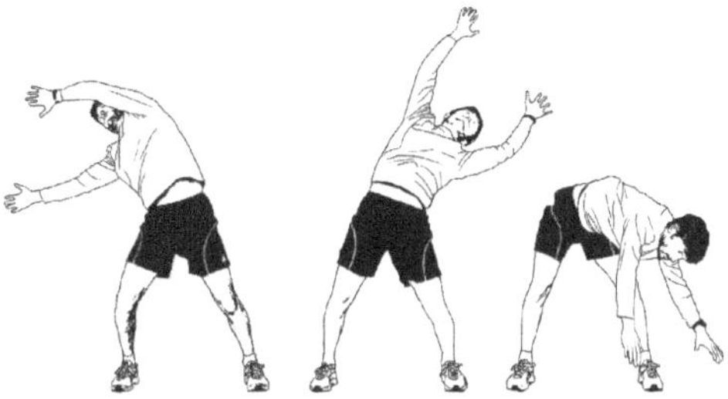

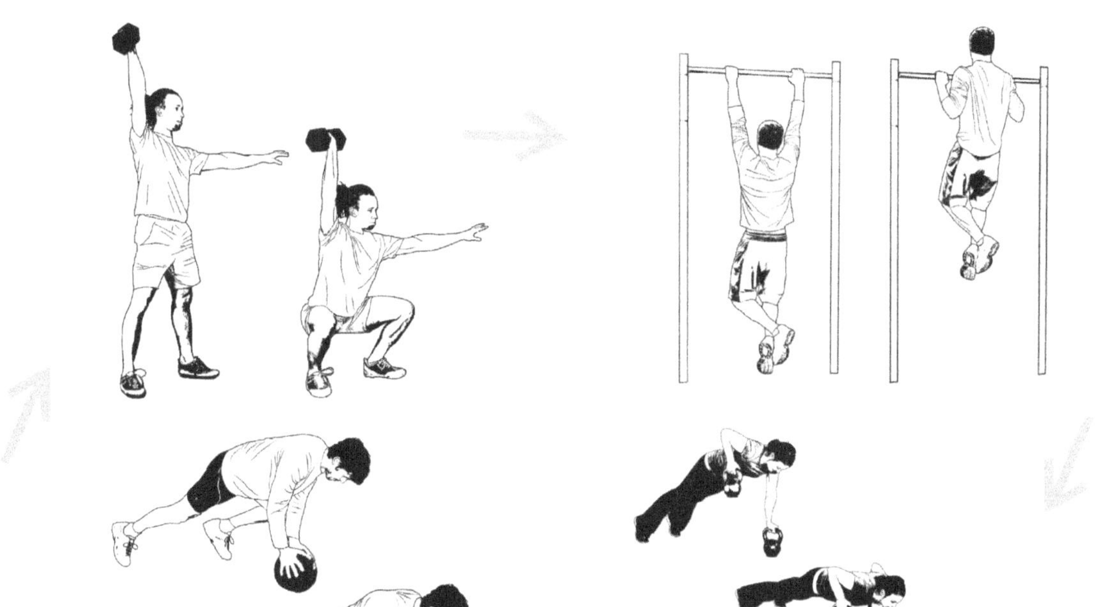

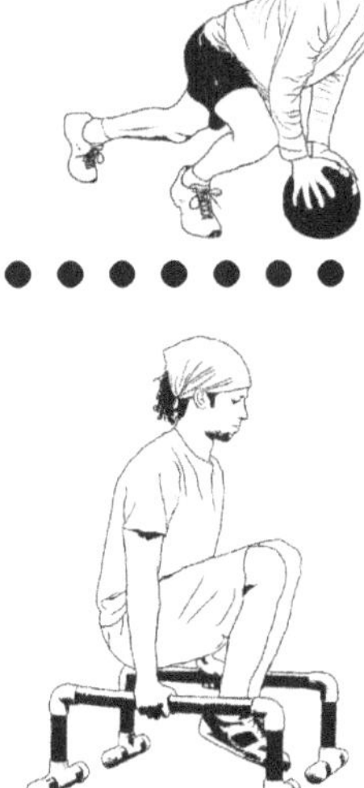

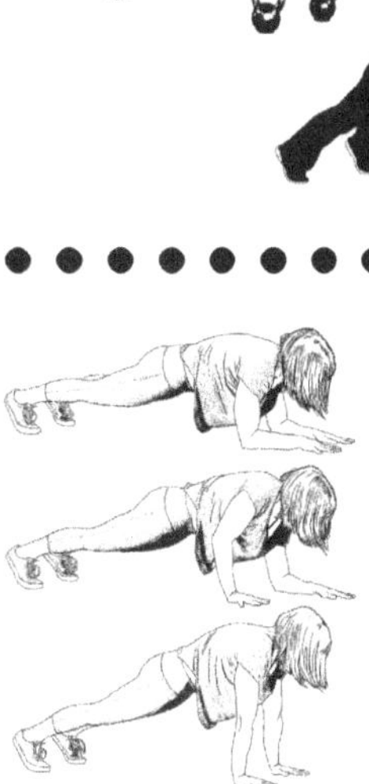

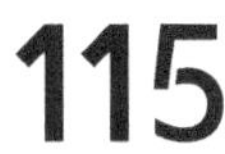

Hungry for more?

Stay to tuned for the next mixtape!

&

See more workouts at:

www.StrengthMob.com

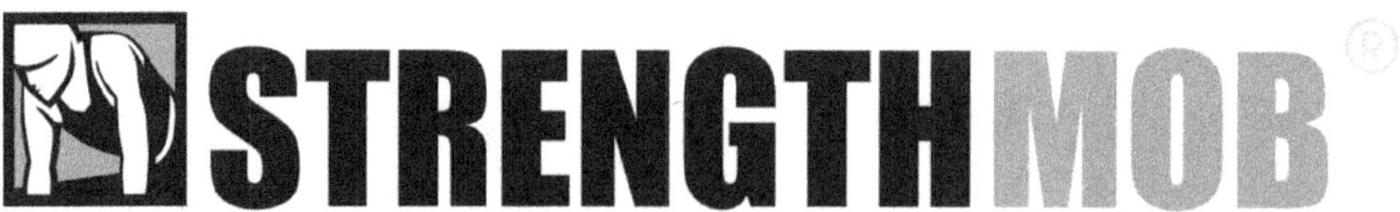

Appendix A
Workout Descriptions

Liner Notes
Appendix A

Key

KB = Kettlebell   WP = Weight Plate
DB = Dumbbell   SB = Stability Ball

"Hold" = The exercise is static, held for time.

"Reps" = The exercise is dynamic, performed for repetitions.

"Distance" = Do the exercise for a set distance across the floor.

Workouts

001.
Warm-up: Jumping Jacks & Butt Kicks
Circuit: DB Single Arm Thrusters, DB Supported Single Arm Rows, Dive Bomber Push-ups
Cool-down: Rowing V-sits & Side Plank (hold)

002.
Warm-up: Split Jumps & Cossack Squats
Circuit: KB Single Leg Romanian Deadlifts, KB Windmills, KB Side Presses, Reverse Flyes
Cool-down: Twisting Toe Touches & Plank Side Crunches

003.
Warm-up: Prisoner Lunges & Arm Circles
Circuit: KB Reverse Lunges, WP Bent-over Rows, Decline Push-ups
Cool-down: Hollow Hold, Plank Splits (reps)

004. Warm-up: Toe Taps & Air Squats
Circuit: KB Good Mornings, KB Goblet Squats, Pike Push-ups, Mountain Climber
Cool-down: Frog Leg Crunches, Side Plank & Knee Tuck (hold)

005.
Warm-up: Jump Rope & Side to Side Lunges
Circuit: DB Step-ups, DB Single Arm Preacher Curls, Narrow Grip Push-ups, Commando Crawl (distance)
Cool-down: Pelvic Thrusts, Prone Leg Extension (hold)
NOTE: If you don't have a bench, use a plyo box or steps to perform the DB Step-ups. You can support your arm on the side of piece of furniture for the Preacher Curl, or substitute with a "Concentration Curl".

LINER NOTES
Appendix A

006.
Warm-up: Twisting Jumps & Donkey Kicks
Circuit: WP Reverse Lunge & Tilts, DB Single Arm Forward Raises, DB Skull Crushers
Cool-down: Russian Twists, Arch Swimmers

007.
Warm-up: Run & Walking Toe Touches
Circuit: Burpees, Bulgarian Split Squats, WP Shoulder Curls
Cool-down: Dynamic Side V-ups, Reverse Hypers
Note: If you don't have a large plyo box, do the Reverse Hypers over the edge of strong piece of furniture. Substitute stairs or a box for the bench if you don't have one.

008.
Warm-up: Speed Skater Jumps & Trunk Circles
Circuit: Single Leg Good Mornings, KB Halos, Side Lunges, Uneven Push-ups (reps)
Cool-down: Dynamic Side Planks, Cossack Squats

009.
Warm-up: Trunk Twists with Bar & Split Jumps
Circuit: KB Kneeling Get-ups, DB Curl & Press, DB Side Bends, Squat Jumps
Cool-down: Twisting Supermans, Roll-ups

010.
Warm-up: Ankle Hops & Reaching Backbends
Circuit: KB Shoulder Presses, DB Single Arm Overhead Squats, Bird Dog Rows
Cool-down: Downward-facing Dog (hold), Cobra Pose (hold)

011.
Warm-up: Squat Kicks & Sprawls
Circuit: Single Leg Deadlift & Plate Raises, Bench Dips, Teaser V-ups, Single Leg - Mountain Climbers
Cool-down: DB Alternating Toe Touches, Side Plank on Elbow (hold)

012.
Warm-up: Sumo Squat Jumping Jacks & Med Ball Trunk Twists
Circuit: Walking Lunges, Burpees, Single Arm Curl & Presses, Quadruped Core Twists
Cool-down: Cossack Stretch (hold), Revolved Lunge (hold)

013.
Warm-up: High Stepping & Deep Lunge + Twists
Circuit: WP Overhead Squats, KB Low Windmill, Butt Scoots, Lateral Raise & Twists
Cool-down: Squat Jumps, Prone Trunk Extension (hold)

Liner Notes
Appendix A

014.
Warm-up: Jumping Jacks & Bent Over Twists
Circuit: KB Turkish Get-ups, T Push-ups, Wall Sit (hold)
Cool-down: Side Plank + Leg Lift (hold) & Twisting Planks

015.
Warm-up: Air Squats & Lateral Leg Swings
Circuit: Resisted Split Jumps, KB Swings, Towel Drags, Triple Stop Push-ups
Cool-down: Twisting Pelvic Thrusts, Box Donkey Kicks

016.
Warm-up: German Arm Swings & Prisoner Lunges
Circuit: Cossack Squat & Presses, Plank Side Hops, DB Hammer Curls, Plank Up Downs
Cool-down: V-sit (hold), Arch Hold

017.
Warm-up: Commando Jacks & Knee Circles
Circuit: KB Head Cutters, DB Lunges, KB Russian
Twists
Cool-down: Plyo Push-ups, Rotated Crunches

018.
Warm-up: Split Jacks & Froggers
Circuit: WP Thrusters, Seated Reverse Flyes, Resisted Side Lunges, Leg Drags (distance)
Cool-down: Twisting Toe Touches, One Arm Plank (hold)

019.
Warm-up: Marching Knee Tucks & Cuban Rotations
Circuit: Step-ups, Shoulder Step-ups, KB Single Leg Romanian Deadlift, KB Figure Eights
Cool-down: Flutter Kicks, Prone Trunk Extension (hold)

020.
Warm-up: Ginga & Cocorinha Squats
Circuit: Squat Jumps, Hip Thrusts, Diagonal Shoulder Press, Single Leg Bicep Curl
Cool-down: 3-Point Plank, Straddle (aka Leg Spread) Toe Touches

021.
Warm-up: Butt Kicks & Side Crawl
Circuit: WP Squats, Jackknife Push-ups, Single Arm Clean & Presses, Tuck-ups
Cool-down: Bird Dog (hold), Hollow Hold

022.
Warm-up: Med Ball Mountain Climbers & Table Top Extensions
Circuit: Offset DB Lunges, Saxon Side Bends, Lateral Raises, Push-up Arm Raises
Cool-down: Oblique Crunches (reps), Glute Bridge (hold)

023.
Warm-up: Run & Grappler Scoots
Circuit: KB Snatches, Prisoner Squats, Pike Push-ups
Cool-down: Supine Plank (hold), Feet-elevated Side Plank (hold)

024.
Warm-up: Inchworms & Hip Circles
Circuit: KB Front Squats, Single Leg Corkscrews, KB Windmills
Cool-down: Russian Push-ups, Rotated Plank (hold)

025.
Warm-up: Backward Run & Kangaroo Crawls
Circuit: DB Deadlift, WP Rows, Broad Jumps, Spiderman Push-ups
Cool-down: Tuck Hollow Hold, Arch Swimmers

026.
Warm-up: Walking Toe Touches & Crab Walk
Circuit: Reverse Lunge & Chops, Single Arm Curl & Presses, DB Side Bends, DB Front Squats
Cool-down: Side to Side Push-ups, Semi-reclined Side Crunches

027.
Warm-up: High Stepping & Hip Rotations
Circuit: Box Pistol Squats, KB Halos, KB Renegade Push-ups
Cool-down: 2-point Plank (hold), Raised Knee Crunches (reps)

028.
Warm-up: Walking Lunges & Trunk Twists
Circuit: KB Sots Presses , Air Squats, Incline Push-ups, Single Leg Good Mornings
Cool-down: Side Plank Leg Swings, Marching Bridges (hold bridge)

029.
Warm-up: Cossack Squats & Knee to Faces
Circuit: Corkscrew, KB Twisting Crunches, Sissy Squats, Decline Push-ups
Cool-down: Bent Over Twists, Extended Puppy Pose (hold)

030.
Warm-up: Carioca & Grappler Scoots
Circuit: Sandbag Overhead Squats, Single Arm Reverse Flyes, Standing Plate Presses, Shoulder Tap Push-ups
Cool-down: Windshield Wipers, Prone Leg Extension (hold)
NOTE: Substitute a loaded duffle bag or backpack if you don't have sandbag to use.

031.
Warm-up: Skip & Side Crawl
Circuit: KB Split Squats, DB Twisting Shoulder Presses, KB Get-up Sit-ups
Cool-down: Cartwheel Push-ups (reps), Saw

032.
Warm-up: Lunge Kicks & Sprawl
Circuit: Wood Chop Lunges, Cross-over Step-ups, KB Presses, Double Leg Raises
Cool-down: Leg Twist Push-ups, Resisted Sit-ups

033.
Warm-up: Split Jumps & Single Leg Toe Touches
Circuit: KB Reverse Lunges, DB Burpees, Lateral Raise & External Rotation
Cool-down: Dead Bugs, Pike Compressions

034.
Warm-up: High Stepping & Butt Scoots
Circuit: Crouched Single Leg Squats, DB Clean & Presses, DB Single Leg Rows,
Speed Skater Jumps
Cool-down: Hollow Arch Rolls, Scissors

035.
Warm-up: Jumping Jacks & Quadrupedal Movement
Circuit: KB Goblet Squats, Reverse Lunge & Tilts, Push-up Plusses
Cool-down: Reverse Crunches, 3-point Plank on Elbows

036.
Warm-up: Toe Taps & Squat to Stands
Circuit: Squatting Calf Raises, Butterfly Hip Thrusts, Alternating Forward Raises,
Breakdance Push-ups
Cool-down: 3-point Supine Plank (hold), Butterfly Sit-up

037.
Warm-up: Jump Rope & Supine Scorpions
Circuit: Single Arm DB Snatches, DB Step-ups, KB Waist Circles, Leg Raise Push-ups (reps)
Cool-down: Twisting Crunches, Arch Swimmers

038.
Warm-up: Butt Kicks & Pelvis Circles
Circuit: Single Arm KB Swings, KB Push Presses, Cossack Squats, Alligator Crawls
Cool-down: Plank Side Hops, Twisting Sit-ups

LINER NOTES
Appendix A

039.
Warm-up: Twisting Lunges & Prone Scorpions
Circuit: DB Swing (single arm), KB Side Presses, Plank KB Drags
Cool-down: Double Leg Raises, 3-point Plank (hold)

040.
Warm-up: Crouched Walk & Deep Lunge + Twists
Circuit: Sandbag Shoulder Clean, Squat Jumps, DB Diagonal Shoulder Presses,
Standing Crunches
Cool-down: Dynamic Side Planks, Fish Hook Crunches

041.
Warm-up: Twisting Jumps & Side Crawls
Circuit: Alternating KB Swing, Air Squat, Supported Plank Rows, Pike Push-ups
Cool-down: Sprinting V-sits, One Arm Plank (hold)

042.
Warm-up: Carioca & Side Step Squats
Circuit: KB Single Arm Front Rack Squat, KB Press Crunches, Supported Bent Over
Rows, KB Reach and Twists
Cool-down: Prone Alternating Arm & Leg Lifts, Twisting Pelvic Thrusts

043.
Warm-up: Shadow Box & Knee Bends
Circuit: DB Suitcase Deadlifts, Rotate Push-ups, Box Squat Jumps, DB Single Arm
Forward Raises
Cool-down: Floor Trunk Twists, 2-point Plank on Elbows

044.
Warm-up: Split Jacks & Hip Cradles
Circuit: Kneeling Overhead Thrusts, Cossack Squats, Single Arm Skull Crusher, KB
Bent Over Rows
Cool-down: Med Ball Trunk Twists, Arch Rocks

045.
Warm-up: High Stepping & Bear Crawls
Circuit: KB Single Leg Romanian Deadlifts, KB Shot Put Presses, Elevated Front Foot
Split Squats, Twist & Lateral Raises
Cool-down: Side Plank & Leg Lift, Toe Touch Crunches

LINER NOTES
Appendix A

046.
Warm-up: Knee Circles & Prone Scorpions
Circuit: DB Forward Lunges, Wood Chops, Alternating DB Shoulder Presses,
DB Hammer Curls
Cool-down: Split Leg Crunches, Table Top Extensions

047.
Warm-up: Forward Leg Swings & Arm Circle
Circuit: DB Single Arm Thrusters, Lateral Leg Raise Push-ups, DB Cross Curls,
KB Figure Eights
Cool-down: Tuck-ups, Plank on Elbows (hold)

048.
Warm-up: Prisoner Lunges & German Arm Swings
Circuit: DB Front Squats, KB 3-point Rows, Jackknife Push-ups, Russian Twists
Cool-down: Semi-reclined Side Crunches, Arch Hold

049.
Warm-up: Jumping Jacks & Side to Side Lunges
Circuit: Sandbag Cleans, Burpees, Canoe Squats
Cool-down: Straddle Hollow Hold, Twisting Supermans

050.
Warm-up: Ankle Hops & Mountain Climbers
Circuit: KB Deadlifts, Pike Push-ups, Lateral Raises, Dynamic Side Planks
Cool-down: Roll-ups, Side Plank on Elbow (hold)

051.
Warm-up: Twisting Lunges & Pelvis Circles
Circuit: DB Single Arm Overhead Squat, Resisted Split Jumps, Push-ups
Cool-down: Rowing Crunches, Prone Trunk Extension (hold)

052.
Warm-up: Jumping Jacks & Marching Knee Tucks
Circuit: Sandbag Alternating Squat Presses, KB Bent Over Rows, Walking Lunges,
Spiderman Push-ups
Cool-down: Hollow Rocks, Sit-up Wall Balls

053.
Warm-up: Squat Kicks & Froggers
Circuit: DB Single Arm Clean & Presses, Horse Stance Squats, DB Single Arm Skull
Crushers, KB Waist Circles
Cool-down: Teaser V-ups, Outrigger Push-ups

LINER NOTES
Appendix A

054.
Warm-up: Butt Kicks & Trunk Circles
Circuit: KB Single Arm Front Squat, DB Single Arm Reverse Flyes, KB Single Arm Push Presses
Cool-down: Feet-elevated Russian Twists, 3-point Plank (hold)

055.
Warm-up: Commando Jacks & Inchworms
Circuit: KB Swings, KB Get-up Sit-ups, Pike Push-ups, DB Cuban Rotations
Cool-down: Plank Splits, Hundreds

056.
Warm-up: Bent Over Twists & Ankle Circles
Circuit: KB Cleans, Bodyweight Chest Flyes, KB Bottoms-up Curls, Squatting Calf Raises
Cool-down: 3-point Supine Plank (hold), Rowing V-sits

057.
Warm-up: Split Jacks & Trunk Twists
Circuit: Reverse Lunge & Tilts, DB Sumo Deadlifts, KB Bottoms-up Carries, DB Side Bends
Cool-down: Stacked Feet Push-ups, Flutter Kicks (reps)

058.
Warm-up: High Stepping & Donkey Kicks
Circuit: KB Kneeling Get-ups, KB Good Mornings, Diamond Push-ups (reps), DB Overhead Lateral Raises
Cool-down: Horizontal Scissors, Prone Leg Extension (hold)

059.
Warm-up: Lateral Leg Swings & Burpees
Circuit: KB Goblet Squats, Scapular-plane Raises, Bench Dips, DB Toe Touches
Cool-down: Hollow Hold, Quadruped Skiers

060.
Warm-up: Speed Skater Jumps & Kangaroo Crawls
Circuit: WP Single Leg Deadlift, Standing Plate Presses, WP Hammer Curls
Cool-down: Scorpion Push-ups, Sit-ups

061.
Warm-up: DB Swings & Med Ball Mountain Climbers
Circuit: WP Clean & Presses, WP Rows, Commando Pull-ups, Stability Ball Jackknifes
Cool-down: Med Ball Push-ups, Side Plank – Feet Elevated (hold)

062.
Warm-up: Indian Club Overhead Swings & Indian Club Back Strokes
Circuit: Med Ball Squat Cleans, Ring Rows, Parallette Push-ups
Cool-down: SB Skiers, Plank Splits
Note: If you don't have Indian Clubs, substitute with light dumbbells (1-2 lbs), or water bottles. Also, the more horizontal your body is during ring rows, the harder they become.

063.
Warm-up: Split Jumps & Single Arm KB Swings
Circuit: WP Squats, Single Arm DB Chest Press, Knees to Elbows, Single Arm DB Preacher Curl
Cool-down: Frog Leg Crunches, Box Donkey Kicks

064.
Warm-up: Twisting Jumps & Standing Crunches
Circuit: WP Overhead Squats, Ring Push-ups, DB Bench Pull-Overs, KB Waist Circles
Cool-down: Overhead Weighted Sit-ups, Plank Arm Raises
Note: The more horizontal your body is during ring push-ups, the harder they are.

065.
Warm-up: Swing Squats & Hip Circles
Circuit: Box Jumps, Dive Bomber Push-ups, Chin-ups
Cool-down: Straddle Hollow Hold, Twisting Supermans

066.
Warm-up: Sumo Squat Jumping Jacks & Plank Walks
Circuit: Single Leg Deadlift & Plate Raises, Side to Side Pull-ups, Jackknife Push-ups, Side to Side Lunges
Cool-down: Reverse Hyper Kick-outs, Uneven Push-ups (reps)

067.
Warm-up: Toe Taps & Gingas
Circuit: Med Ball Slams, Bulgarian Split Squats, Ring Tuck Hold, WP Truck Drivers
Cool-down: SB Roll-out, SB Push-up

068.
Warm-up: Skier Raises & Ankle Circles
Circuit: Broad Jumps, DB Single Arm Thrusters, DB Step-ups, Narrow Grip Chin-ups
Cool-down: Dynamic Side Planks, Quadruped Core Twists

069.
Warm-up: Swing Squats & Wrist Circles
Circuit: Staggered Push-ups, Parallette Tuck Hold, KB American Swings, Counter Balance Pistols
Cool-down: Russian Twists, Prone Leg Extension (hold)

070.
Warm-up: Jump Rope & Standing Side Bends,
Circuit: WP Curl & Presses, Hanging Trunk Twists, KB Cleans, Cossack Squats
Cool-down: SB Back Extensions, Plank of Elbows

071.
Warm-up: Walking Toe Touches & Mountain Climbers
Circuit: SB Single Leg Presses, Chin-ups, Sandbag Get-ups, Narrow Grip Push-ups
Cool-down: Bicycle Crunches (reps), Side Plank & Leg Lift (hold)

072.
Warm-up: High Stepping & Air Squats
Circuit: Ring Dips, Alternating Rows, Resisted Side Lunges
Cool-down: Tuck Hollow Hold, 3-point Plank on Elbows (hold)

073.
Warm-up: Jumping Jacks & Quadruped Skiers
Circuit: Parallette Dips, Ring Bicep Curls, DB Overhead Lunges, SB Skiers
Cool-down: Windshield Wipers, SB Stir the Pot (reps)

074.
Warm-up: Jump Rope & Marching Knee Tucks
Circuit: Suspension Trainer Pistol Squats, WP Curl & Raises, SB Decline Push-ups,
Parallette Kick-outs
Cool-down: Rowing Crunches, Side Plank Leg Swings

075.
Warm-up: Carioca & Side Crawls
Circuit: Suspension Trainer Bulgarian Split Squats, Wall Balls, SB Punches, WP Halo
Cool-down: Pelvic Thrusts, Flutter Kicks

076.
Warm-up: Commando Jacks & Bear Crawls
Circuit: KB Suitcase Deadlift, KB Reach & Twists, SB Walk-outs, L Hang (hold)
Cool-down: Stability Ball Passes, Straddle Hollow Hold

077.
Warm-up: Run & Knee Circles
Circuit: KB Single Arm Swings, Ring Pull-ups, Squat Jumps, Parallette L-sit (hold)
Cool-down: Pike Compressions, Push-up Hold

078.
Warm-up: Butt Kicks & Pelvis Circles
Circuit: DB Burpees, KB Single Arm Front Squats, WP Curl and Presses
Cool-down: SB Back Extensions, Plank Up Downs

079.
Warm-up: Squat Kicks & SB Mountain Climbers
Circuit: SB Leg Press, Resisted Split Jumps, WP Shoulder Curls, Ring Tuck Hold
Cool-down: Shoulder Tap Push-ups, Hanging Leg Scissors

080.
Warm-up: Split Jumps & Knee Bends
Circuit: Elevated Front Foot Split Squats, Wide Grip Pull-ups, Bodyweight Skull Crushers, KB Low Windmills
Cool-down: SB Oblique Crunches

081.
Warm-up: Sumo Squat Jumping Jacks & Karate Skips
Circuit: Med Ball Thrusters, Parallete Shoot Throughs, KB Single Leg Romanian Deadlifts, Dive Bomber Push-ups
Cool-down: SB Pikes, Russian Twists

082.
Warm-up: Split Jacks & Bear Crawls
Circuit: DB Goblet Squats, Supported Plank Rows, Twisting Shoulder Presses
Cool-down: Reverse Hypers, Hollow Rocks

083.
Warm-up: Jumping Jacks & Med Ball Mountain Climbers
Circuit: KB Snatches, Parallette Push-ups, Reverse Flyes, L Pull-ups
Cool-down: Straddle V-ups, Side Plank Leg Swings

084.
Warm-up: High Stepping & Table Top Extensions
Circuit: KB Front Squats, Bench Dips with Ball, Farmer Carries, WP Hammer Curls
Cool-down: Plank Side Hops, Modified Crunches

085.
Warm-up: Squat to Stands & Side Crawls
Circuit: DB Offset Lunges, DB Concentration Curls, Jackknife Push-ups, Parallette Tuck Hold
Cool-down: SB Push-ups, Straddle Toe Touches

086.
Warm-up: Forward Leg Swings & Shoulder Dislocates
Circuit: DB Step-ups, DB Alternating Bicep Curls, DB Single Arm Shoulder Press, Ring Tuck Hold
Cool-down: Toes to Bar (reps), Prone Leg Extension (hold)

Liner Notes
Appendix A

087.
Warm-up: Prisoner Squats & Lateral Bench Hops
Circuit: Toenail Pistols, KB Bent-arm Bottoms-up Carries, Decline Push-ups, Inverted Rows
Cool-down: Plank Side Crunches, V-sit (hold)

088.
Warm-up: KB Swings &Twisting Jumps
Circuit: WP Overhead Squats, DB Shot Put Presses, Archer Pull-ups
Cool-down: Twisting Planks, Knee Grab Sit-ups

089.
Warm-up: Trunk Twists with Bar & SB Hip Thrusts
Circuit: WP Single Leg Deadlift & Overhead Raises, Chin-ups, Ring Chest Flyes, Parallette Single Leg L-sit
Cool-down: Towel Drags, Twisting Supermans
Note: Make the Chest Flyes easier by starting in a more vertical position.

090.
Warm-up: Speed Skater Jumps & Forward Lunges
Circuit: DB Front Squats, Box Jumps, Ring Rows, Uneven Push-ups (reps)
Cool-down: Semi-reclined Side Crunches, Straddle Hollow Hold

091.
Warm-up: Cariocas & Plank Side Steps
Circuit: DB Single Arm Clean & Presses, Elevated Feet Wall Push-ups, Wall Sit & Med Ball Raise (hold), Ring Bicep Curls
Cool-down: Ab Roller, Reverse Hyper Kick-outs

092.
Warm-up: Ankle Hops & Walking Lunges
Circuit: Atlas Squats, KB Bottoms-Up Curl, WP Forward Raises, Mountain Climbers
Cool-down: SB Hip Rolls, 3-point Plank (hold)

093.
Warm-up: Butt Kicks & Sprawls
Circuit: Ring Dips, KB Suitcase Carries, KB Deadlifts, KB Halos
Cool-down: Plank Splits, Twisting Pelvic Thrusts

094.
Warm-up: Jump Rope & Burpees
Circuit: DB Single Arm Split Snatches, Ring Archer Push-ups, Resisted Side Lunges
Cool-down: Arch Hold, Roll-ups
Note: Scale back the archer push-ups with regular ring push-ups. Remember, the more vertical you are, the easier they become.

095.
Warm-up: Tiptoe Squats & Bent Over Twists
Circuit: Single Bar Dips, KB Kneeling Get-ups, DB Single Arm Reverse Flyes, Squat Jumps
Cool-down: KB Twisting Crunches, SB Punches
Note: If you can't do it or have access to a bar to perform a single bar dip, substitute with ring dips.

096.
Warm-up: Split Jumps & Quadrupedal Movement
Circuit: Rotating Lunges, Decline Push-ups, Straddle L-sit (hold), KB 3-point Rows
Cool-down: Rope Climbing V-sit, Plank on Elbows

97.
Warm-up: Jumping Jacks & Plate Pushes
Circuit: KB Goblet Squats, DB Alternating Toe Touches, Single Arm Hang (hold), Pike Push-ups
Cool-down: Frog Leg Raises, Side Plank on Elbow
Note: If you don't have a plate to push, use a towel or anything else that will slide along the ground.

98.
Warm-up: Med Ball Mountain Climbers & Reaching Backbends
Circuit: Ring L-sit (hold), Twisting Shoulder Presses, Dumbbell Lunges
Cool-down: Fist Push-ups, Horizontal Scissors

099.
Warm-up: Marching Knee Tucks & Trunk Circles
Circuit: DB Step-ups, KB Double Windmills, Parallette Push-ups, DB Supported Single Arm Rows
Cool-down: Arch Swimmers, Raised Knee Crunches (reps)

100.
Warm-up: KB Swings & Single Leg Mountain Climbers
Circuit: Reverse Lunge & Tilts, Ring Rows, KB Side Press
Cool-down: Ballistic Push-ups, Towel Floor Clean

101.
Warm-up: Indian Club Overhead Swings & Pelvis Circles
Circuit: DB Single Arm Overhead Squats, WP Rows, KB Reach & Twists, Cossack Squats
Cool-down: Pseudo Planche Push-ups, Fish Hook Crunches

LINER NOTES
Appendix A

102.
Warm-up: Prisoner Lunges & Arm Circles
Circuit: Parallette Tuck Hold, Ring Push-ups, Inverted Rows, Sandbag Front Squats
Cool-down: Dynamic Planks, Russian Twists - Feet Elevated

103.
Warm-up: High Stepping & Dive Bomber Push-ups
Circuit: KB Snatches KB Renegade Push-ups, Pull-ups
Cool-down: Overhead Weighted Sit-ups, Prone Trunk Extension (hold)

104.
Warm-up: KB Waist Circles & Side Step Squats
Circuit: Ring Dips, KB Single Leg Romanian Deadlifts, Med Ball Mountain Climbers, Seated Reverse Flyes
Cool-down: Toe Touch Crunches, Reverse Hypers

105.
Warm-up: Cossack Squats & Indian Club Lateral Raises
Circuit: Ballistic Push-ups, WP Overhead Squats, Spiderman Pull-ups
Cool-down: Toes to Bar (reps), Straddle Hollow Hold

106.
Warm-up: KB Alternating Swings & Overhead Squats
Circuit: Mixed Grip Pull-ups, DB Chest Flyes, DB Single Arm Thrusters
Cool-down: SB Single Leg Pikes, Single Leg Push-ups

107.
Warm-up: Toe Taps & Karate Skips
Circuit: WP Squats, WP Overhead Carries (distance), Prone Leg Extension (reps), Ring Rows
Cool-down: Push-ups, Teaser V-ups

108.
Warm-up: Squat Kicks & Inchworms
Circuit: DB Diagonal Shoulder Presses, KB Goblet Squats, Wide Grip Pull-ups, KB Russian Twists
Cool-down: Flutter Kicks, Prone Alternating Arm & Leg Lifts

109.
Warm-up: Commando Jacks & Lunge Kicks
Circuit: DB Thrusters, Corkscrews, Diamond Push-ups, Knees to Elbows
Cool-down: Dynamic Side Planks, Plank Arm Raises

110.
Warm-up: Prisoner Squats & Lateral Leg Swings
Circuit: KB Split Squats, Squat Jumps, SB Weight Rolls, DB Bent Over Rows
Cool-down: Rotated Crunches, Leg Twist Push-ups

111.
Warm-up: Single Leg Toe Touches & Knee to Face (reps)
Circuit: WP Curl & Press, DB Stiff Leg Deadlift, T Push-up
Cool-down: Hanging Windshield Wipers, SB Single Leg Hip Thrusts

112.
Warm-up: High Stepping & Prone Scorpions
Circuit: Ring Pull-ups, DB Side Bends, DB Supported Single Arm Rows,
KB Single Arm Front Squats
Cool-down: Twisting Planks, Pelvic Thrusts

113.
Warm-up: Commando Jacks & Froggers
Circuit: DB Single Arm Tricep Kickback, Reverse Lunge & Chop, SB Jackknifes,
DB Alternating Bicep Curls
Cool-down: Side Plank Knee Tucks, Hollow Hold

114.
Warm-up: Crouched Walk & Tip Toe Squats
Circuit: Bulgarian Split Squats, Ring Bicep Curls, KB Side Presses
Cool-down: Uneven Push-ups (reps), Plank Side Crunches

115.
Warm-up: Split Jumps & Trunk Circles
Circuit: DB Overhead Squats, Pull-ups, KB Renegade Push-ups,
Med Ball Mountain Climbers
Cool-down: Parallette Tuck Hold, Plank Up Downs

Appendix B
EXERCISE PROGRESSIONS

These progressions are suggestions only. Your baseline mobility or strength could make a more "advanced" movement seem easier than its predecessor. Proceed with an open mind.

Liner Notes
Appendix B

Squat Progression

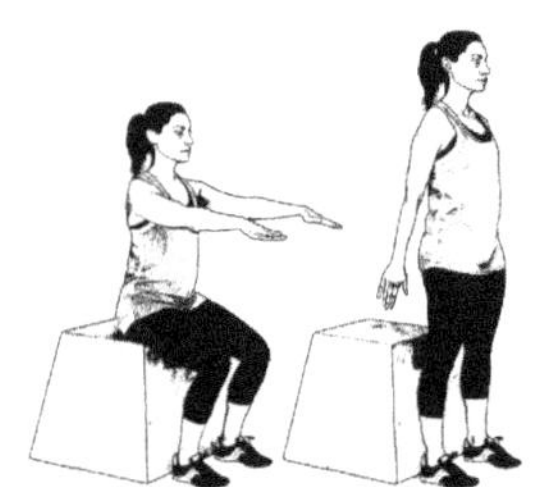

1.

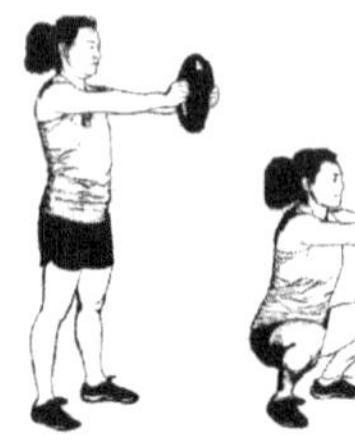

2.

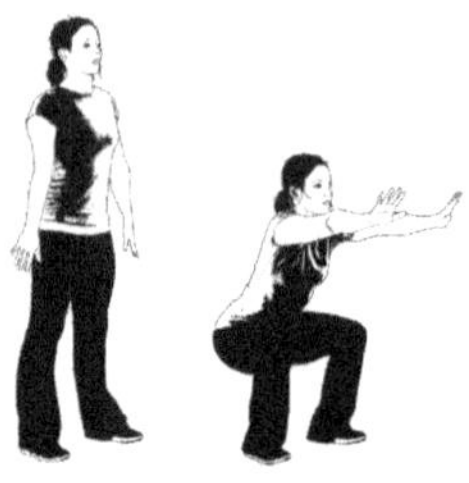

3.

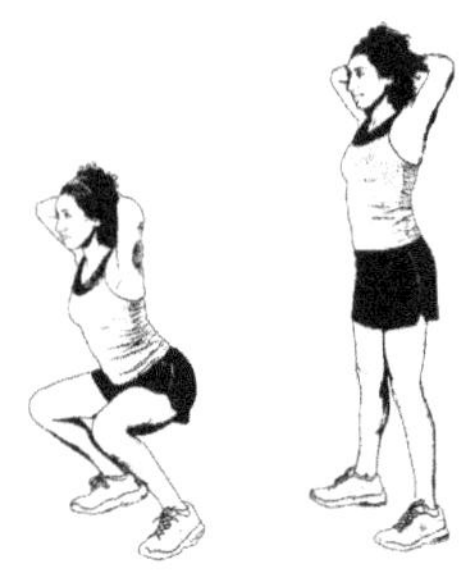

4.

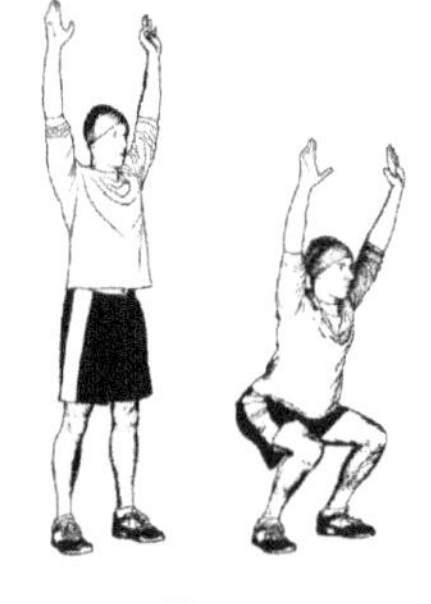

5.

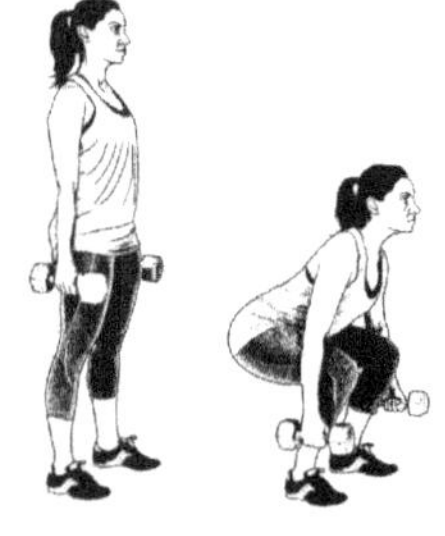

6.

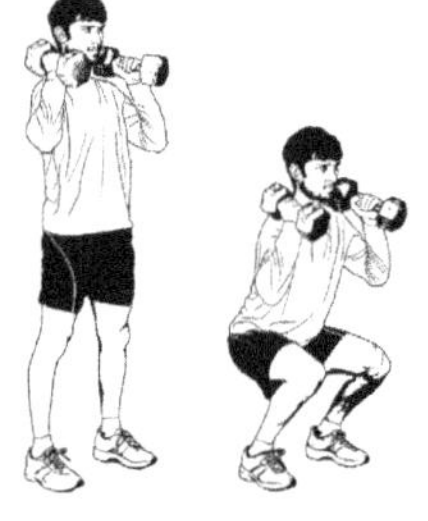

7.

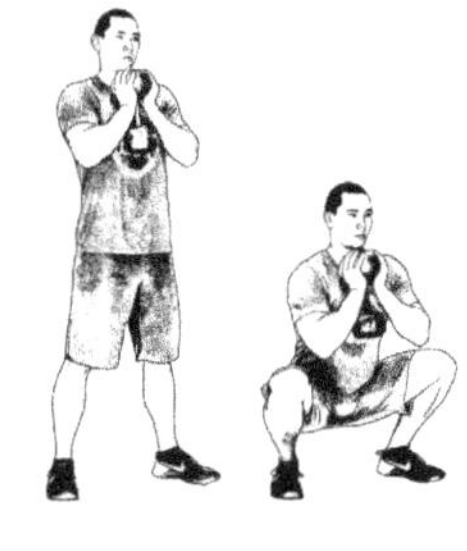

8.

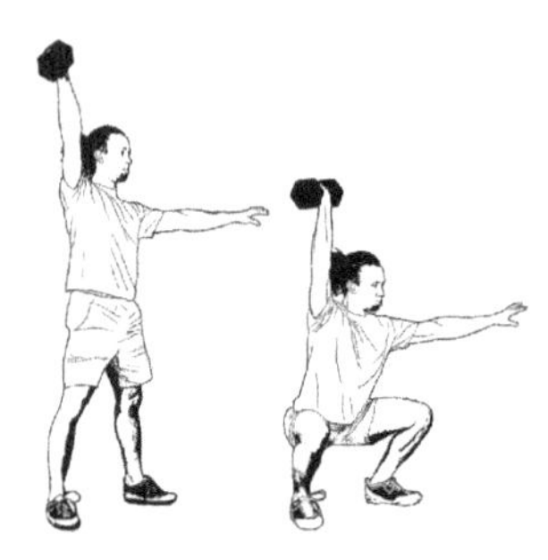

9.

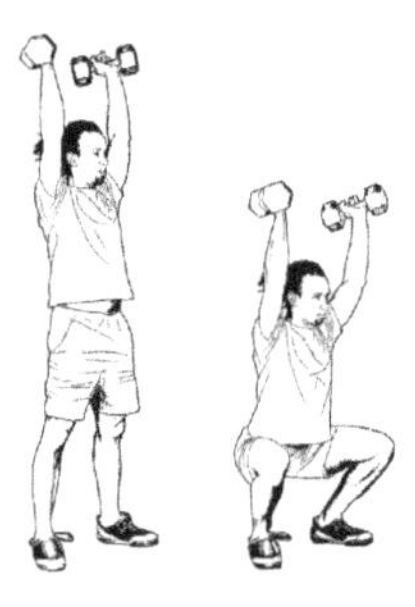

10.

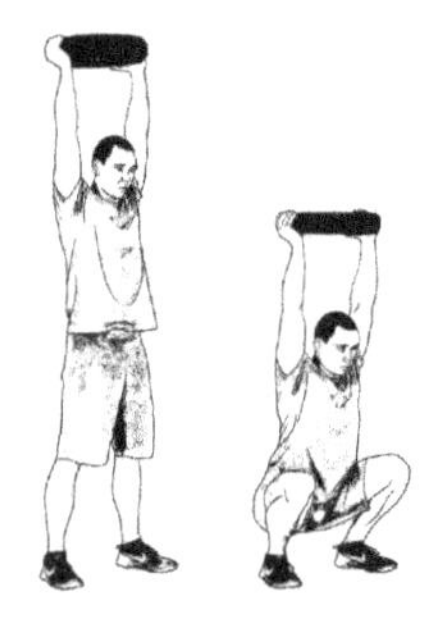

11.

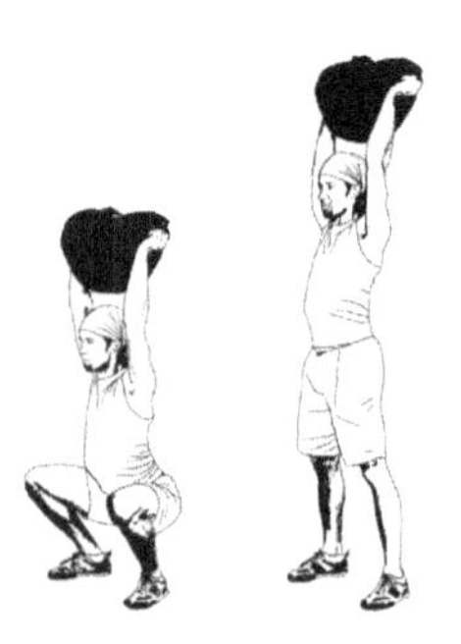

12.

AB-01

LINER NOTES
Appendix B

Pistol Progression

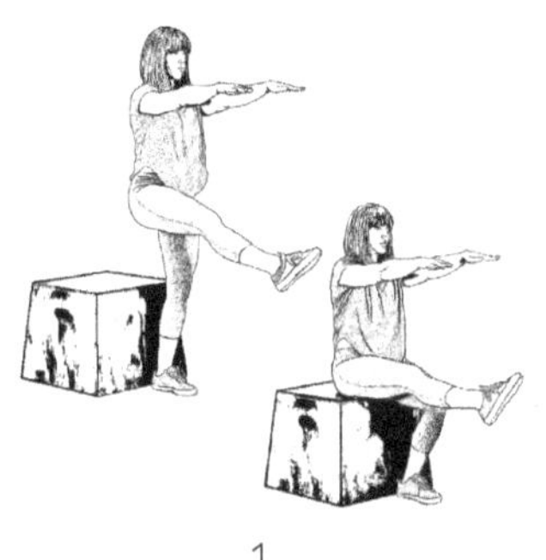

1.

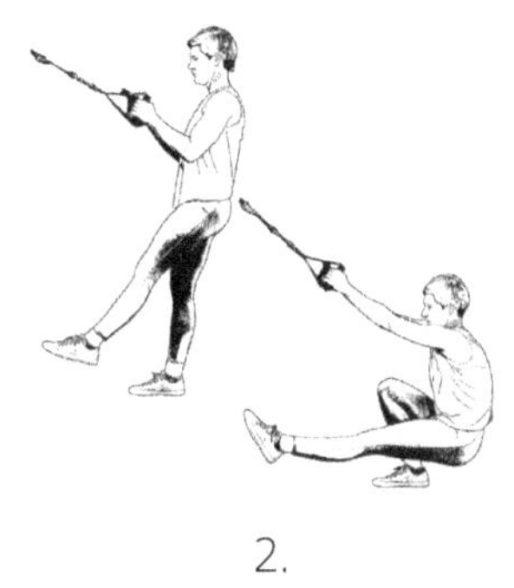

2.

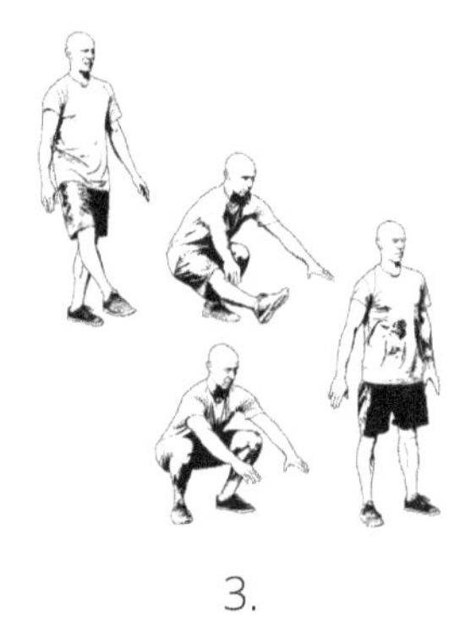

3.

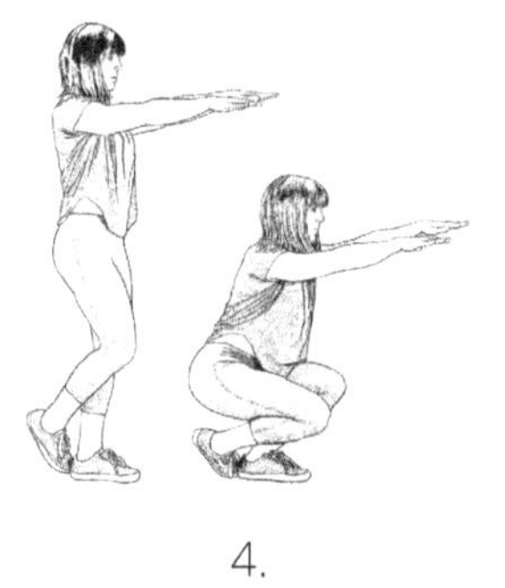

4.

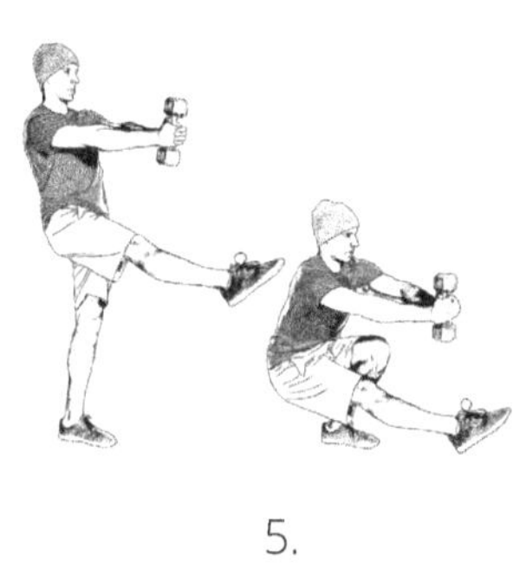

5.

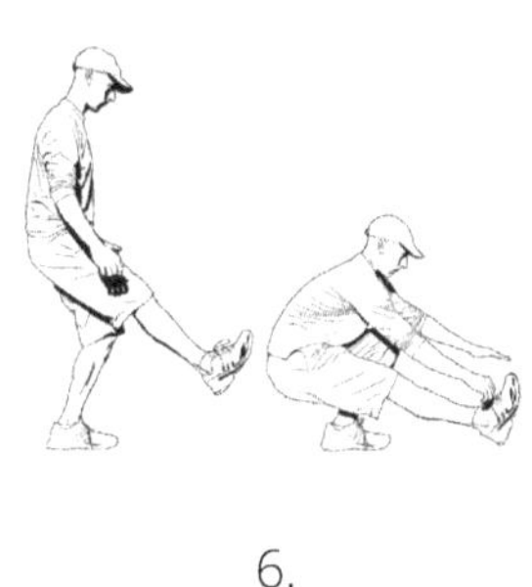

6.

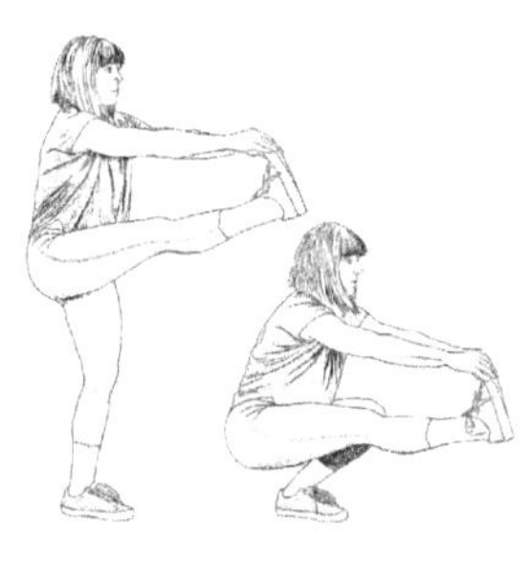

7.

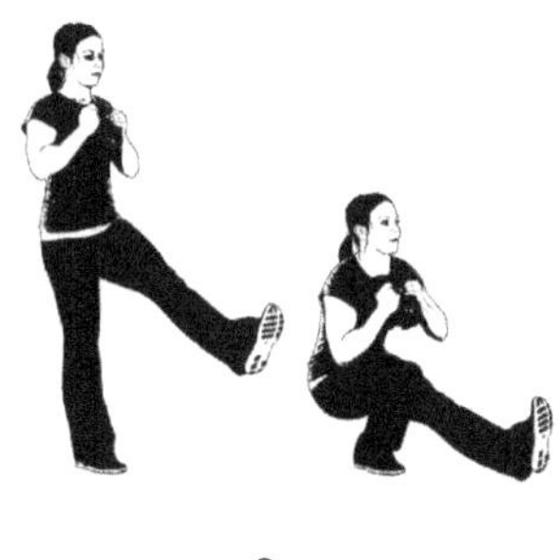

8.

Liner Notes
Appendix B

Push-up Progression

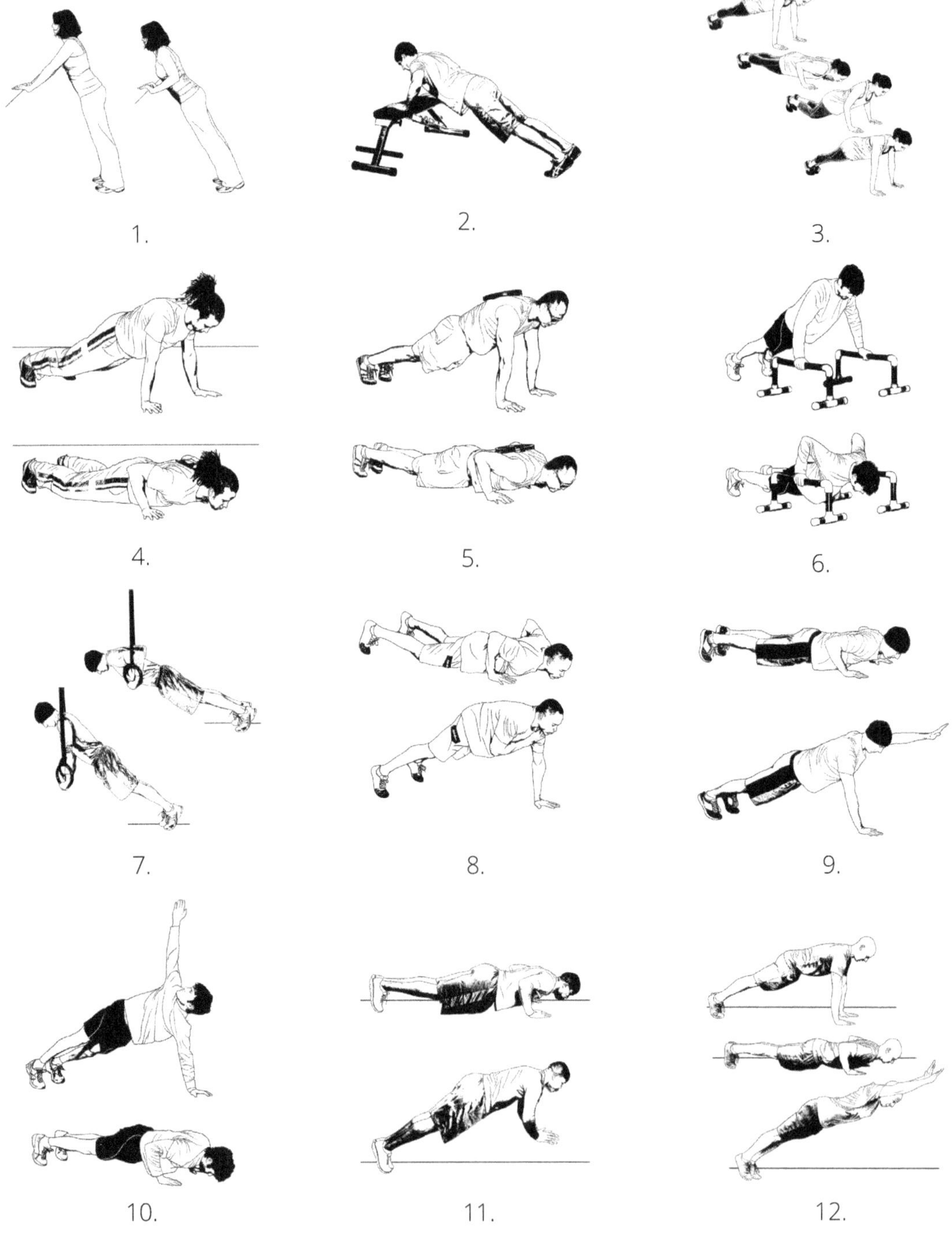

AB-03

Appendix B

Pull-up Progression

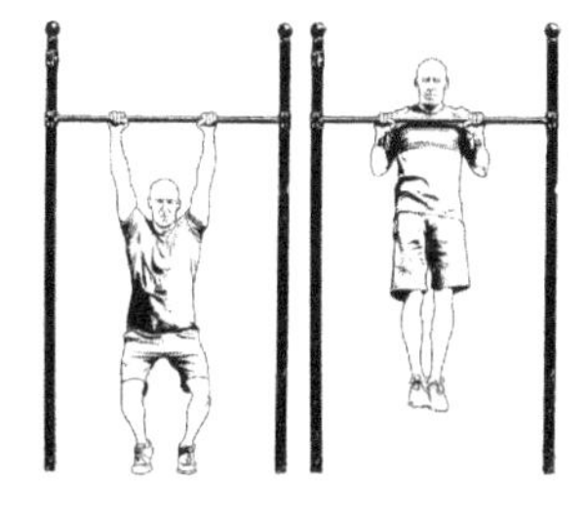

1.

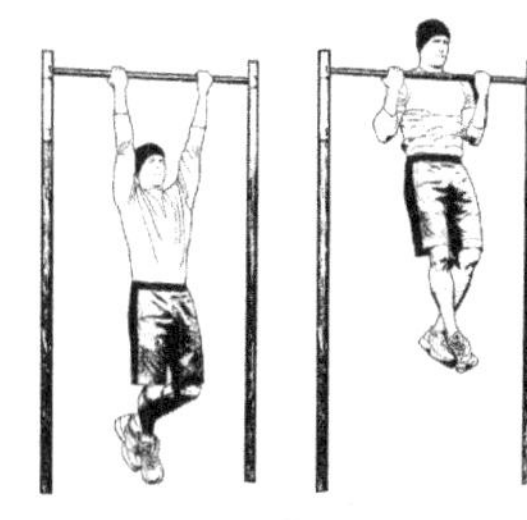

2.

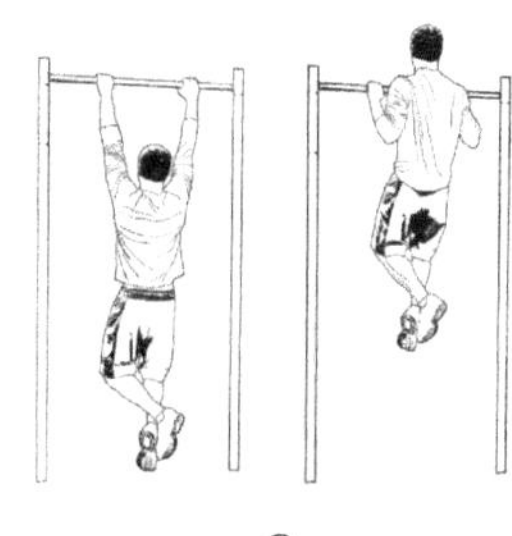

3.

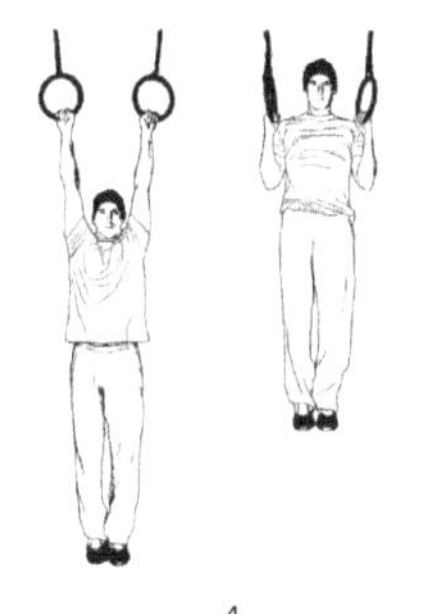

4.

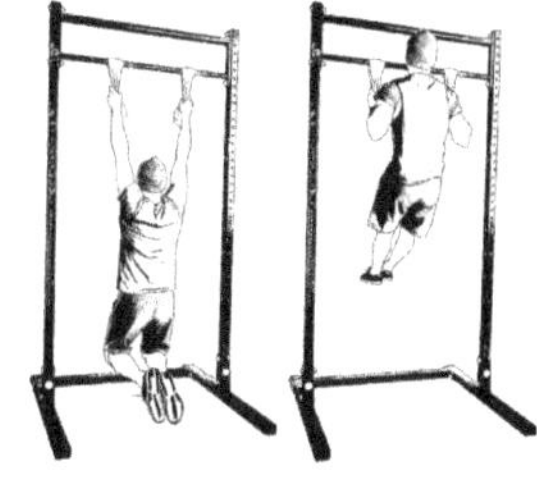

5.

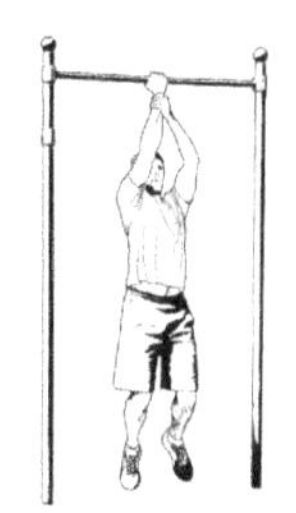

6.

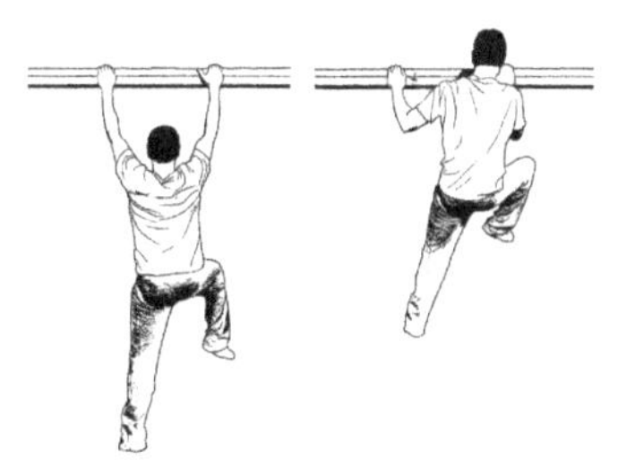

7.

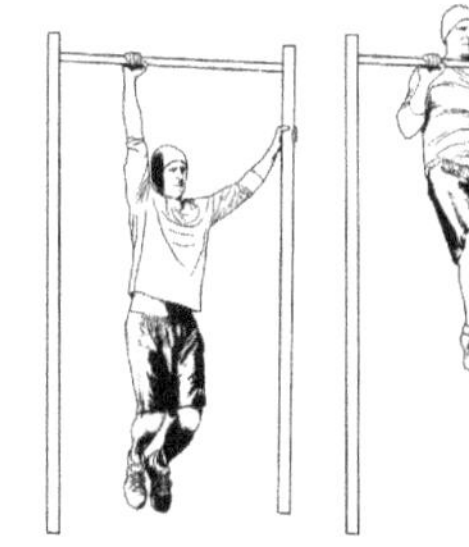

8.

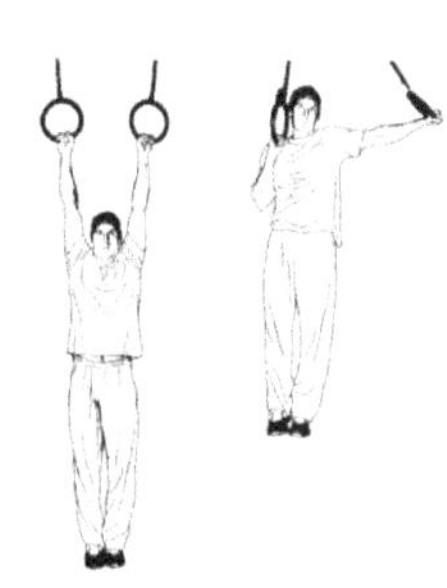

9.

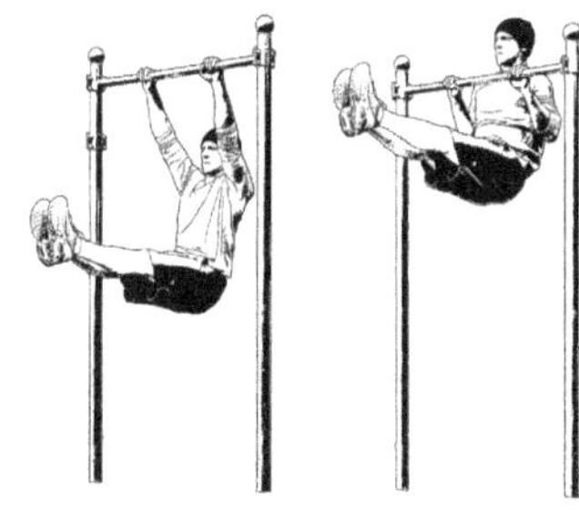

10.

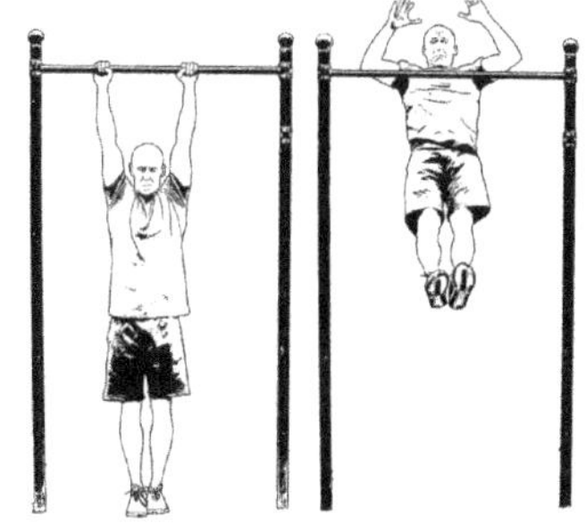

11.

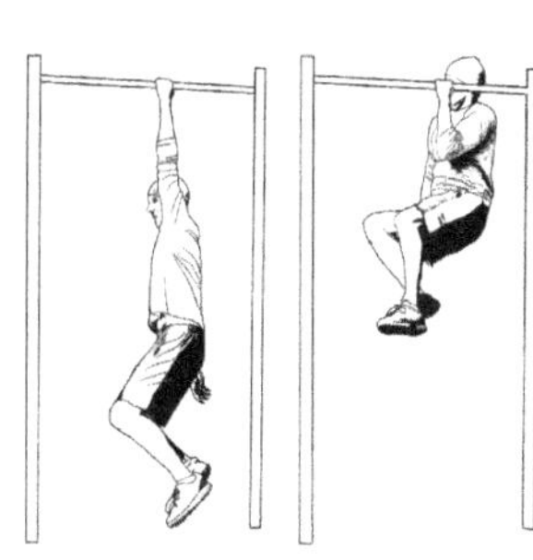

12.

LINER NOTES
Appendix B

Leg Raise Progression

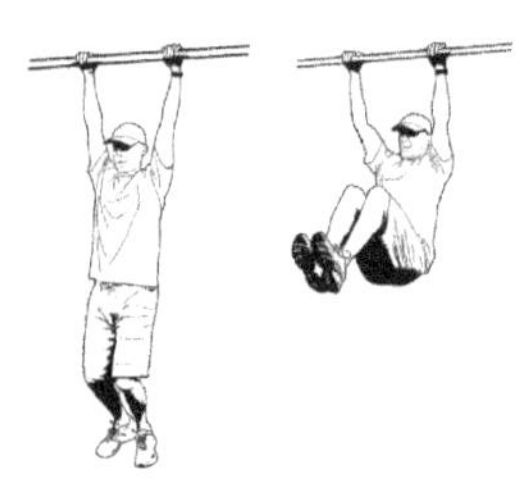

1.

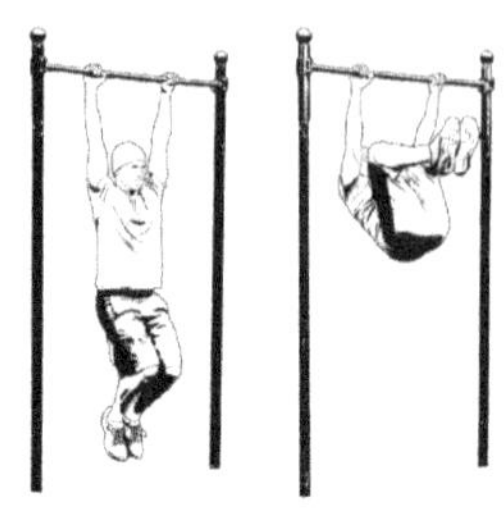

2.

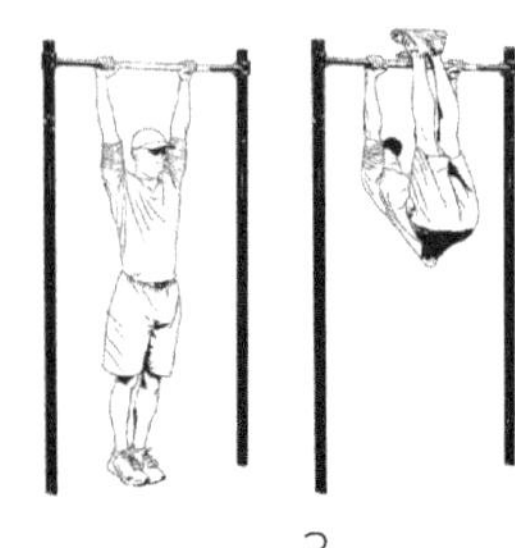

3.

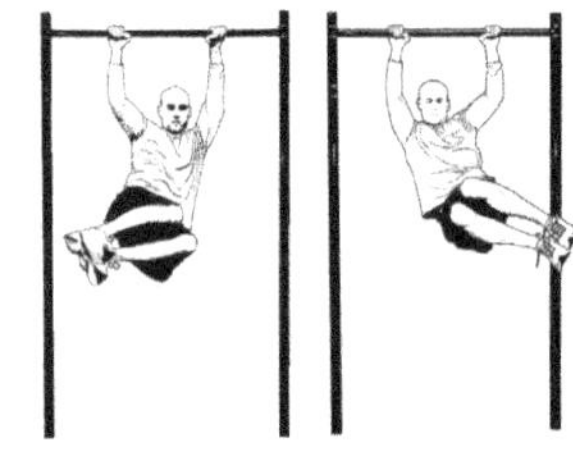

4.

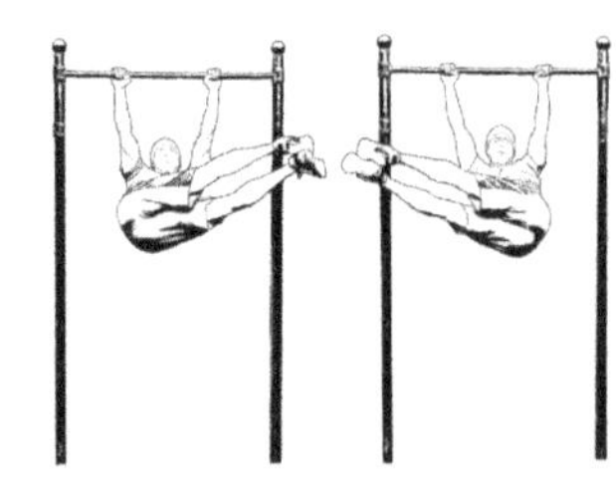

5.

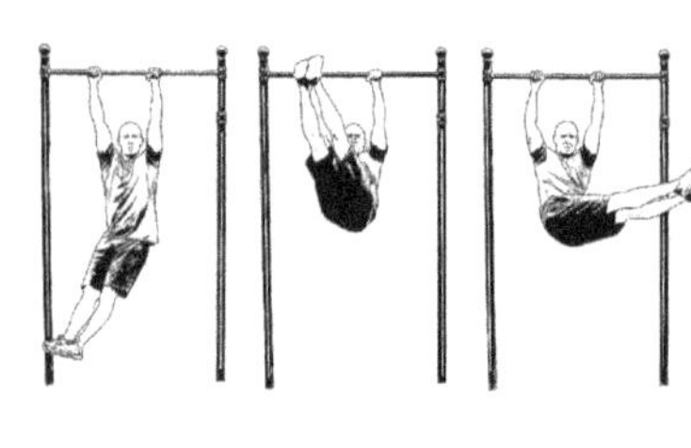

6.

V-sit Progression

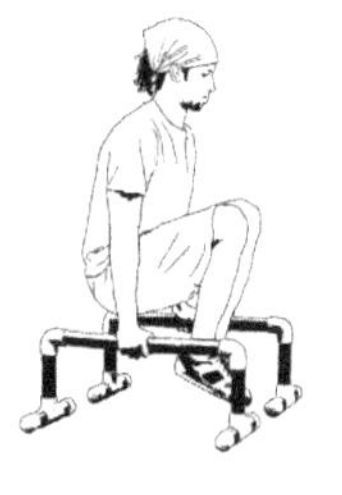

1.

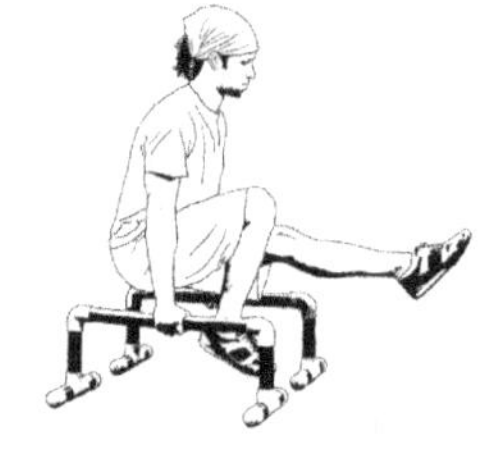

2.

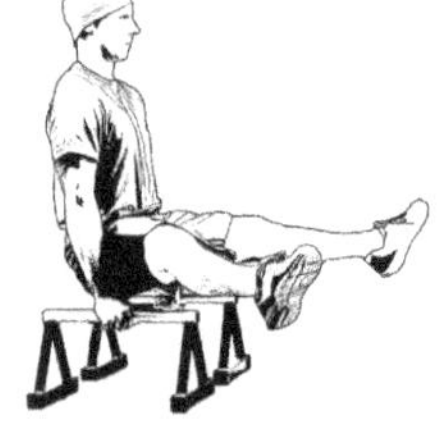

3.

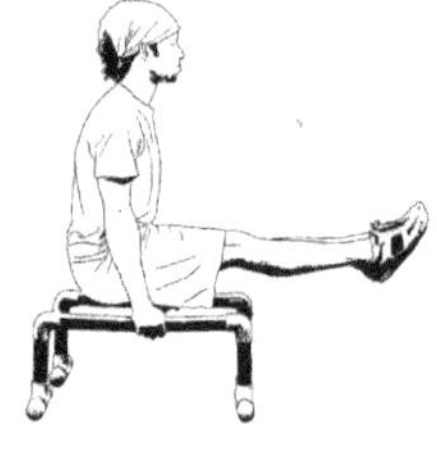

4.

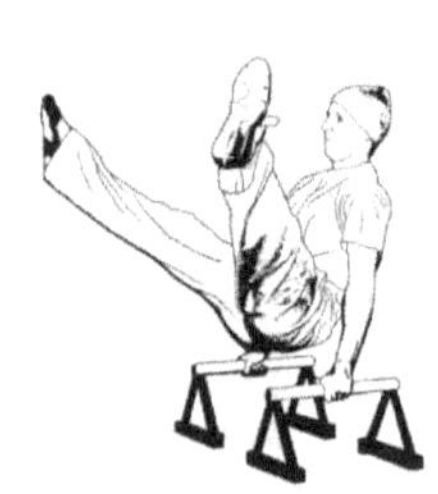

5.

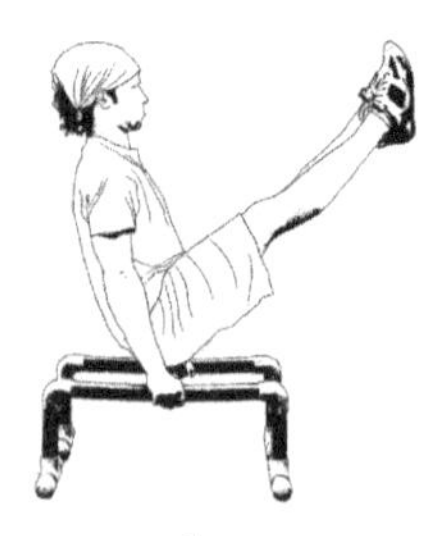

6.

AB-05

LINER NOTES
Appendix B

Handstand Push-up Progression

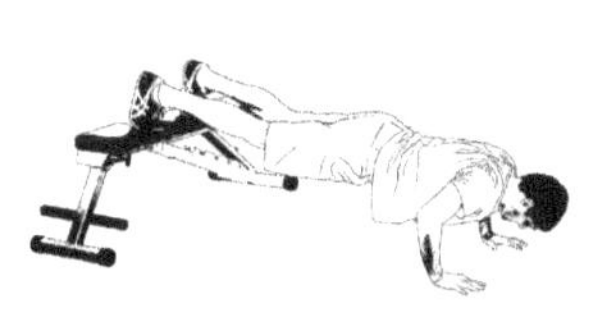

1.

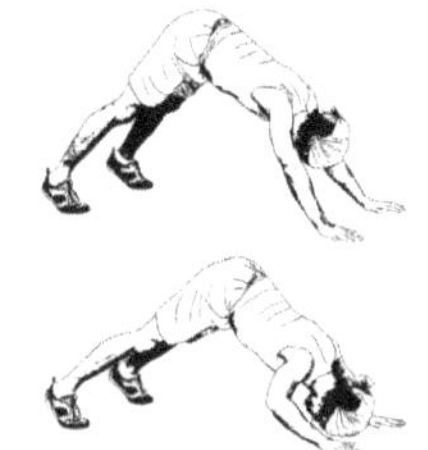

2.

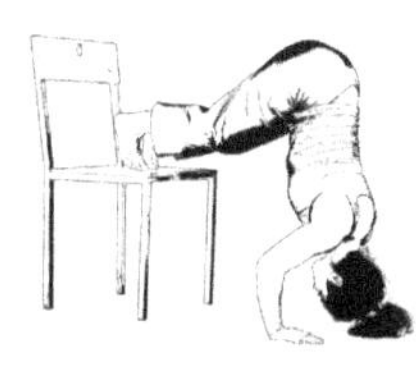

3.

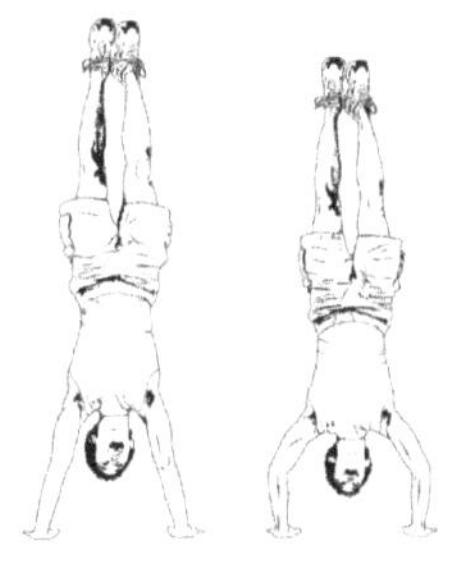

4.

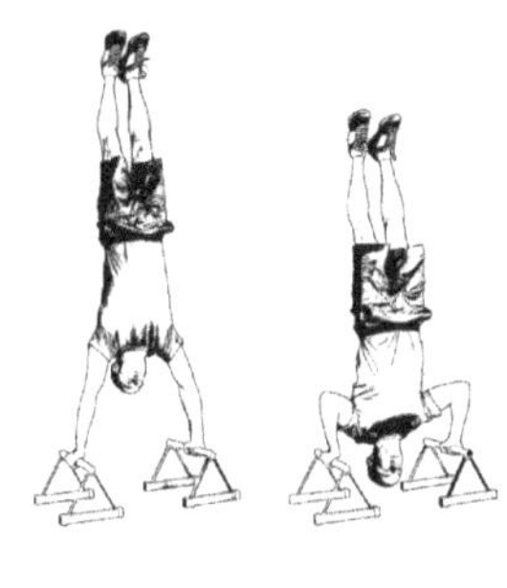

5.

Plank Progression

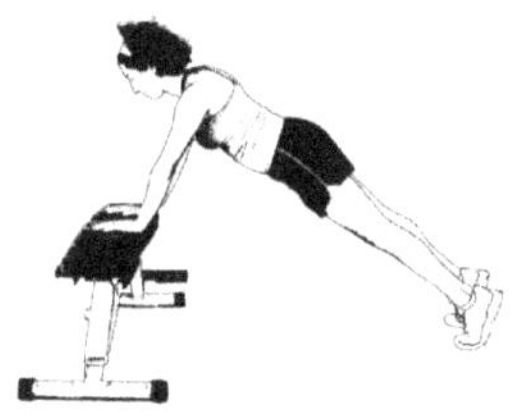

1.

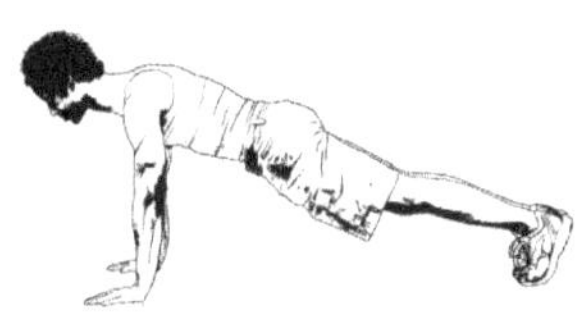

2.

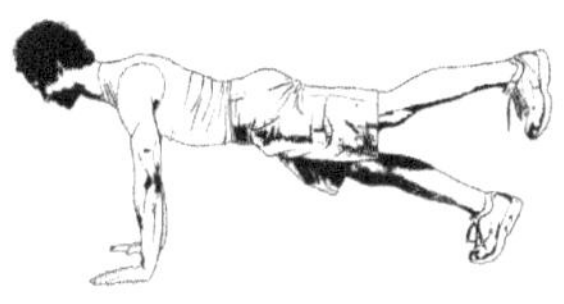

3.

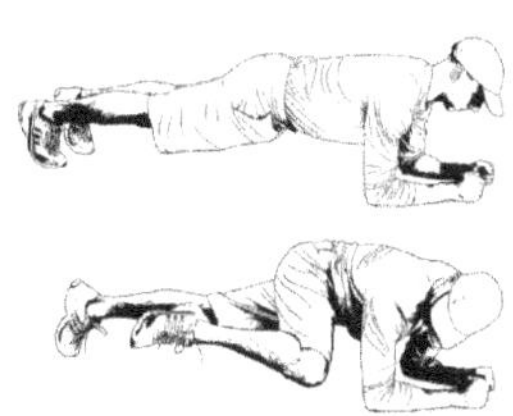

4.

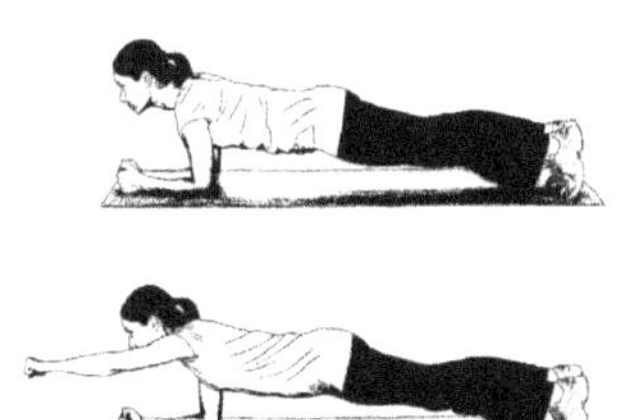

5.

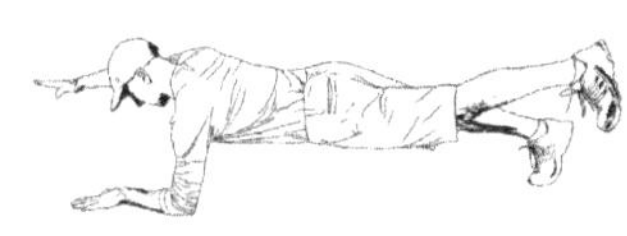

6.

More books by this publisher

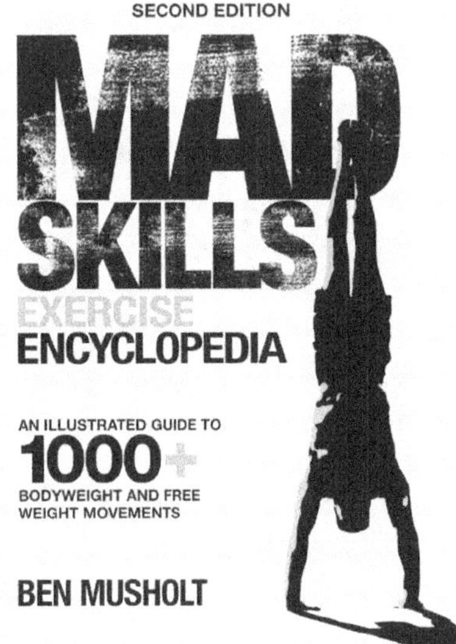

Are you hungry for more variety in your training?
Do you want to become a more well-rounded athlete?

Get ready because **Mad Skills** will help you:
- Warm-up before a training session
- Master bodyweight and calisthenics-type exercises
- Learn classic weight lifting techniques
- Build strength with barbell and kettlebell lifts
- Challenge yourself with whole body movements
- Incorporate single arm and double leg drills
- Fashion a rock-solid core for better athletic performance
- Improve your mobility with yoga postures and stretching variations.
- Have fun with partner-based skills
- Design killer at-home and garage gym workouts
- Never be boerd with fitness again!

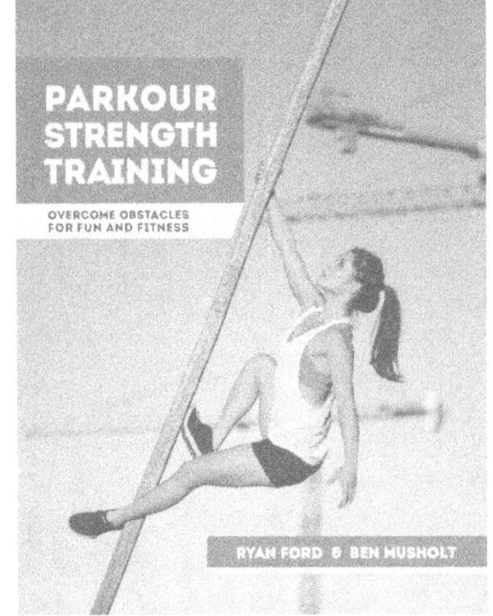

In **Parkour Strength Training,** you will learn how to:
- Accelerate your athletic development with three fundamental bodyweight exercises
- Promote the flexibility and mobility necessary for safe obstacle-based fitness
- Prepare and condition your joints to avoid injuries
- Train safely outdoors
- Remedy the common faults and errors that plague parkour newcomers
- Incorporate ground-based exercises, such as quadrupedal movement, bounding, and jumping into your workouts
- Use low obstacles such as benches, handrails, and walls for full-body strength training
- Fly over barriers using three basic vaults
- Mount, traverse, and overcome head-high walls and bar structures
- Master proper climb-up technique using many supplemental exercises
- Design an effective strength training program
- Combine skill-based drills and games to become a more well-rounded practitioner
- Dominate obstacle courses

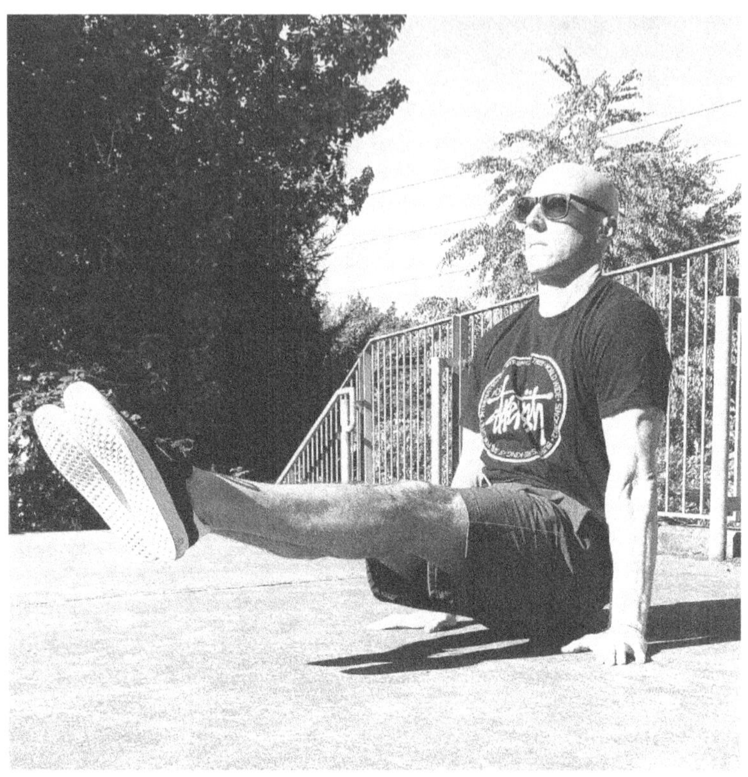

Ben Musholt is an athlete and physical therapist in Portland, Oregon. He co-authored Parkour Strength Training in 2016, and he first published the Mad Skills Exercise Encyclopedia in 2013. When not coaching or helping his clients move better, he can be found exploring the Pacific Northwest wonderland.

His goal is to do 3 fun physical activities per day.
Good luck keeping up!

www.BenMusholt.com

Instagram: @benmusholt
Facebook: madskillsbook